MW01641109

MOLECULAR GENETICS IN MEDICINE

PROGRESS IN MEDICAL GENETICS
Arno G. Motulsky, Barton Childs, Charles J. Epstein, *Series Editors*

PROGRESS IN MEDICAL GENETICS
New Series, Vol. 7

MOLECULAR GENETICS IN MEDICINE

Editors

Barton Childs, MD
Professor Emeritus

Neil A. Holtzman, MD
Professor

Haig H. Kazazian, Jr., MD
Professor

David L. Valle, MD
Professor

Department of Pediatrics
Johns Hopkins University School of Medicine
Baltimore

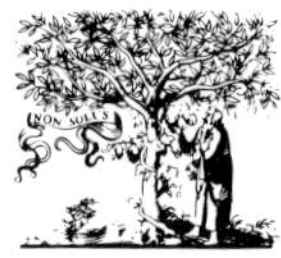

Elsevier
New York • Amsterdam • London

No responsibility is assumed by the Publisher for any injury and/or damage to persons or property as a matter of products liability, negligence or otherwise, or from any use or operation of any methods, products, instructions or ideas contained in the material herein. No suggested test or procedure should be carried out unless, in the reader's judgment, its risk is justified. Because of rapid advances in the medical sciences, we recommend that the independent verification of diagnoses and drug dosages should be made. Discussions, views and recommendations as to medical procedures, choice of drugs and drug dosages are the responsibility of the authors.

Elsevier Science Publishing Co., Inc.
52 Vanderbilt Avenue, New York, New York 10017

Distributors outside the United States and Canada:

Elsevier Science Publishers B.V.
P.O. Box 211, 1000 AE Amsterdam, the Netherlands

Library of Congress Cataloging-in-Publication Data

Molecular genetics in medicine.

(Progress in medical genetics; v. 7)
Includes index
1. Medical genetics. 2. Molecular genetics.
3. Recombinant DNA. 4. Genetic disorders – Diagnosis.
I. Childs, Barton, II. Series. [DNLM: 1. DNA – analysis.
2. Genetics, Medical. 3. Hereditary Diseases – diagnosis.
W1 RP6709 v.7 / QZ 50 M7185]
RB155.P7 vol. 7 616′.042] s[616′.042] 87-22215

ISBN 0-444-01254-0

Current printing (last digit):
10 9 8 7 6 5 4 3 2

Manufactured in the United States of America

Contents

Preface

That the conventional medical aims of diagnosis, treatment, and prevention have been forwarded by technological advances is a commonplace. Our insights into the causes and pathogenesis of disease are also based on that same technology. In pursuing their aims, investigators have employed a reductionist strategy, moving from physiologic explanations to biochemical descriptions of pathways, enzymes, and other proteins, then to molecular descriptions of structure and function of cellular mechanisms, and finally to detailed analyses of the genes themselves.

The questions asked by the participants in these discoveries are mainly categorical: how is the genetic message transcribed and translated? how are the peptides aggregated to form enzymes or cell surface receptors? how do these proteins work? or, apropos of disease, what are the molecular mechanisms of the pathogenesis of, say, diabetes or rheumatoid arthritis? Individual variation in all these processes has not been a salient concern.

But the study of the molecular basis of individuality and variation, although commanding less attention, has capitalized on the same technological progress to provide some understanding of differences (including different diseases) between individuals. Now, recombinant DNA and allied techniques make it possible to examine the individuality of disease by detecting the mutants involved, characterizing them, locating them in the chromosomes, and studying their role in pathogenesis. The tempo of this research suggests an impending avalanche of such information about all sorts of diseases, not only those we call genetic—information physicians cannot afford to ignore. This book provides the reader with a review of the impact of recombinant DNA analysis on molecular genetics and shows how information derived thereby is likely to become an important basis for understanding and discussion of all aspects of disease. Specifically, the authors examine the methods themselves and how they are being used to study the structures of the genes, the nature of mutations, and gene linkage and mapping. Information of this kind is useful in diagnosis as well as in prevention, at present in antenatal diagnosis, and potentially in screening for disease predisposition. New treatment strategies are discussed, as well as the participation of the new biotechnology companies in basic and applied research. The theme of the book is that categorical descriptions of disease processes are not enough; diseases afflict individuals individually. Recombinant DNA analysis is revealing how extensive this individuality is and how it makes a difference in the pursuit of medical aims.

The Editors

Contributors

Stylianos E. Antonarakis, MD
Associate Professor, Pediatrics, The Johns Hopkins University School of Medicine, Baltimore

Norman Arnheim, PhD
Professor of Molecular Biology, Department of Biological Sciences, University of Southern California, Los Angeles

Corinne D. Boehm, BS, MS
Assistant Professor, Pediatrics, The Johns Hopkins University School of Medicine, Baltimore

David Botstein, PhD
Professor of Genetics, Department of Biology, Massachusetts Institute of Technology, Cambridge, Massachusetts

Barton Childs, MD
Professor of Pediatrics, The Johns Hopkins University School of Medicine, Baltimore

Helen Donis-Keller, PhD
Senior Research Director, Department of Human Genetics, Collaborative Research, Inc., Bedford, Massachusetts

Henry A. Erlich, PhD
Senior Scientist and Director, Human Genetics Department, Cetus Corp., Emeryville, California

Neil A. Holtzman, MD, MPH
Senior Analyst, Office of Technology Assessment, Washington, D.C.

Haig H. Kazazian, Jr., MD
Professor of Pediatrics, The Johns Hopkins University School of Medicine, Baltimore

Grant A. Mitchell, MD
Research Fellow, Pediatrics, The Johns Hopkins University School of Medicine, Baltimore

Arno G. Motulsky, MD
Professor of Medicine, University of Washington, Seattle

Stuart H. Orkin, MD
Associate Professor, Pediatrics, Harvard Medical School, Division of Hematology, Childrens Hospital, Boston

John A. Phillips, III, MD
Professor of Pediatrics and Director, Division of Genetics, Vanderbilt University School of Medicine, Nashville, Tennessee

David L. Valle, MD
Professor of Pediatrics, Medicine and Molecular Biology and Genetics, The Johns Hopkins University School of Medicine, Baltimore

David A. Williams, MD
Assistant Professor of Pediatrics, Harvard Medical School, Division of Hematology/ Oncology, Childrens Hospital, Boston

CHAPTER 1

Introduction

Barton Childs, MD

> . . . If an equally close linkage were found between the genes determining blood group membership and that determining Huntington's Chorea we should be able, in many cases, to predict which children of an affected parent would develop the disease and to advise on the desirability, or otherwise, of their marriage. (Bell J Haldane JBS *Proc Roy Soc* 1936;123:119–150.)

It has become almost a cliché to speak of the "revolution" in molecular biology and genetics brought about by the use of recombianant DNA and allied techniques. Although the definition of the word revolution has proved more elusive than it once seemed, there is no doubt that these methods represent entirely new ways of investigating biologic problems. The scope and versatility of these techniques make it possible to test ideas previously open only to speculation, and there is something exponential in the rate at which ideas are tested and in the accumulation of information about each. Along with other aspects of biology, every medical field participates: immunology and infectious disease, endocrinology, oncology, and genetics, to name only some. And as for the conventional missions of medicine—the discovery of cause and pathogenesis, diagnosis, management, prognosis, and prevention of disease—each is served.

So there is general agreement that something quite new has been added to the technology of medical research, something with exceptional powers of inference and analysis. But the aims toward which the methods are used are not new; revolutionary means are being used to evolutionary ends. For example, among the genetic questions for which molecular strategies are providing answers are many that have been asked since the rediscovery of Mendel 87 years ago. The reference above is merely one example made timely by the current focus on Huntington's disease in consequence of the discovery and mapping to chromosome 4 of restriction fragment length polymorphisms (RFLP) that segregate with the disease phenotype.[1] The point was made tellingly by Robson, who wrote an editorial on the occasion of the 50th year of publication of the Annals of Human Genetics entitled "Fifty years of human genetics: Plus ça change, plus c'est la même chose."[2] In the first volume of the Annals, just under one-third of the articles were concerned with new ways of doing linkage analysis, statistical maneuvers made necessary by the special qualities of human family data. In the 50th anniversary volume, a little more than half of the articles dealt with chromosome mapping based on linkage analysis, a strategy to which recombinant DNA methods have brought a new dimension of resolving power.[3] (See Chapter 2.)

Mendel's predecessors could not imagine how traits could be transmitted independently, and so they were unable to conceive of any relationship between qualities that were plainly inherited and any genetically transmitted particle. That was Mendel's contribution. The drosophilists, in turn, showed how segregation and independent assortment could be accounted for by the behavior of the chromosomes in meiosis. Linkage was first suggested by Bateson in 1902, and the details were later worked out by the drosophilists. By 1910 the genes of drosophila were localized to specific chromosomes, and by 1913 there was a rudimentary map showing the linear arrangement of several genes in the X chromosome. Later, in the 1930s, when the physical basis of heredity was well established, attention was turned to physiological genetics, or what the genes do, and a strategy was established that we still use in resolving, layer by layer, the affinities between concretely defined phenotypes and abstract genes (Fig. 1.1). Even after the identification of deoxyribonucleic acid (DNA) as the genetic material and the discovery of the genetic code, the gene remained an abstraction, defined in genetic experiments by its inferred properties as units of function, each divisible into smaller units of recombination and mutation. Estimates of the size of each of these units were provided by Benzer, who showed, as a result of matings of strains of the bacteriophage T_4, that the various units could be measured in angstroms, allowing so many base pairs for each; for example, the unit of mutation could be as small as a single base.[4] But it remained for recombinant DNA analysis to give molecular reality to the genes, to make them all but palpable, to make it possible to locate them and to define the functional units in sequences of base pairs in strands composed of exons, introns, regulatory elements, and flanking sequences. The extraordinary versatility and power of these molecular strategies resulted from the discovery of bacterial enzymes (restriction enzymes) that cleave DNA at sites specific to each enzyme.[5] These remarkable properties enable the investigator, after isolating DNA from test subject, to choose how to cut the strands and then to manipulate the products

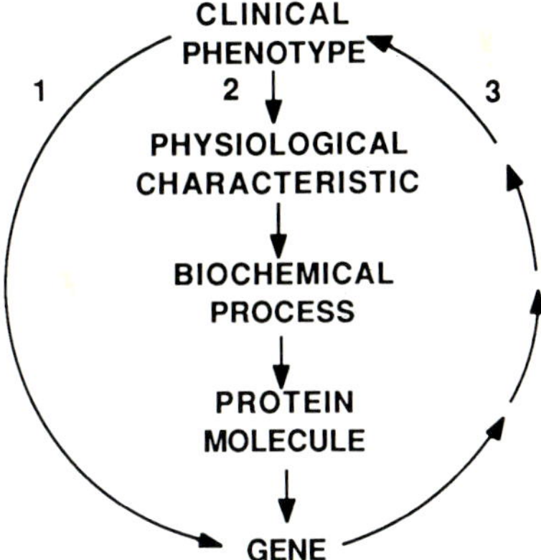

FIGURE 1.1 Strategies for relating phenotypes and genes. (1) Mendelian segregation reveals a relationship between a phenotype and a gene even when nothing is known of how the gene action is mediated. (2) The gene–phenotype relationship may be described at several levels, each a consequence of a previous one. (3) "Reverse genetics" is a mirror image of process 2. The structure of a gene may suggest a protein that may be found to have a biochemical function that plays a role in some homeostatic system accounting for the phenotype.

appropriately to test hypotheses that cannot otherwise be tested. For example, human genes can be transferred to other organisms where their functions can be studied under conditions not permissible in intact human beings. And in such experiments the person who is the source of the DNA, and whose genetic identity is to be defined with such precision, is merely a bystander, an observer who is thereby spared the intrusion of human clinical research.

WHAT DO THE METHODS DO?

General Applications

The methods have uses in all biologic investigations in which gene action and genetic variation are issues for study. Although only prokaryotic organisms produce the restriction enzymes upon which the techniques depend, the specific sequences they cleave are widely distributed. This means that the scope for the use of recombinant DNA techniques is limitless; obviously, only some aspects of the work are applicable to medicine. But medicine partakes of two kinds of information, some of general biological interest, some germane only to the pursuit of the practical aims of diagnosis and treatment. For example, mutation, polymorphism, and gene mapping have implications for all biology, but information generated in such investigations can be turned to practical account in tests for genetic heterogeneity, the elucidation of pathogenesis, population screening, antenatal diagnosis, treatment, and prevention.

Mutation

Germ-line Mutation: Prior to the advent of recombinant DNA methods, our concepts of mutation were limited to what could be observed at the level of amino acid sequences; point mutations including missense, nonsense, and frameshifts were all known, as well as deletions and the consequences of unequal crossing over. "Regulatory" mutations were presumed to exist, of course, but their exact nature could not be imagined. But the ability to examine the DNA directly has added greatly to this list (see Chapter 3). Mutations that interfere with protein synthesis rather than amino acid sequence have been described; some involve the promoter or other regulatory elements, some the processes of RNA cleavage and splicing. Others, appearing in introns and flanking sequences, and so never translated, are both frequent and harmless. Furthermore, the fine structure of chromosomal mutations has been described. Deletions, translocations, and other aberrations too small to be seen with the light microscope but easily observed by restriction enzyme analysis have turned out to account for mendelizing phenotypes previously presumed to be due to single gene differences, but actually involving several contiguous genes.[6] Clearly, the adjective *mendelian* is indefinite as to what is segregating, an ambiguity the recombinant DNA methods may be expected to resolve. Also likely to yield to this kind of analysis is the identity of genes in the limited segments of chromosome 21 which, when trisomic, apparently account for Down's syndrome.

Somatic Mutation: There are mutations in somatic cells as well as in the germ line; DNA replication occurs in mitosis, so point mutations and chromosomal aberrations are to be expected. Recently, somatic mutation has been demonstrated; for example, it explains variation in immunoglobulins beyond that accountable to gene shuffling; point mutations have been found in the variable elements of both light and heavy chains.[7]

For many years somatic mutation has been invoked to account for malignant change. Mutagenic agents are usually carcinogenic too, and although there are familial cancers, even mendelizing forms, the age-dependent incidence of most cancers is most easily accounted for by somatic change in response to something in the environment.[8,9] But, apart from the observation of aneuploidy in many tumors and the translocated Philadelphia chromosome in chronic myeloid leukemia, it was not clear just what the mutagens did. Now, as a result of the new molecular methods we know that we all possess proto-oncogenes, genes that produce important regulators of cellular replication and that in their nucleotide sequences bear close resemblance to genes in retroviruses that are involved in the cancer of some animals and are capable of malignant transformation of mammalian cells.[10,11] (See Chapter 5.) And it has been demonstrated that somatic mutations activate the proto-oncogenes by subverting their normal processes of regulation. Clearly, this conversion of proto-oncogenes to oncogenes is not the only step in the generation of malignancy, nor is it the only mechanism, but it does seem evident that the actions of carcinogens in producing malignancies are mediated by genes at several loci.[10,11]

Polymorphism

Restriction enzyme analysis has a major contribution to make in estimates of the extent of human genetic variation. Such estimates are essential for population genetics and for our understanding of evolutionary processes.[12,13] And, as things are turning out, the discovery of the genetic variants by which such estimates are made has significance for medicine as well; they are useful as markers of susceptibility to disease and as genetically linked surrogates for genes as yet unidentified. (See Chapters 2, 4, 5, and 10.)

Until recently, such markers consisted entirely of protein variants—enzymes, serum proteins, blood group substances, and the like. To be useful as such, the marker gene must be "polymorphic," that is, it must be relatively common in the population. So a locus is defined as polymorphic when there are two or more alleles, the least common of which exists at a frequency of 1% or more. This somewhat arbitrary figure was chosen because it exceeds that which could be accounted for by mutation alone. That is, an appeal must be made to natural selection, random drift, founder effect, or some other cause to explain the presence of genes at such frequencies. Studies of electrophoretic migration of proteins of many organisms, including man, have revealed that about 30% of the loci qualify by this definition as polymorphic.[12,13] A determined search will turn up mutants in lower frequencies also, perhaps 0.5 percent or less, at most, if not all loci, and such mutants certainly contribute some share of the variation, perhaps more than we know. Each of us possesses an unknown number of them; but it is the 30% of polymorphic loci that furnish the bulk of this kind of genetic variation exhibited by individuals. The remaining 70% of the loci that, apart from rare mutants, are invariant, determine the qualities that distinguish the species—in our case our humanness. They supply the background upon which the polymorphic alleles stamp that variable effects.

The degree of polymorphism varies from one locus to another. Some have a principal allele with a frequency of nearly 90%, with one or two others at a few percent each; obviously, most people would be homozygous for the principal allele and, therefore, uninformative with regard to differences within families. At the opposite extreme are the HLA loci, each with numerous alleles in frequencies such that nearly everyone is heterozygous.[14] The ABO and other blood groups, some complement loci and a few others lie in between these limits. Obviously, the more polymorphic the locus, the more useful it will be in providing marker alleles; that is, the more likely it will be to be useful in distinguishing individuals in both populations and families.

Marker genes are of two kinds: (1) those associated with the disease, whether in cause or pathogenesis, and (2) those that are genetically linked but functionally independent, that is, they are situated in the chromosome so near to the gene in question as seldom to be parted by recombination.[15] Indeed, a linked gene may act as a stand-in for a gene of unknown location or even of unknown function, and such a surrogate could be of value in diagnosis, perhaps especially in the antenatal diagnosis of conditions of unknown pathogenesis. But as long as we were dependent upon protein polymorphism, progress in the discovery of linkages and associations, to say nothing of their use in medicine, was disappointing; although there were some successes, particularly the association of HLA alleles with autoimmune diseases. But this limitation should be no surprise; phenotypic variation, even at the level of protein difference, is likely to be subject to selective constraint. First, there is that 70% of loci that are invariant, except for the rare mutants that are not useful as markers. Then the degree of variation for most of the polymorphic loci is just not enough to make many families informative. What is needed to make the use of linkage for diagnosis prosper is an exuberant variation, less constrained by selection. And that is just what has been exposed by restriction-enzyme analysis of the DNA; a restriction fragment length polymorphism (RFLP) is encountered on an average of once in every few hundred bases. Further, they appear mainly in the noncoding parts of the DNA, the introns and flanking sequences, and often in such population frequencies as to make them very likely to distinguish individuals in families. So they have increased enormously the potential use of such markers.

Mapping the Chromosomes

The details of how DNA polymorphisms are discovered and how they are used in linkage analysis and in mapping of human chromosomes are given in Chapter 2. It is enough here to point out the virtues of such maps for medical use.[16] First, the mapping is proceeding at a furious pace; the number of mapped genes and arbitrary DNA segments doubles about every 2 years, having reached a total of nearly 1,500 by 1985.[17] And there is no reason to suppose that the pace will slacken. Indeed, it may accelerate, because the greater the density of the map, the more easily is a new gene or fragment to be mapped. In the end, it is anticipated that there will be enough markers spaced throughout the whole genome to facilitate quick location of any gene or fragment.[16]

Medical uses are obvious. A marker may be used to make a diagnosis in cases where the identity of the disease is in doubt or to strengthen a probable diagnosis, or merely to stand as one among other evidences for or against. More often they are likely to be used as evidence of susceptibility; a signal of some homeostatic vulnerability predisposing to a disease commonly precipitated by some experience. In any of these instances the presence of the marker is seldom *proof* of the presence of disease or even of susceptibility. Although the sib of a patient with Huntington's disease who shares the marker for that disorder may have a high probability of having it, for other diseases the pathogenesis may be too complex to be initiated by a single gene.

Reverse Genetics

No one is ready to stop with the detection of RFLP markers, however useful they may be. Such a discovery is merely a preliminary to efforts to find the relevant gene itself. For purely diagnostic purposes a very tightly linked RFLP may serve the purpose, but there are rewards for finding the gene itself.[6,18,19] That is, there may be ways to explain the phenotype in reverse order, inferring a protein from the base sequence of the gene and then drawing conclusions as to the role of the latter in homeostasis, perhaps by comparing the sequence of its amino acids with those of proteins of known function. The point of the exercise, after discovering the role of the gene in cause or pathogenesis, is to devise some strategy to reverse or to neutralize it. To attempt to direct treatment according to cause is conventional medical practice. What is unprecedented here is the idea of a genetic analysis that proceeds from the bottom up, rather than from the top down. (See Chapters 4 and 5.)

The process seems to close a circle, the first arc of which was described by Mendel. That is, reverse genetics is a mirror image of Mendelian analysis. In the latter, a phenotype is explained by physiological, biochemical, and molecular accounts of gene action (Fig. 1.1). But the properties of phenotypes often fail to give direction to such an effort, so there remain many phenotypes, for example, most of the disease entries in *Mendelian Inheritance in Man,* that are undistinguished by attributes suggestive of the mechanisms of the genes from which they originate. Recombinant DNA methods will expose the genes for many such phenotypes so that physiological explanations can be pursued in the opposite direction, that is, from the gene to a protein and on to the clinical phenotype (Fig. 1.1). But, in addition, genes will be discovered in the absence of phenotype, so we will have genes in search of phenotypes as well as phenotypes in search of genes.

Medical Applications

What are other impacts of these methods on medicine?

1. More aspects of diagnosis may be displaced from the patient to the laboratory
2. The methods offer ultimate resolution of the question of genetic heterogeneity
3. They make possible prenatal identification of the relevant gene in any genetic disorder
4. They may lead to simplified methods of population screening.

Diagnosis

Before the advent of recombinant DNA methods, genetic diagnosis always had to be by indirection. Mendelian segregation helps materially in drawing the diagnostician's attention to the probability of genetic causes, but the presence and quality of particular mutants always had to be inferred by the detection of metabolites in body fluids, by tolerance or other stress tests, or by biopsies, endoscopies, radiographs, or other procedures, often invasive and uncomfortable. At best, an assay of enzyme activity or other test of molecular specificity may suggest the nature of the mutant, but too often the enzyme presumed to be culpable cannot be examined directly because it is limited to inaccessible tissues. At worst, and most stressful, it may be necessary simply to await the onset of some premonitory expression; only then can the presence of the gene be inferred. Recombinant DNA tests are more versatile. (See Chapters 4 and 5.) For example, leukocytes will serve as a source of DNA, even when the putative mutant has its action only in, say, the CNS or kidney. Further, the tests can be done in the patient's absence; it is not uncommon for DNA analyses yielding important diagnostic information to be done on patients living on the opposite side of the globe.

So we may expect an enormously increased diagnostic capability in which specific genes or gene markers will be used. Knowledge of how the gene works to produce the signs and symptoms, however desirable, is not actually necessary, so the principal limits in the development of such diagnostic tests will be the availability of appropriate probes and the interest of competent and well-financed investigators. Some of this development, especially for relatively common genetic disorders—cystic fibrosis is an example—is being undertaken by biotechnology companies, some of which are exploring the feasibility of rapid, specific, and sensitive tests.[20] (See Chapters 9 and 10.)

Heterogeneity

It may be said with justice that in demonstrating the inheritance of alternative forms of a character, Mendel introduced the issue of genetic heterogeneity. Since then, because the genetic specificity of phenotype has always had to be inferred, some residual suspicion of heterogeneity, in even the best of circumstances, has necessarily remained. For example, deficiency of enzyme activity may be due in one case to a defect in the active site and in another to insensitivity of the enzyme to a cofactor, or the same phenotype may be due in different families to defects in different enzymes, and these variations cannot always be inferred on clinical grounds. Even immunologic specificity, which we suppose to establish molecular identity, is suspect; identical HLA phenotypes have been found to vary genetically and in ways that have clinical significance.[21] So it is clear that in laying open the DNA to inspection, restriction enzyme analysis must be the final arbiter of genetic homogeneity or variation, providing at best information that may be influential in the choice of treatment or prevention, and at the least imparting an unaccustomed accuracy to genetic counseling. (See Chapter 5.)

Treatment

It is axiomatic that knowledge of cause and pathogenesis of a disease will suggest a plausible treatment. This belief is based on the dazzling therapeutic successes of vaccines and antibiotics in the prevention and treatment of infections and of essential nutrients in nutritional deficiencies. In both, the treatments were directed specifically to cause: in the infections to destroying the invading organisms and in the nutritional disorders to supplying the deficiency. And it has been suggested that these triumphs are exemplary of what is to come once we learn to "think our way around" the biologic mechanisms of other categories of disease.[22] That is, it is presumed that as our insights into the details of cellular and organ homeostasis become increasingly comprehensive, and as we learn more and more of the mechanisms of pathogenesis, we should be able to see a way to prevent, or even to cure, anything, possibly leading to a more or less disease-free life for nearly everyone. In this scenario, which has informed medical thought for perhaps 100 years, it is the knowledge of structure and function that is central, a knowledge that is to be elaborated through molecular technology.

It is true that recombinant DNA methods may make it possible to discover the position and identity of any gene that exerts a major effect in the cause of a disease, and although it may prove more difficult, it should be possible in time to describe the role of such genes in pathogenesis. So it is likely that the future will bring an elucidation at the molecular level of cause and pathogenesis for any disease that commands enough attention. There may be problems in sorting out the environmental agencies and experiences that act across genetic variability in engendering diseases, but although these conditions and events may never be appraised with the precision of molecular technology, there is no reason why such influences cannot be discovered. Then, with all the information in hand, and given the extraordinary scope and analytic power of recombinant DNA and other molecular expedients, it will be possible, disease by disease, to test the hypothesis of the equation of knowledge of cause and pathogenesis with treatment. The questions that molecular biology will allow us to begin to test is whether or not, in which instances, and in what degree, a disordered homeostasis *can* be influenced when we know in detail how and where it has gone wrong. It is an exciting prospect, but the outcomes, which could well turn out to be various, are unpredictable.

Some of the difficulties, however, may be foreshadowed by present performance. The case of sickle cell anemia is well known; knowledge of the nucleotide and amino acid substitution in the β chains of hemoglobin has not led to an effective treatment. But as an alternative, discovering some way to increase the amount of fetal hemoglobin at the expense of the abnormal S hemoglobin could represent a cure, and efforts are afoot to test that possibility.[23] The present state of treatment for other inborn errors also reveals a need for inventive thinking. A review of the treatment of 65 such diseases in which a deficient enzyme was recognized revealed reasonably good control for 12%, some amelioration for 40%, and no change at all in 48%.[24] And of those ameliorated, the improvement was only marginal for more than half.

Some improvement of this record may be expected to follow better insights into pathogenesis, but so indifferent a success with conventional strategies has caused investigators to try such alternatives as enzyme therapy and organ or bone marrow transplantation.[25,26] Of these, bone marrow transplantation after total body irradiation has produced the best outcomes, mainly when the defect is expressed in the marrow cells themselves. The limitations of all these methods has prompted serious thought to be given to gene therapy in which a normal gene could be added in the expectation of restoring deficient enzyme activity. Such gene substitutions are frequently employed in the study of microorganisms and experimental animals (indeed, in bacteria they occur spontaneously) and will no doubt have some successes in human beings as well, perhaps at first in disorders that can be managed by transformation of the patient's own bone marrow. For this, the experience with allogenic bone marrow transplantation will supply some invaluable guidance by having shown which disorders, among those in which the defective enzyme is normally expressed only in other organs, say the liver or brain, have been helped by the transplant.[26] The prospects for success and the obstacles still to be surmounted are reviewed in Chapter 6.

All this is not to say that there are not already some important advances in treatment. Recombinant DNA methods have a surpassing advantage in the fabrication of useful peptides and proteins. Some of these can substitute for animal products that regularly immunize the patient. Examples are insulin, interferon, interleukin-2, Factor VIII, growth hormone, and α-1-antitrypsin, all of which have been produced and are being tried. Human erythropoeitin is perhaps the most recent arrival,[27] and vaccines for malaria and other diseases are in the offing.[28] The only apparent limitation is the isolation of cloned genes, and this obstacle is likely to give way to a determined effort wherever the need for the product is overriding.

The commercial potential of such products has stimulated some of the biotechnology companies to finance and carry out their development.[29] No doubt many problems remain, but the prospects, like so much else in this field, seem limitless. Still, the future is likely to be defined in the long run by the variable and uncertain responses of human homeostasis. (See Chapter 9.)

Prevention

It cannot be said that any of these treatments is simple and easy to apply. Only a successful transfer of a normally functioning gene could effect an actual cure; other treatments make a chronic disease, albeit a more tolerable one, out of an acute disorder. Even bone marrow transplants that "cure" the enzyme deficiency require immunosuppression. So the virtues of prevention have become appealing. Prevention of genetic disease takes three forms: (1) antenatal diagnosis followed by abortion of affected fetuses, (2) changes in dietary or other habits after discovery of some quality that indicates risk, and (3) other actions consequent upon genetic counseling. Recombinant DNA methods are relevant to the first two forms.

Antenatal Diagnosis: Until recently, antenatal diagnosis depended upon karyotyping or assay of enzyme activity or other metabolic abnormality; occasionally ultrasound has been used to visualize anomalous development. But restriction-enzyme analysis has increased immeasurably the scope for detection of diseased fetuses by bypassing the disease process altogether and making a diagnosis at the gene level, either directly or by showing the mutant to be closely linked to an RFLP. (See Chapter 7.) This capability may be expected to expand in direct proportion to the density of the gene map, and it should be possible, eventually, to link to a discernable marker, and so to localize, anything that mendelizes.[16,30] So it may become common to make an antenatal diagnosis of genetic conditions without knowing much of how the mutant effect is mediated. Indeed, just such a service is now available to those at risk for Huntington's disease who might wish, even should they turn out to be carriers, to have children who would never grow up with the prospect of a premature and horrible death.[31]

Of course, it will always be better to be able to examine the relevant gene itself. First, when the gene is known it may be possible to gain some revealing insights into pathogenesis. Then, it should be possible to resolve the uncertainties of heterogeneity. Some mutants may lead to severe expression, others to mild expression, and the decision for or against abortion may hinge on the expectation of severity. And finally, RFLP identification is generally useful only in families marked by at least one bona fide case of the disease in question.

Genetic Risk Factors: The second form of prevention involves discovery of genetic variation that constitutes risk or susceptibility, to be followed by changes in the environment or in habits and experiences that are calculated to diminish the hazard. (See Chapter 10.) This search for genetic risk factors may be carried out either in families marked by an affected person or in whole populations. There are advantages and disadvantages to each of these strategies. First, the family approach is more likely to turn up people with the gene, and such people are more likely actually to be at risk. For example, relatives who share an HLA allele with a patient who has an autoimmune disease are more likely to be affected than are unrelated persons with (ostensibly) the same allele who are discovered in a population survey. Perhaps genes other than the HLA allele are required, and these are more likely to be represented in affected families, or there may be genetic heterogeneity distinguishable only by recombinant DNA analysis. Or, the probability of family aggregation of affected persons may be heightened by shared habits or other precipitating conditions.

But although more likely to discover susceptibles or affected patients, the family screening approach has the limitation of focusing only on families brought to attention by an affected patient. In contrast, for population screening there is no need for such a signal; possessors of the marker are discovered without prior knowledge of susceptibility. But this strategy has its limitations too. It is more expensive; the marker should be the mutant itself, not an RFLP; its population frequency is likely to be far less than that in a family marked by an affected patient; and there is far more uncertainty about its significance to any particular individual discovered without reference to an affected person.

Recombinant DNA methods will improve the sensitivity and specificity of the tests for these genetic risk factors. By reducing the ambiguity of heterogeneity they will define the genes, and therefore the risks, more precisely, and in determining risks for single-gene diseases, especially in relation to antenatal diagnosis, recombinant DNA analysis should raise the precision of diagnosis to a maximum. But, although population risk defines genes that contribute to multifactorial diseases, it may not do so for all individuals. That is, where other factors beyond one well-defined gene are required to precipitate the disease, including other genes, special experiences, habits, and conditions, then the actual risk to a specific individual must depend upon the presence or absence of, or particular concentrations of, such other factors. So, while recombinant DNA analysis will help in defining the *genetic* elements among those other factors, thus further refining the risk attributable to each, the true risk must remain incalculable until something is known of the nature, prevalence, and exact mechanism of interactions of the non-genetic elements. And the complexity of these interrelationships, especially if occurring through development, or in relation to aging processes, may make the practice of prediction a precarious one. (See Chapter 8.)

IMPACT ON MEDICAL CONCEPTS

Finally, we may ask some questions of more general content: What is (and what will be) the impact of the uses of recombinant DNA methods on the way we view disease and on the context in which we discuss their illnesses with patients? How will these new insights influence the medical curriculum? How will knowing the fine structure of genes and chromosomes modify our understanding of human illness? There are several ways. Among them are

a. A new grasp of the extent to which genetic variation underlies disease
b. A new understanding of the individuality of disease
c. A greatly enhanced insight into the implications of gene-environment interactions.

Genes and Disease

Restriction enzyme analysis has greatly increased our perception of the store of human genetic diversity and its association with disease. Our present experience is that nearly all diseases recur in relatives at above population frequencies and monozygotic twin concordance nearly always exceeds that of dizygotic pairs. And we are increasingly accustomed to the discovery of RFLPs either within, or in close association to, genes that specify proteins clearly involved in pathogenesis. Thus, it turns out that there is no qualitative difference in the nature of causes between multifactorial and mongenic diseases; it is only quantitative. So the question to be asked is no longer, "Is it a genetic or an environmental disease?" but rather "What is the contribution of genetic variation to the cause of this disease?" Or, it might be asked, "Is everyone equally susceptible, or only some or a very few, and who are they?"

Since this final question carries a significant message for patients, their relatives, and the public in general, it must influence physicians' attitudes to prevention and must inform their counseling. And the pervasive influence of genetic variation in differential susceptibility to disease must have impact on teaching, both in medical school and in postgraduate training.

The Individuality of Disease

We have been accustomed to thinking of disease as something a patient "has" or "comes down with" and we usually describe each one in terms of the "typical" or "classical" case, as if the disease had some sort of identity independent of the individuals it afflicts. But there is a growing dissatisfaction with such classical case descriptions as the heterogeneity of both cause and expression of most diseases has become evident. Now we are more likely to think of disease as a consequence of a faltering homeostasis with dynamics that reflect the individuality of the homeostatic components and their organization. Obviously, this transition has been given impetus by the recognition of human genetic diversity and its contribution to the origins of diseases. So, more and more, we are coming to see the qualities of each patient's illness—age at onset, severity, duration, response to treatment, indeed, whether or not he has it at all—as a manifestation of individuality, itself a property of the actions of genes through many experiences, and that has evolved over a lifetime. It is in the molecular characterization of the genetic contribution to this individuality that recombinant DNA methods are proving so useful; a description that must help to explain not only the clinical features experienced by each patient, but individual susceptibility as well.

Biological-Cultural Relationships

We often speak of gene-environment interaction, by which we refer to the conditional effect of a gene on a phenotype. For example, it has been observed that certain apolipoprotein variants, defined by restriction analysis, are concentrated in patients with coronary artery disease, and there is the implication that the variants, perhaps in conjunction with other genes as well, have made their possessors more susceptible to the potentially adverse effects of dietary fat or smoking or other still undescribed experiences.[32] Although not usually emphasized, such interactions account for variation in monogenic disorders as well; phenylketonuria (PKU) is ameliorated by dietary control, and it has been suggested that the age at onset of Huntington's disease is influenced by aging processes.[33] No doubt aging is influenced by the genes, but there is ample evidence of non-genetic elements as well.[34] So what gene-environment interaction means is that, in addition to local and internal environments, cellular and organ homeostatic systems, there are elements of cause residing in social and cultural organization, causes that derive from incongruences between the biologic properties of particular people and the way society is structured. But such a view of the causes of disease is not new. What *is* new is that recombinant DNA analysis is beginning to reveal how complex the biologic side of such interrelationships is. So long as susceptibility is simply an abstract quality, strongly likely to be assigned to someone else, it can be ignored. But if a range of molecular variants can be shown to be associated with a range of degrees of susceptibility in a substantial fraction of the population, and if most diseases can be shown to partake of such variability, then we may want to begin to think deeply about how we want to organize ourselves for more healthful living; it may turn out that making each person responsible for his own health is not enough. And recombinant DNA methods promise to show us just how extensive and pervasive such variation is. Detailed descriptions of these methods and of how they are being used in the pursuit of the various medical aims outlined above are provided in the chapters of this book.

REFERENCES

1. Gusella JF: DNA polymorphism and human disease. *Ann Rev Biochem* 1986;55:831–834.
2. Robson EB: Fifty years of human genetics: Plus ça change, plus c'est la même chose. *Ann Hum Genet* 1986;50:1–2.
3. Smith CAB: The development of human linkage analysis. *Ann Hum Genet* 1986;50:293–311.
4. Benzer S: Genetic fine structure. *Harvey Lectures* 1961;56:1–21.
5. Nathans D, Smith HO: Restriction endonuclease in the analysis and restructuring of DNA molecules. *Ann Rev Biochem* 1975;44:273–290.
6. Schmickel RD: Contiguous gene syndromes: A component of recognizable syndromes. *J Pediat* 1986;109:231–241.
7. Baltimore D: Somatic mutation gains its place among the generators of diversity. *Cell* 1981;26:295–296.
8. Knudson AE Jr: Genetics of human cancer. *Ann Rev Genet* 1986;20:231–252.
9. Cairns J: The origin of human cancers. *Nature* 1981;209:353–357.
10. Varmus HE: The molecular genetics of cellular oncogenes. *Ann Rev Genet* 1985;18:553–612.
11. Klein G, Klein E: Evolution of tumours and the impact of molecular biology. *Nature* 1985;315:190–195.
12. Lewontin RC: Population genetics. *Ann Rev Genet* 1985;19:81–102.
13. Harris H: *Human Biochemical Genetics,* ed 3. New York, Elsevier, 1980.
14. Bodmer WF: HLA today. *Human Immunol* 1986;17:490–503.
15. Ott J: Analysis of Genetic Linkage in Human Families. Baltimore, Johns Hopkins University Press, 1986.

16. Botstein D, White RL, Skolnick M, et al: Construction of a genetic linkage map in man using restriction fragment length polymorphisms. *Am J Hum Genet* 1980;32:314–331.
17. de la Chapelle, A: The 1985 human gene map. Human Gene Mapping 8. *Birth Defects Original Article Series.* 1985;21 No. 4:1–7.
18. Orkin SH: Reverse genetics and human disease. *Cell* 1986;47:845–850.
19. Royer-Pokora B, Kunkel LM, Monaco AP, et al: Cloning the gene for an inherited disorder —chronic granulomatous disease—on the basis of its chromosomal location. *Nature* 1986;322:32–38.
20. Saltus R: Biotechnology firms compete in genetic diagnosis. *Science* 1986;234:1318–1320.
21. Stetler C, Grumet FC, Erlich HA: Polymorphic restriction endonuclease sites linked to the HLA-DR gene: Localization and use as genetic markers of insulin-dependent diabetes. *Proc Natl Acad Sci* 1985;82:8100–8104.
22. Thomas L: The future place of science in the art of healing. *J Med Ed* 1976;51:23–29.
23. Charache S, Dover GJ: Hydroxyurea-induced augmentation of fetal hemoglobin production in patients with sickle cell anemia. *Blood* 1987;69:109–116.
24. Hayes A, Costa T, Scriver CR, et al: The effect of mendelian disease on human health: II. Response to treatment. *Am J Med Genet* 1985;21:243–255.
25. Desnick RJ, Paul N: Enzyme therapy in genetic diseases. *Birth Defects Orig Series* 1980;16 No. 1.
26. Parkman R: The application of bone marrow transplantation to the treatment of genetic diseases. *Science* 1986;232:1373–1378.
27. Eschbach JW, Egrie JC, Downing MR, et al: Correction of the anemia of end-stage renal disease with recombinant human erythropoeitin. *N Eng J Med* 1987;316:73–78.
28. Miller LH, Howard RJ, Carter R, et al: Research toward malaria vaccines. *Science* 1986;234:1349–1356.
29. Entage JS: DNA makes protein makes money. *Nature* 1985;317:185–186.
30. Skolnick MH, Bishop DT, Cannings C, et al: The impact of RFLPs on human gene mapping, in Rao DC, Elston RD et al (eds): *Genetic Epidemiology of Coronary Heart Disease.* New York, AR Liss, 1984, pp 271–292.
31. Martin JB, Gusella JF: Huntington's disease. Pathogenesis and management. *N Eng J Med* 1976;315:1267–1276.
32. Deeb S, Failor A, Brown BG, et al: Molecular genetics of apolipoproteins and coronary heart disease. *Cold Spring Harbor Sym Quant Biol* 1987;51:403–409.
33. Farrer LA, Conneally M: Predictability of phenotype in Huntington's disease. *Arch Neurol* 1987;44:109–113.
34. Fries JF, Crapo LM: Vitality and Aging. San Francisco, WH Freeman, 1981.

CHAPTER 2

Recombinant DNA Methods: Applications to Human Genetics

Helen Donis-Keller, PhD, and
David Botstein, PhD

The past decade has seen a revolution in molecular biology due mainly to the introduction of recombinant DNA methods. These methods have allowed the isolation and characterization of genes from any organism and the determination of the DNA sequence and any encoded protein sequences. It has become possible as well to follow genes through families, and indeed, over evolutionary changes. The ability to isolate and analyze human genes has had, if anything, an even more profound effect on the field of human genetics than on most areas of biology. The new technology has already made possible the understanding of many inherited diseases at the molecular level. Perhaps more important, recombinant DNA methods, for the first time, have permitted direct general application of mendelian ideas to human families, through the use of restriction fragment length polymorphisms (RFLPs).

The purpose of this chapter is to review briefly the technology in a way that makes for better understanding by non-specialists, rather than to introduce actual techniques. For the latter purpose, several extremely helpful technical manuals and other publications[1,2,3,4] are available for those interested in laboratory work; for linkage analysis at the technical level the reader is referred to Ott (1985).[5] In what follows we will describe very briefly principles underlying the use of restriction endonucleases, DNA sequence analysis, gel-transfer hybridization (Southern blotting), gene cloning, and library construction, as well as the principles of genetic mapping using RFLPs. The last-named subject will take us into a description of the statistical ideas and methodologies required to make and use a linkage map of the human genome.

ISOLATION AND CHARACTERIZATION OF GENES AND DNA FRAGMENTS

Restriction Enzymes Cleave Double-Stranded DNA

The era of recombinant DNA methods can be thought of as beginning with the discovery and purification of sequence-specific endonucleases. These are bacterial enzymes that recognize specific nucleotide sequences in DNA from all organisms and cleave the DNA within that sequence or very nearby it. They are called *restriction enzymes* because they apparently evolved in bacteria as defenses against the invasion of foreign DNAs in the form of viruses or plasmids. Each of the enzymes is associated with a modification activity (usually a methylase) that protects the bacterial cell's own DNA against cleavage: a cell carrying a specific restriction/modification system will modify the restriction sites in its own DNA, whereas foreign intruding DNA, being unmodified, will be cleaved upon entry.

Through the pioneering work of Nathans and Smith (1975),[6] it became clear that, whatever role these enzymes played in nature, they could be used as reagents to characterize the sequences of DNAs. Many enzymes with different sequence specificities have been found, some recognizing sequences only 4 base pairs (bp) in length (thus cutting DNA every 256 bp on average, ie, 4^4), others recognizing 6 bp sites (cutting on average every 4,096 bp, ie, 4^6). Recently, enzymes recognizing sites as large as 10 bp have been found. Convenient, up-to-date summaries of available enzymes are the catalogs of the manufacturers (eg, New England Biolabs). Since the enzymes read bits of DNA sequence, the number and arrangement of restriction sites is characteristic of a given DNA sequence: this is called its *restriction map*. One maps DNA molecules for three major purposes: first, as a "signature," since each sequence has a unique map; second, as an aid to manipulations, such as subcloning and RFLP analysis; third, as a prelude to determination of the nucleotide sequence.

The restriction map of a DNA molecule is deduced in practice from the pattern of fragment sizes produced after digestion with a number of different restriction enzymes, separately or in combination. The pattern can conveniently be analyzed by separating the fragments by electrophoresis through an agarose gel; the DNA is stained with ethidium bromide or visualized by hybridization in situ. In most systems of electrophoresis, fragment mobility is inversely proportional to the logarithm of molecular length, allowing easy comparison of lengths. Use of standards of known length allows routine determination of molecular length to a precision of about 5%. A large number of restriction enzymes are commercially available, and the apparatus for agarose gel electrophoresis and visualization of the fragments is simple to use.

Cloning DNA Sequences

The direct determination of the restriction map of a DNA sequence requires its isolation in bulk. For anything beyond small virus genomes, it is necessary to clone the sequences of interest in order to create restriction maps of them directly. There are many systems of cloning, and their basis is beyond the scope of this article. However, it should be borne in mind that DNA clones consist of a *vector,* that is, a DNA segment that contains means of replication and selection in bacteria, and an *insert,* that is, the cloned DNA that has been joined to the vector and replicated in bacteria with it. The means of replication may be simply a site ("origin of replication") recognized and used by the bacterial host DNA synthesis machinery, or else it may involve both a viral origin of replication and additional viral enzymes required for replication. The selection system is usually a gene conferring resistance to an antibiotic such as ampicillin or tetracycline. These elements, when attached to insert DNA, allow the selection for bacteria carrying the composite "clone." The clone will replicate and, by expressing drug resistance, be able to withstand the applied selection. There are three general vector types: (1) plasmid vectors, (2) viral vectors, and (3) cosmid vectors. *Plasmid vectors* are relatively small (2–5 kilobases [kb]) self-replicating circles of double-stranded DNA that accommodate all sizes of insert (0–40 kb) and are frequently used as vectors when large segments of DNA are subdivided or "subcloned." *Viral vectors* may be mammalian viruses such as SV40 or bacteriophages, for example, bacteriophage λ, that have been modified by removing regions of their genomes not essential for replication or packaging, and replacing this DNA with insert DNA (up to 20 kb). The cloning of human genomic DNA into such vectors is schematically represented in Figures 2.1 and 2.2. *Cosmids* are combination vectors with bacteriophage λ and plasmid elements that allow the efficient insertion and replication of very large segments of DNA (up to 40 kb). The advantages of cosmid systems are in the efficiency of cloning (packaging of cloned DNA in viral capsids): the end result is a population of plasmid clones with very large inserts.

The source of inserts can be the DNA of the target organism (in which case the clones are called *genomic* clones), or it can be a messenger RNA copied into DNA by reverse transcription, in which case the clones are called complementary DNA (*cDNA*) clones. Since most human genes are split by intervening sequences that are removed by the cell in the process of making the mRNA, a cDNA clone of very modest length (say, 1000 bp) may contain sequences spanning 200,000 bp in the human genome. A schematic representation of the cDNA cloning procedure is shown in Figure 2.3.

A major difference between cDNA and genomic clones is the presence in the latter of repeated sequences that abound in the genome, but are rarely

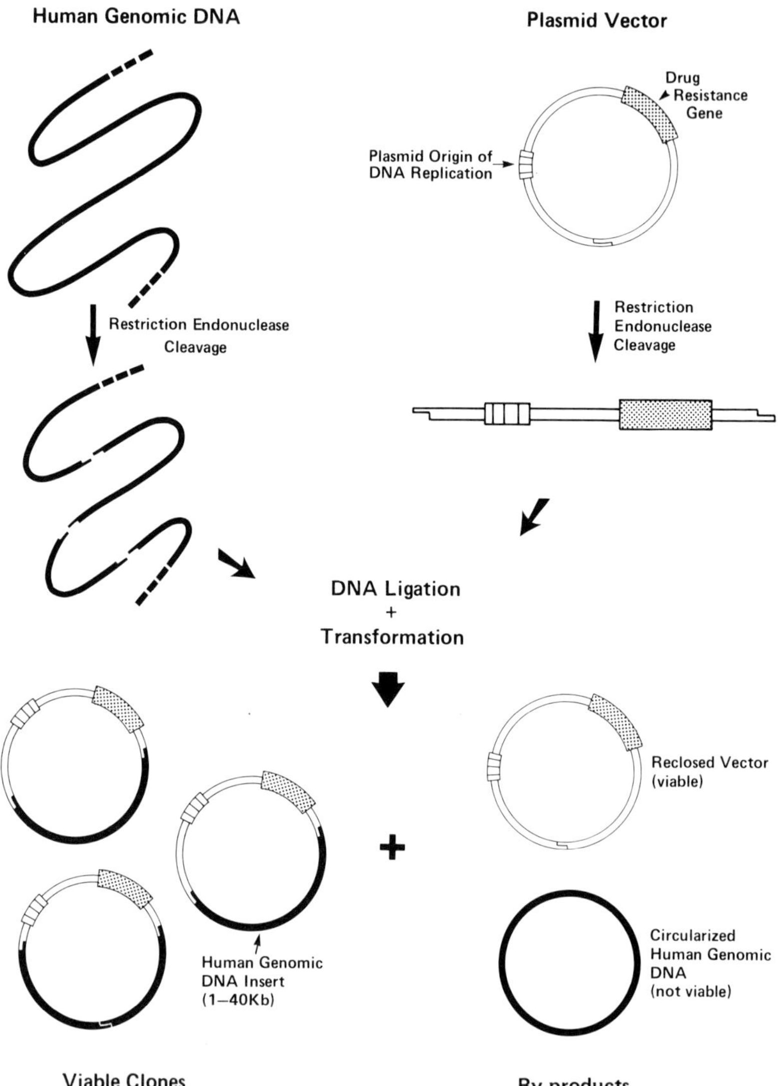

FIGURE 2.1 Cloning human DNA into a plasmid vector. Human genomic DNA is cleaved with a restriction endonuclease and inserted into a standard plasmid vector that contains a means of replication and a selectable marker. Various by-products of the procedure (closed vector and circularized human DNA) are also represented.

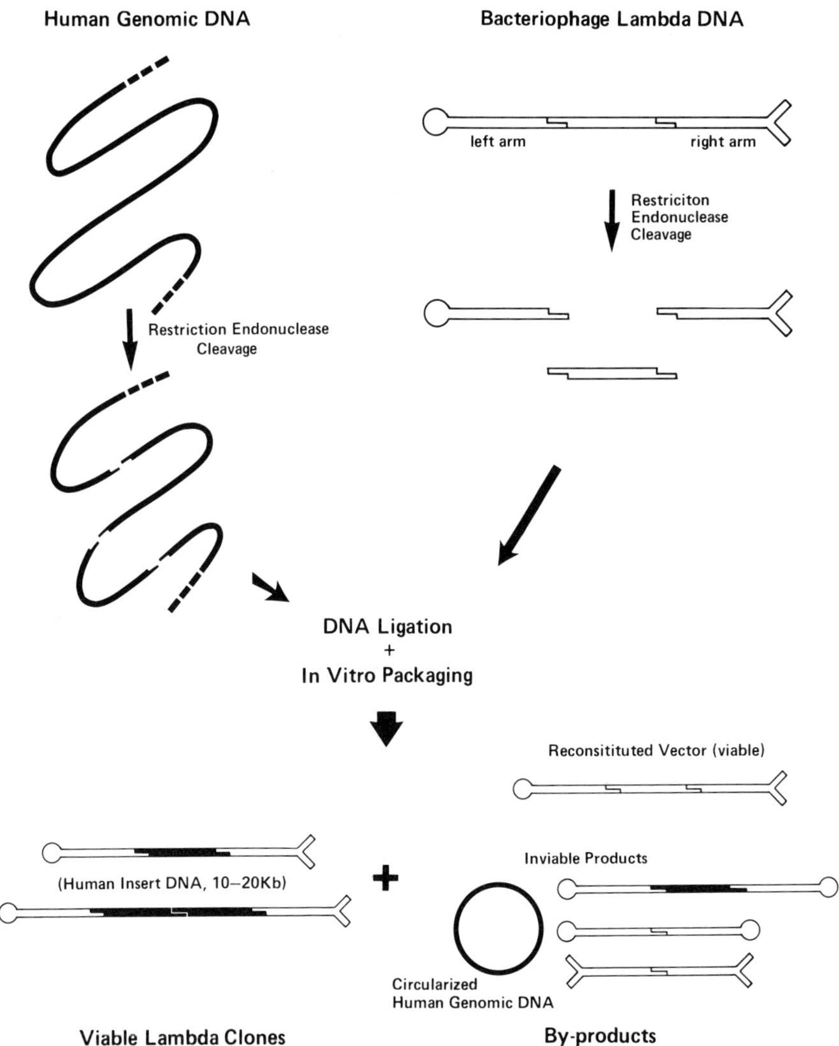

FIGURE 2.2 Cloning human DNA into a bacteriophage λ vector. Human genomic DNA is cleaved with a restriction endonuclease and inserted into a bacteriophage λ vector. The recombinant vector is then packaged into bacteriophage capsid particles in an in vitro reaction. Various by-products of the procedure are also pictured.

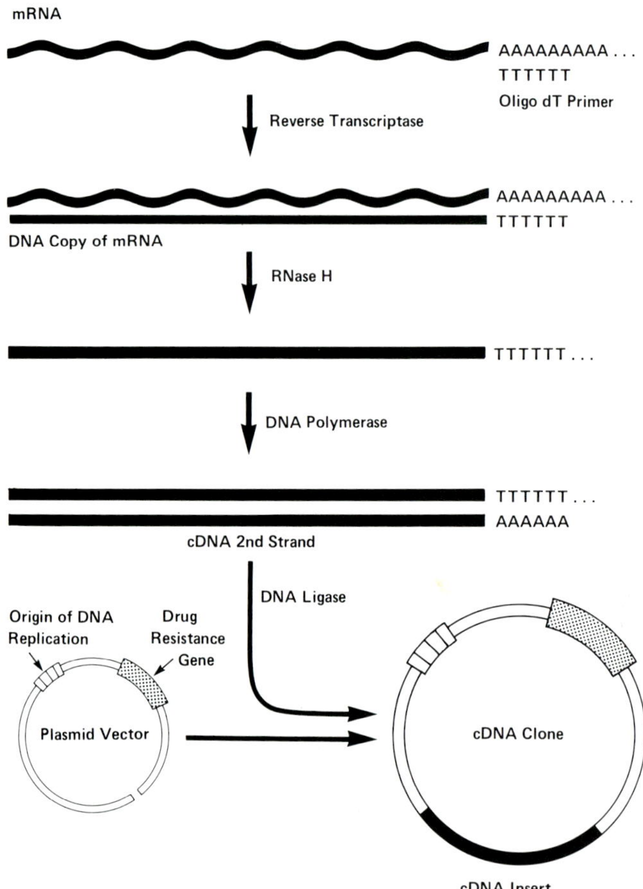

FIGURE 2.3 cDNA cloning. Schematic representation of the in vitro reactions that result in the production of cDNA clones.

transcribed and even more rarely included in the final processed mRNA. A random genomic clone is thus overwhelmingly likely (98%) to contain heavily repeated sequences, whereas a cDNA clone will be repeated, in general, only if the protein specified is a member of a gene family, such as the globins or the immunoglobulins.

In general, particular human genes have been cloned by the cDNA route, in which the protein specified by the gene is known. In such cases the mRNA is isolated from the tissue in which the gene is expressed, copied into DNA using the viral enzyme reverse transcriptase, and ligated into a suitable vector. Genomic clones are then obtained by using the cDNA clone as a hybridization "probe" in order to retrieve corresponding genomic sequences from "libraries" of genomic sequences.

Constructing DNA Libraries

Since all nucleated cells contain essentially the entire genome (which represents all the human genetic material except mitochrondrial DNA), DNA to be used in the construction of genomic libraries can be easily obtained from lymphocytes isolated from a peripheral blood sample. Such libraries are made by fragmenting randomly the genomic DNA by partial digestion with a restriction enzyme and cloning the fragments into a vector such that enough clones are generated to make it overwhelmingly probable that all sequences are represented several times. Thus, one good genomic library, for example, the Maniatis human genomic library in a λ vector,[7] suffices for virtually all genomic cloning purposes.

A genomic library will contain different types of sequences aside from those that code for genes. Unique sequence DNA is estimated to comprise 70% of the human genome (reviewed in Lewin, 1980),[8] while the remainder consists of moderately repetitive DNA segments like ribosomal genes and others that are highly repeated such as the "Alu" or "Kpn" families.[9,10] Some highly repeated sequences are difficult to clone because they frequently recombine and are lost during standard cloning procedures and therefore may not be represented in genomic libraries.[11,12] It is also possible to construct chromosome-specific libraries by using as a source of insert physically separated chromosomes or hybrid cell lines (originating from fusions of rodent with human cells)[13] that are thought to contain a single human chromosome.[14]

In contrast, cDNA libraries reflect the tissue of origin, being made of copies of mRNAs that vary according to tissue type; different genes are expressed in liver and in brain, for example, and thus different mRNAs are present. In summary, the human geneticist has available two kinds of cloned human DNAs: cDNA, representing particular genes or the expressed genes of particular tissues, and genomic DNA, containing a continuous segment of the human genome. Both kinds of clone have uses in human genetics, many of which involve the examination of human DNAs and their restriction maps indirectly by hybridization.

DNA Sequencing

The ultimate characterization of a DNA molecule is, of course, its complete nucleotide sequence. Since the simultaneous development of the chemical and enzymatic approaches,[15,16,17] each method has been refined and extended so that it has become routine to determine sequences of genes as they are cloned (See Fig. 2.1).

The chemical method employs the idea of radiolabeling a fragment of DNA just at one end and then chemically cleaving in a base-specific manner. A partial reaction, in that case, will contain a nested set of molecules whose different lengths correspond to the positions of the base at which cleavages were made. The lengths of labeled fragments from four such reactions suffice to indicate the relative positions of each of the bases in the sequence. Figure 2.4 shows a diagrammatic representation of these concepts. A recent extension of the chemical methods allows the determination of sequences without cloning, by using highly radioactive DNA probes directly on genomic DNA cleaved and separated by size instead of direct end labeling.[18]

The enzymatic method[17] is similar to the chemical method except that the DNA to be sequenced is copied in vitro with DNA polymerase and the reaction stopped in a base-specific manner, usually by the addition of chain-termination dideoxynucleotide analogs as substrates. Methods for applying enzymatic methods to DNA from whole genomes by amplification of specific segments have also been published.[19,20]

DNA sequencing is very labor intensive, whether one uses chemical or enzymatic methods. For this reason there is great interest in methods of automation of this process. A prototype automatic system has been announced.[21]

RECOMBINANT DNA METHODS IN GENETIC ANALYSIS

Genetic Markers

The ability to follow the inheritance of marker traits in humans is of particular importance in medical genetics for diagnostic applications, and, in addition, may constitute the initial steps toward the identification and characterization of the genes for which the molecular mechanisms are unknown. Furthermore, even complex disorders in which environmental and genetic factors combine can in principle be studied by following the inheritance of any one or more genetic loci that might be responsible for the phenotype. In addition to the contribution of environmental factors, identification of the genetic loci important in such a disorder may allow the subdivision of the phenotype into different classes, each of which may be effectively treated with a therapy tailored to the subtype. Classical genetic markers, for example, protein polymorphisms such as ABO blood groups and HLA antigens, have found practical benefit for blood and tissue typing, but have limited usefulness in genetic mapping in humans because they are too few in number

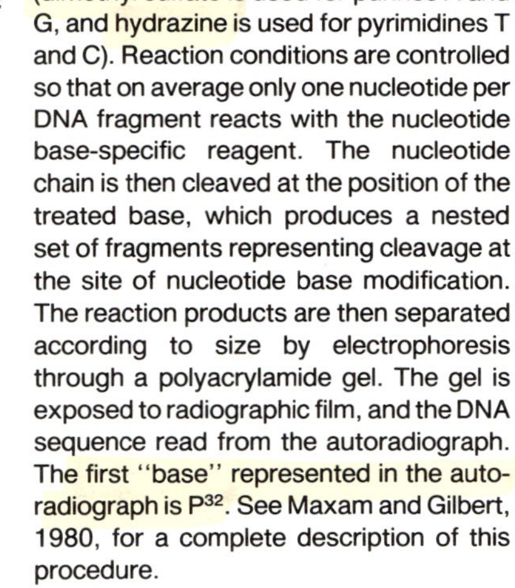

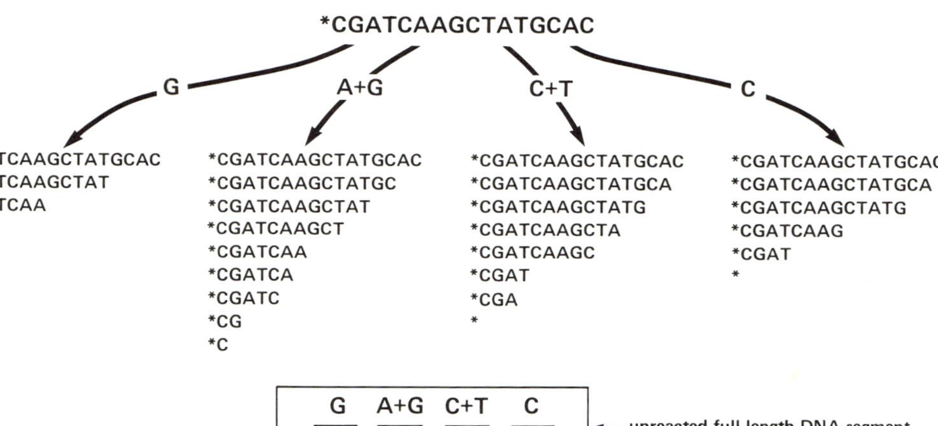

FIGURE 2.4 Maxam Gilbert DNA sequencing. A unique-sequence DNA fragment labeled at the 5′ end with P^{32} is treated with nucleotide base-specific reagents in four separate chemical reactions (dimethyl sulfate is used for purines A and G, and hydrazine is used for pyrimidines T and C). Reaction conditions are controlled so that on average only one nucleotide per DNA fragment reacts with the nucleotide base-specific reagent. The nucleotide chain is then cleaved at the position of the treated base, which produces a nested set of fragments representing cleavage at the site of nucleotide base modification. The reaction products are then separated according to size by electrophoresis through a polyacrylamide gel. The gel is exposed to radiographic film, and the DNA sequence read from the autoradiograph. The first "base" represented in the autoradiograph is P^{32}. See Maxam and Gilbert, 1980, for a complete description of this procedure.

The principle of other sequencing methods is similar except that the differences are in the method of interrupting the chain in a base-specific manner or the method of labeling the 5′ end of the molecule specifically.

and, except for HLA, are insufficiently polymorphic. The advent of recombinant DNA technology opened the way to the development of an entirely new system of genetic markers for humans that enable the mapping of virtually any inherited trait. These markers, RFLPs, exploit the variation in DNA sequence among individuals. The examination of sequence variation at particular regions of the genome allows distinctions to be made among individuals with a resolution much greater than any preexisting method. It has been estimated that sequence differences among individuals occur on average every 50 to 100 nucleotides.[22] Such regions of variation can be sampled by the use of restriction enzymes since they recognize and cleave unique sequences in DNA.*

Detecting RFLPs by Southern Blotting

The methodology most commonly employed to visualize sequence polymorphism is by gel transfer and hybridization of size-fractionated enzyme-cleaved genomic DNA to labeled cloned DNA; this procedure is also known as *Southern blotting*[22] (Southern, 1975). The procedure is carried out as follows (Fig. 2.5):

1. Genomic DNA from a set of unrelated individuals (A–E in Fig. 2.5) is cleaved with a restriction enzyme and fractionated according to size by electrophoresis through an agarose gel.
2. The DNA is denatured to separate the strands and transferred to a solid support such as a nitrocellulose or nylon membrane.
3. A cloned segment of DNA is radioactively labeled and hybridized to the genomic DNA attached to the membrane in the presence of a solution that facilitates the formation of hydrogen bonds. The cloned DNA hybridizes, or anneals with, its complementary sequence present in the genomic DNA. The membrane is then washed to remove any nonspecifically bound labeled DNA and exposed to radiographic film.
4. Any polymorphism is inferred from the differences, if any, between individuals in the pattern of restriction-fragment lengths displayed on the autoradiograph.

*A note on the word *polymorphism* is in order. In classical population genetics a locus is said to be polymorphic when it displays at least one alternative allele present at a frequency of at least 1% in the population. In modern DNA work, one is interested mainly in the likelihood of heterozygosity at a locus, which will be usefully high only when the locus is very polymorphic (minor allele frequencies of 10% or greater, and multiple alleles). The way in which DNA polymorphisms are now employed has resulted in a subtly different usage of the word, although no formal change in definition is required. In RFLP analysis stress is put on the expected degree of *heterozygosity* at a locus, not, as was classically the case, on the absolute frequency in a population of the particular alleles at a locus.

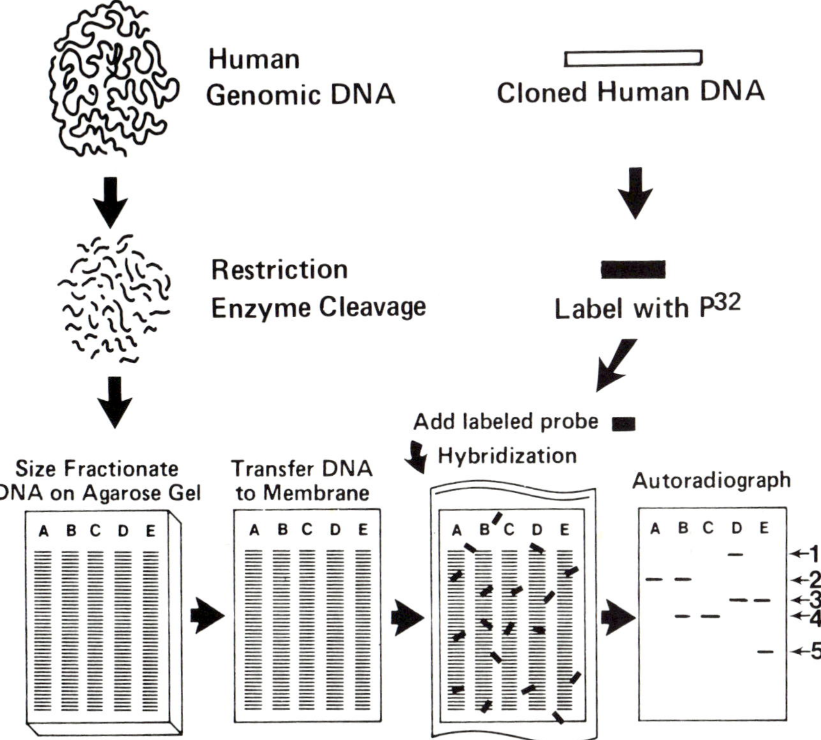

FIGURE 2.5 Detection of polymorphism by gel transfer. A cloned human DNA segment is tested for its ability to reveal polymorphism by hybridization to size-fractionated genomic DNA from five unrelated individuals (A,B,C,D,E) cleaved with a restriction enzyme. Five different fragment lengths (alleles 1–5) are detected with the radioactively labeled human DNA probe. The genotypes of the individuals are A 2,2; B-2,4; C-4,4; D-1,3; E-3,5.

As Figure 2.5 shows, five different patterns are seen among the five unrelated individuals. Since everyone inherits two copies of each chromosome, one from the mother and one from the father, except for the sex chromosomes, one would expect to see two fragment lengths, or alleles, in each individual. Individuals *A* and *C* in Figure 2.5 each have two alleles that are the same length, thus showing only one band, are therefore termed *homozygotes*. Individuals *B, C,* and *E* have a different fragment length for each allele and are termed *heterozygotes*. Therefore, this region of DNA displays polymorphism in DNA fragment length: this is a good RFLP locus. There are five alternative fragment lengths (*alleles*) at this locus. In some cases, more than one fragment length constitutes a single allele at a locus and thus the set of fragments is inherited according to mendelian principles (see Knowlton et al, 1986,[24] and Schumm et al, 1987,[25] for examples). The geneticist recognizes as a "locus" any length of DNA within which recombination (see below) is so small as to be negligible.

A genomic library with relatively large inserts (10–20 kb) is a good source of cloned DNA probes to test, as above, for polymorphism. Since most of the clones will contain repeated DNA, it is necessary to prehybridize the clones with total genomic DNA so that only unique sequence regions of the clones are available to be tested for polymorphism in the gel transfer experiment[25,26] (Litt et al, 1985; Schumm et al, 1987). Alternatively, about 1% of the human DNA clones in λ vectors contain entirely single-copy DNA and therefore can be tested for polymorphism without the prehybridization step.[27] The cloned DNA sequences are compared as above to genomic DNA from a variety of unrelated individuals.

A set of restriction enzymes that survey different sequences are tested with each genomic clone. It has been observed that the enzymes Taql and Mspl are especially useful in revealing polymorphism in humans because they contain as part of their recognition sequence the dinucleotide CG, which is apparently highly mutable.[25,28] Other restriction enzymes that are particularly useful in revealing polymorphism are Rsal, Hindlll, Bglll, Pstl, EcoR1, and BamH1.[25]

Figure 2.6 shows an examle of a typical screening blot in which the genomic DNA of five unrelated individuals is cleaved with six restriction enzymes and tested for polymorphism with a cloned DNA probe, CRI-RL4-117. All of the individuals apparently share the same sequences at the sites tested with five of the enzymes. However, a polymorphism is visualized with the enzyme Mspl. This is a simple two-allele polymorphism that is caused by a single base pair difference at the recognition site of the enzyme. Polymorphism may also occur as a result of DNA rearrangements, that is, by the insertion or deletion of DNA segments. Figure 2.7 shows an example of a rearrangement polymorphism. Polymorphisms at single genetic loci can be much more complicated than the simple ones illustrated here and may consist of clustered site changes and/or multiple DNA rearrangements with a number of fragment lengths that characterize each allele. The most useful polymorphisms have a large number of alleles represented at equal frequencies in the population. With such markers it is likely that most individuals will be heterozygous at the locus and that the alleles contributed by each parent can be identified in the offspring. The usefulness of a polymorphism in an inheritance study is represented by its polymorphism information content (PIC)* value.[22]

*The PIC is a mathematical measure of the usefulness of a polymorphism in linkage studies. It is the probability of identifying in any given offspring the parental chromosome contribution. Some authors use the mean heterozygosity (simply the frequency of heterozygotes) as a measure of polymorphism. The difference between PIC and heterozygosity is that the former estimates

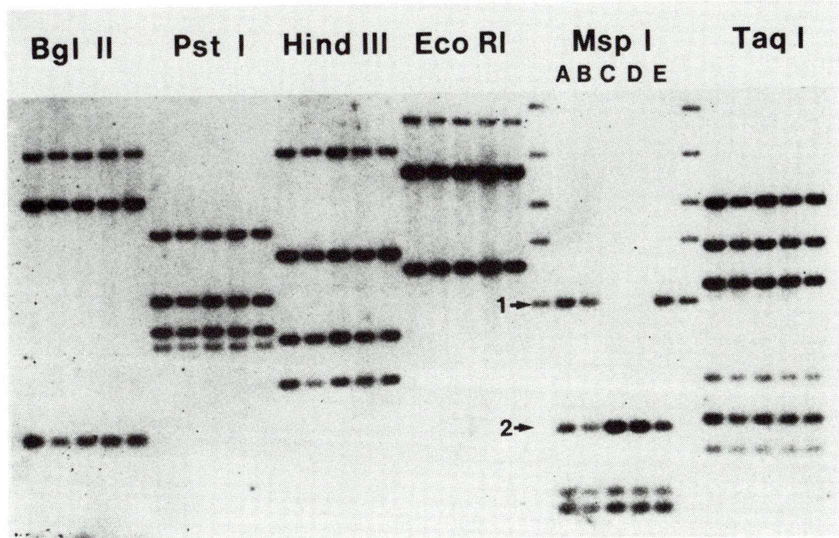

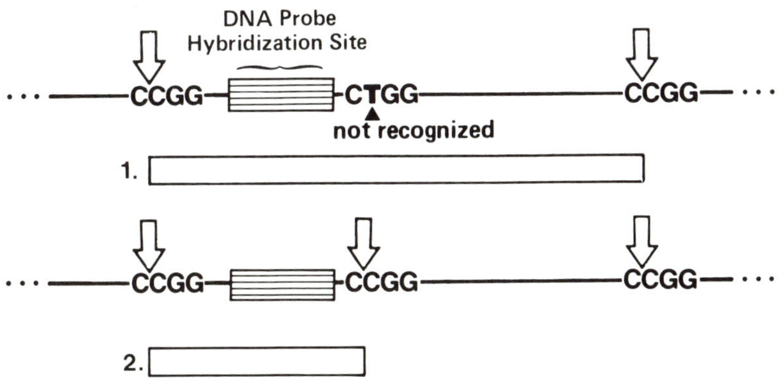

FIGURE 2.6 Screening for polymorphism: base change polymorphism. Southern transfer of genomic DNA from five unrelated individuals (A,B,C,D,E) cleaved with the restriction enzymes indicated and probed with genomic clone CRI-RL4-117. A site change polymorphism is revealed by the enzyme MspI. Individuals A,B, and E are heterozygous at the locus, whereas individuals C and D are homozygous for allele 2 (*arrows*). The recognition site of the enzyme and resulting fragment lengths (alleles) are shown below the autoradiograph. Note: DNA probe hybridization site is not drawn to scale, and only the top strand of the duplex DNA molecule is illustrated with the restriction endonuclease cleavage sites.

more exactly the probability that a marker will be informative in practice when used in an inheritance study of a random family. The heterozygosity overestimates the usefulness of a marker at low values; at high values the PIC and heterozygosity converge. A polymorphism with a PIC value of 1 is fully informative for any mating (ie, the parental chromosome contribution can be unambiguously determined in the offspring). Figure 2.8 shows the inheritance of an RFLP fully informative in a three-generation family. Four distinguishable alleles at the locus are present in the parents, and it is easy to trace the inheritance of the alleles in the offspring.

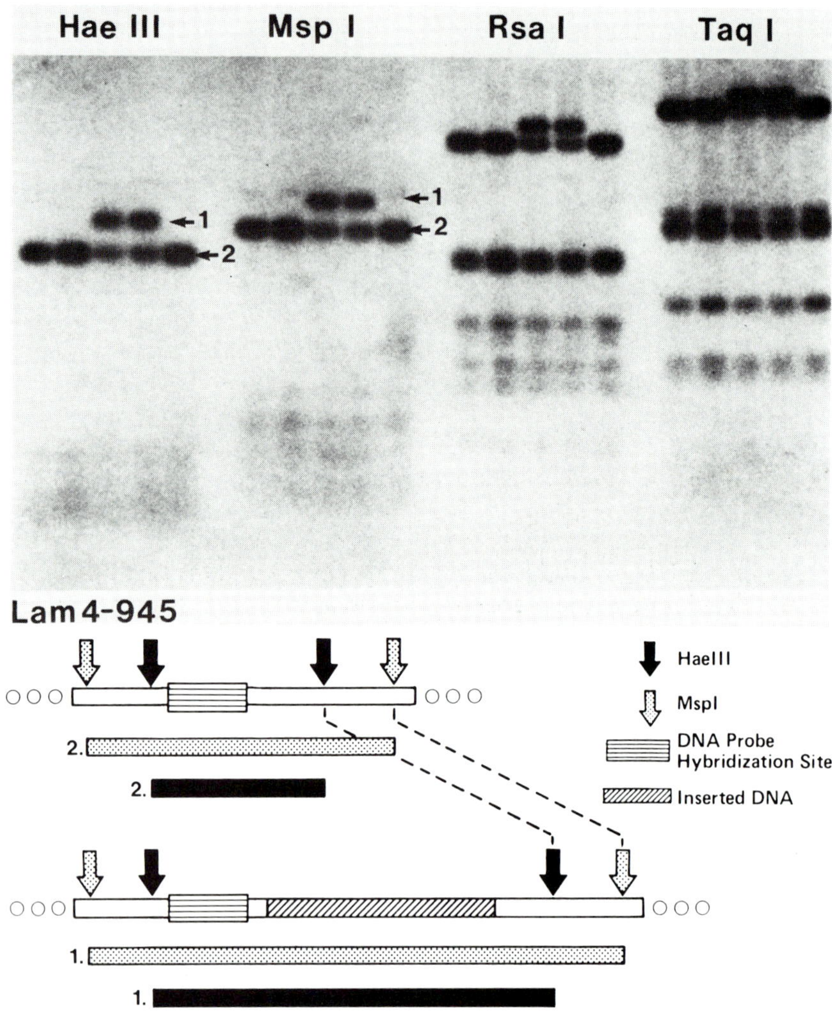

FIGURE 2.7 Screening for polymorphism: DNA rearrangement polymorphism. Southern transfer of genomic DNA from five unrelated individuals cleaved with the restriction enzymes indicated and probed with the genomic clone CRI-Lam4-945. An insertion/deletion polymorphism is indicated from comparison of the similarity of patterns from each of the enzymes; the alleles differ in molecular weight by an absolute amount in the various restriction digests, as indicated by the drawing shown below the autoradiograph.

The examples shown demonstrate polymorphism of DNA fragments that range in length from 1 to 20 kb. It is also possible to resolve smaller and much larger fragment lengths by using different gel systems and electrophoresis conditions. Polymorphisms have been identified with fragments that range in length from ten to several hundred nucleotides,[29] and in principle polymorphisms should be identifiable with fragments in the hundreds of kilobases resolved by orthogonal field gel electrophoresis (OFAGE)[30] or field inversion electrophoresis systems (FIGE).[31]

Other Methods for Detecting Sequence Variation

Another method of detecting sequence variation that does not rely on restriction enzymes is the use of denaturing gradient gel electrophoresis.[32] This method, which in principle can detect heterozygosity at any sequence (not just restriction sites), has yet to be applied on a large scale to the detection of polymorphisms suitable for use as genetic markers. It has been used, however, to detect many known mutations in the globin genes.

Synthetic nucleotide probes can also be used to identify sequence variation. In this case small oligonucleotide probes are used to test for single base differences. For example, oligonucleotide probes of 17 nucleotides have been used to detect the base change that is responsible for sickle cell anemia.[33] In this case the hybridization conditions were controlled so that even a single mismatch between the sequence of the probe and the genomic DNA resulted in a failure of the probe to hybridize to the corresponding genomic sequence.

Detection Systems

By far the most commonly used method for labeling DNA is nick translation[1,34] using radioactive nucleoside triphosphates in vitro. Random sequence priming and the production of radioactive RNA copies, all in vitro, have also been used to enhance the degree of specificity of radiolabeling.[35] Nonradioactive labeling methods have been suggested. Most notable among these are the ones based on biotinylated nucleosides after nick translation. The biotin can be used to attach avidin coupled to many different detectable materials, including fluorescent compounds and enzymes.[36] Unfortunately, these methods have not yet reached the sensitivity of the radiolabeling method; for the problem of detecting a single copy sequence in the human genome one still needs the high signal-to-noise ratio of the radioactive method.

GENETIC MAPPING

Linkage of Genetic Markers

The indispensable element of any kind of linkage study is heterozygosity. Only if an individual is heterozygous at each of two loci can the linkage relationship between the two loci be established. In the case of humans, the requirement for heterozygosity means that high degrees of polymorphism are required, since one is dependent upon the natural occurrence of heterozygosity in random matings. As described above, RFLPs have provided an essentially inexhaustible supply of polymorphisms particularly suitable for linkage studies, since both alleles can always be determined in heterozygotes.

Given a set of fully informative RFLPs (ie, ones polymorphic enough that each parent in a randomly chosen family is likely to be heterozygous at every RFLP locus), it is possible to follow each of the parental contributions into the children directly and thus to determine linkage (see Figure 2.8). The principle is illustrated in Figure 2.9, where two of each of the parents chromosomes are shown. On one chromosome is shown the RFLP marker A, and the father has distinguishable RFLP alleles A1 and A2 while the mother has alleles A3 and A4. The other chromosome carries two other RFLP loci, B and C, each with four alleles (B1 and B2 in the father, B3 and B4 in the mother, C1 and C2 in the father, and C3 and C4 in the mother). All the properties of mendelian inheritance can now be demonstrated:

1. Each of the children receives either A1 or A2 from the father and either A3 or A4 from the mother (Mendel's first law of segregation) so that the four possible genotypes of the children are A1/A3, A1/A4, A2/A3, or A2/A4. Likewise for loci B and C.
2. All combinations of A and B alleles deriving from each parent are found in the children. Thus, following only the contribution from the father, we find that the combinations A1,B1; A2,B1; A1,B2; A2,B2 are equally common. This is Mendel's second law, also called the *rule of independent assortment.* Loci A and C also assort independently.
3. In contrast, only a limited number of combinations of B and C alleles deriving from each parent are found in the children: thus, again following the contribution from the father, we find that the combinations B1,C1 and B2,C2 are found in the children, but the combinations B1,C2 and B2,C1 are not. This principle is called *linkage,* and reflects the fact that B and C are physically close together on the chromosome in the example. When linkage is complete, then the alleles B1 and C1 were inherited from the grandparents together and in turn are passed on together to the children.

Unlike the example in Figure 2.9, however, linkage ordinarily is not an all-or-none phenomenon. Some gene pairs indeed lie so close together that they rarely reassort and thus approximate the limiting case of complete linkage, but linked markers usually lie far enough apart that they can become separated in meiosis by a process called *recombination.* Thus, in the example the allele combinations B1,C2 and B2,C1 are recombinant types, whereas the combinations B1,C1 and B2,C2 are *parental.* Linkage is more generally

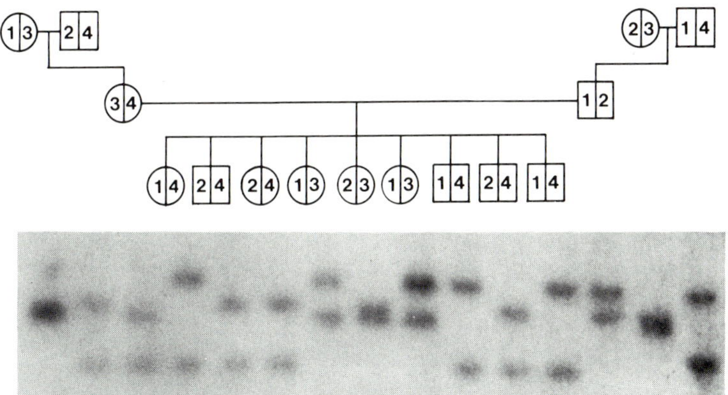

FIGURE 2.8 Inheritance of RFLP alleles. Mendelian inheritance of an RFLP in a three-generation family. A human DNA clone RL4-365 isolated from a human genomic library, labeled with P^{32} by a nick translation reaction and hybridized against the human genomic DNA cleaved with the restriction enzyme BglII detects four alleles (1-4.2kb;2-4.0kb;3-3.8kb;4-3.5kb).

expressed as a deviation from random assortment (ie, equal frequencies [50%] of parental and recombinant types in the progeny, as in loci A and B above) so that the recombinant types appear less frequently than the 50% expected.

It is important to understand that there is nothing in the RFLP pattern or "phenotype" of the parents that indicates whether alleles B1 and C1 lie on the same chromosome (and B2 and C2 on the other) or whether the opposite arrangement (B1 and C2 on one chromosome and B2 and C1 on the other). All we know from examination of their DNA with RFLP probes is that the genotype of the father is B1/B2, C1/C2 and the genotype of the mother is B3/B4, C3/C4. In the example, we know the answer to the question of their chromosomal origin from the way in which the pair was passed on to the children (ie, B1 and C1 together); we could also infer the arrangement (often called the *linkage phase*) from an examination of the DNA of the grandparents.

Yet, as the example shows, when we do not know about linkage in advance, and even when we do not know the linkage phase in advance, it is clear that one can infer both. If there are many children and the RFLPs are informative enough (ie, sufficiently polymorphic to be used in many different families), we can infer linkage by looking for enough data to make the deviation from random assortment statistically significant.

Quantitative assessments of the significance of linkage estimates are made by calculations in which the likelihood that the data observed arose from a particular model (ie, linkage) is compared to the likelihood of observ-

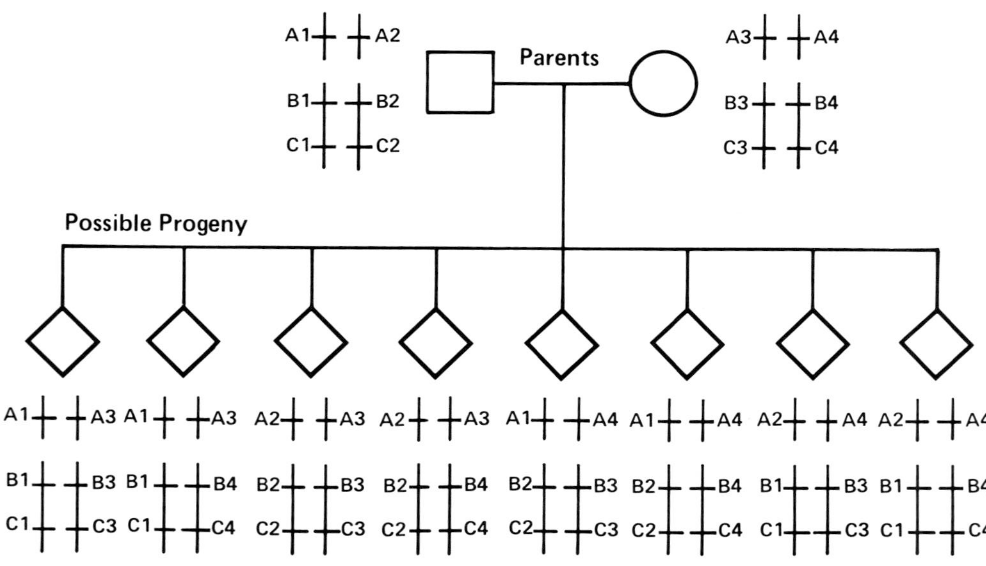

FIGURE 2.9 Using the inheritance of RFLP alleles to determine linkage. Three RFLP loci (A,B,C) on chromosome pairs are shown with possible inheritance patterns in the offspring (see text for details).

ing the same data on the alternative hypothesis (random assortment). By longstanding convention, linkage is regarded as having been demonstrated when the likelihood ratio (often called the odds ratio) reaches 1,000 : 1 in favor of the linkage hypothesis[37] (see Ott, 1985,[5] for a full discussion of likelihood methods as applied to linkage). The statistic usually calculated is the logarithm of the odds ratio (LOD); LOD scores obtained from different families are additive, and, of course, significance is achieved when the LOD reaches a value of 3. The calculation of a LOD score expected for a simple case is given in Figure 2.10, where it can be seen that a single phase-known meiosis will contribute an expected LOD score of +0.16 if the hypothesis of linkage at a distance of 10% recombination is true, and −0.22 if the alternative hypothesis of nonlinkage is true.

The likelihood method is very flexible, and hypotheses much more complex than the one in Figure 2.10 can be accommodated. Uncertainties of linkage phase, for example, can easily be taken into account by altering the hypothesis and thus the calculation of the likelihood that the data was derived from this hypothesis. Of course, ambiguities (such as lack of knowledge of linkage phase) will reduce the magnitude of a given family's contribution to the overall LOD score; conversely, the presence of multiple affected siblings will raise the contribution. LOD scores can be obtained from several different families, and these scores can be added until the score rises to 3 (or, alternatively, declines to −2, the conventional level for rejection of the linkage hypothesis).

Thus, RFLP markers are used to map disease genes by applying them to members of families in which the disease is segregating and trying, for each RFLP marker, to find evidence for linkage as assessed by the LOD scores. As mentioned, the value of different families with respect to their contribution to achieving an LOD of 3 varies: in general, for simple mendelian diseases, the ideal circumstance is a family in which there are several affected siblings (to provide many opportunities to observe crossovers or the lack of crossovers with the RFLP marker) and, if possible, grandparents (who can reduce ambiguities about linkage phase).

Closing in on a Gene

Genetic linkage to several single gene disorders has been discovered over the past few years. For example, the loci responsible for Duchenne muscular dystrophy,[38] Huntington's disease,[39] adult polycystic kidney disease[40] and cystic fibrosis[41–44] have been identified by testing random DNA markers for linkage in families segregating these disorders.

The major virtue of the linkage approach is that one follows, in family studies, the actual biologic defect in inherited disease because presence and absence of the disease phenotype itself is scored. Before beginning, one has

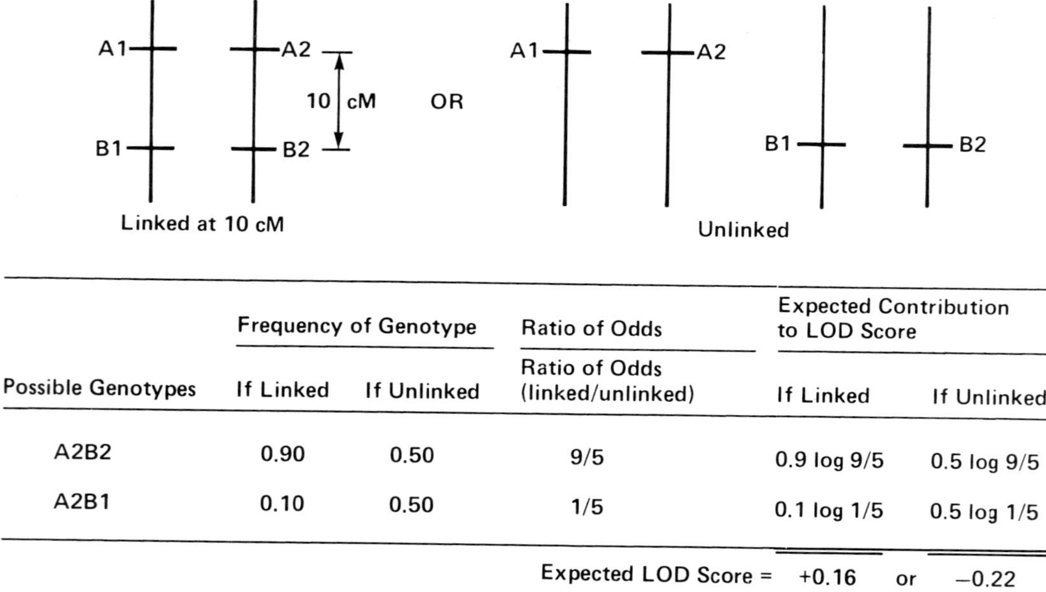

	Frequency of Genotype		Ratio of Odds	Expected Contribution to LOD Score	
Possible Genotypes	If Linked	If Unlinked	Ratio of Odds (linked/unlinked)	If Linked	If Unlinked
A2B2	0.90	0.50	9/5	0.9 log 9/5	0.5 log 9/5
A2B1	0.10	0.50	1/5	0.1 log 1/5	0.5 log 1/5
			Expected LOD Score =	+0.16	or −0.22

FIGURE 2.10 LOD score from a single-phase known meiosis. The contribution of one meiosis to the LOD (log of the odds) score calculation is shown. For the purpose of illustration, 10 cM is taken as exactly 10% recombination.

no idea of the physical location of the disease gene in the genome unless, of course, it is sex linked. However, upon detection of statistically credible linkage to an RFLP marker, a piece of DNA (the probe) is available that can be located physically by conventional methods. Currently these methods are two: mapping by somatic cell hybrids between rodent and human cells[45] and in situ hybridization to human chromosomes.[46]

Somatic cell hybrid panels are constructed by fusion of rodent cells to human cells and continued propagation of the products of fusion. The rodent complement of chromosomes remains stable during this process, but the human chromosomes are somewhat randomly lost during passage of the cells. Thus, one collects a set of individual cell lines that may contain, for example, a cell line with human chromosomes 6,2,X, and the rodent chromosomes (cell line A); another cell line (B) containing human chromosomes 2,5,8,10, and the rodent chromosomes; and another cell line (C) with human chromosomes 5,6,8,10,X, and the normal complement of rodent chromosomes. By characterization of the cell lines as to their human chromosome constitution a panel of cell lines can be assembled such that an uncharacterized segment of DNA can be assigned to a human chromosome based on its ability to hybridize (or fail to hybridize) to human DNA from the hybrid lines. By a process of scoring the hybridization for concordance or discordance, the chromosomal origin of the DNA segment can be deduced. In the example outlined above, the DNA segment could be unambiguously assigned to chromosome 2 if the DNA segment hybridized to the cell lines containing human chromosome 2 (lines A and B) and not to line C, the cell line containing human chromosomes also present in lines A and B (ie, 5,6,8,10,X).

The other method used to assign DNA segments to chromosomes consist of labeling the DNA segment of interest with tritiated hydrogen and hybridizing the segment directly to stained metaphase chromosomes that have been attached to glass slides. Autoradiographs are made of the fixed chromosomes and the "grains," that is, the radioactive decay positions, are counted and scored as to the chromosomal location (the chromosomes are first identified by their characteristic staining pattern).

These two methods are complementary, and each is capable of localizing the marker (and thus the linked gene) to a physical chromosome with a resolution on the order of a few percent of the human genome. In every case where linkage has been detected to an autosomal mendelian disease locus, this physical mapping has followed immediately.[39,42]

Knowledge of the chromosomal location is helpful in trying directly to clone and identify the disease gene. Many approaches are being tested for this purpose: the most promising include direct microdissection of the relevant region from a number of stained chromosomes;[47] the identification of expressed sequences in the region of interest from cDNA libraries from appropriate tissues;[48] the use of natural chromosomal rearrangements in the region of interest.[49,50] More speculative approaches include attempts to produce restriction maps of very large chromosomal fragments using OFAGE and FIGE and the development of methods to jump, hop, or skip along chromosomes over distances of hundreds of kilobases using a continually evolving array of new vectors.[51,52]

Virtually all of these physical methods profit from the identification by further linkage studies of additional polymorphic markers in the region of interest. As a rule of thumb, 1% recombination (a minimally detectable distance) corresponds on the average to about 1 million base pairs. The largest segment of DNA that one can clone is about 50 kb. Therefore, simply trying to "walk" along the chromsome by overlapping clones is formidable by current technology. It is eminently worthwhile, having found linkage at about 5 to 10% recombination, to attempt to saturate the region with polymorphism in the expectation of getting down to the minimal 1% (ie, 1 megabase [mb]) before applying the physical methods. In the case of chronic granulomatous disease, in fact, the availability of many markers in a region allowed the direct detection of the mRNA product of the disease gene as well.[48]

Efficient Genetic Mapping Using a Genome RFLP Map

The way in which RFLP markers are used also has an influence on the efficiency with which disease genes can be mapped. If, instead of trying markers randomly one at a time, one first maps the markers with respect to each other, multilocus mapping methods can be applied in which the LOD score contributed by a single meiosis can be twice or more that obtained for the same markers scored singly.[53,54] Maps of RFLP loci with respect to each other are made in the same way as linkage to diseases, using families with many siblings and, where possible, grandparents. Maps of several chromosomes already exist, notably the X chromosome[55] and chromosome 7.[56,57] Although these maps are made, in part, with RFLPs of limited informativeness, their existence clearly indicates the strong likelihood that a complete useful RFLP map of the human genome is at most a few years away.

Applications of the Human RFLP Map

Using a complete RFLP map instead of markers singly has advantages beyond efficiency in mapping simple mendelian traits. It recently has been found that use of a complete map offers the possiblity of mapping much more complex genetic diseases. Among the situations that clearly can be dealt with are *genetic heterogeneity* (in which a disease is caused by any of several genes); some kinds of multifactorial or polygenic diseases (in which several genes must cooperate to produce the disease); and instances in which the gene(s) involved provide not a certainty of disease, but only a predisposition to it.[54,58]

The informativeness, number, and distribution of RFLPs required to make a useful RFLP map can be calculated as well. In summary, a map of completely informative RFLPs (PIC greater than about 0.8) evenly spaced at intervals of 40 centimorgans (cM) (ie, less than 100 RFLP loci for the whole genome, which is 3300 cM in length) will be nearly optimal for efficient mapping of single-gene diseases in as few as 10 families with two or more affected sibs. Where the RFLPs are less informative, more markers per centimorgan will be required. To achieve even spacing, of course, many more markers will have to be mapped than the number that, in the end, would delimit the even intervals.[59] More complicated genetic problems will require better maps.

It is clear that there are many more diseases in which inheritance plays a major part than just the simple mendelian ones. The complete RFLP map affords an opportunity for studying the inherited components of this larger group of diseases. Theoretic studies[54,58,60] indicate that inherited diseases in which any of as many as five genes can cause a disease (genetic heterogeneity) are susceptible to analysis with a complete map. Such diseases include ataxia telanglectasia and xeroderma pigmentosa and possibly many other conditions. Furthermore, similar calculations suggest that diseases in which more than one gene participates in a given family can also be analyzed successfully.[58] Thus, it seems likely that progress can be made in that very large area in which positive evidence (eg, twin studies or family clustering) for inherited components exists but for which a simple genetic hypothesis does not suffice. This class of diseases is very large and includes bipolar affective disorder (manic depression), many forms of cancer, and diabetes.

We have seen that the use of recombinant DNA methods in clinical medicine has already become a reality, especially in the diagnosis of inherited diseases. The number of inherited diseases[61] makes it inevitable that many more diagnositically useful tests will emerge in the very near future. The extension of linkage methods (especially the completion of the RFLP map) promises to make possible in the not-too-distant future the application of linkage methods to common diseases not simply caused by the inheritance of a single dominant or recessive gene. It is too early to tell exactly how useful genes defining the inherited components of such diseases will be. It seems certain, however, that the continued application of these methods in research will result, at the minimum, in a much better understanding of the relationship between heredity and other factors.

ACKNOWLEDGMENTS
We thank Gita Akots, Valerie Brown, and Cindy Helms for use of the autoradiographs shown in Figures 2.6, 2.7, and 2.8, respectively.

REFERENCES

1. Maniatis T, Fritsh EF, Sambrook J: *Molecular Cloning: A Laboratory Manual.* New York, Cold Spring Harbor Laboratory, Cold Spring Harbor, 1982.
2. Wu R (ed): Recombinant DNA, in *Methods in Enzymology,* New York, Academic Press, 1979, vol 68.
3. Wu R, Grossman L, Moldave K: Recombinant DNA: Part B, in *Methods in Enzymology.* New York, Academic Press, 1982, vol 100.
4. Wu R, Grossman L, Moldave K: Recombinant DNA: Part C, in *Methods in Enzymology,* New York, Academic Press, vol 101.
5. Ott J: *Analysis of Human Genetic Linkage.* Baltimore, Johns Hopkins University Press, 1985.
6. Nathans D, Smith HO: Restriction endonucleases in the analysis and restructuring of DNA molecules. *Ann Rev Biochem* 1975;44:273–290.
7. Lawn R, Fritsch E, Parker R, et al: The isolation and characterization of linked delta and beta globin genes from a cloned library of human DNA. *Cell* 1978;15:1157–1174.
8. Lewin B: Eukaryotic chromosomes, in *Gene Expression,* ed 2. New York, John Wiley & Sons, 1980, vol 2, pp. 503–569, 861–930.
9. Schmid CW, Deininger L: Sequence Organization of the Human Genome. *Cell* 1975;6:345–358.
10. Schmid CW, Jelinek WR: *Science* 1982;216:1065–1070.
11. Wyman AR, Wolfe LB, Botstein D: Propagation of some human DNA sequences in bacteriophage lambda requires mutant *Escherichia coli* hosts. *Proc Nat Acad Sci USA* 1985;82:2880–2884.
12. Wyman AR, Barker D, Wertman KF, et al: Factors which equalize the representation of genome segments in recombinant libraries. To be published.
13. Van Dilla MA, Dearen LL, Albright RL, et al: Human chromosome-specific libraries: Construction and availability. *Biotechnology* 1986;4:537–552.
14. Saxon PJ, Srivatsan ES, Leipzig CV, et al: Selective transfer of individual human chromosomes to recipient cells. *Mol Cell Biol* 1985;5:140–146.
15. Maxam AM, Gilbert W: A new method for sequencing DNA. *Proc Natl Acad Sci USA* 1977;74:560–564.
16. Maxam AM, Gilbert W: Sequencing endlabeled DNA with base-specific chemical cleavages. *Meth Enzymol* 1980;65:499–560.
17. Sanger F, Nicklen S, Coulson AR: DNA sequencing with chain-terminating inhibitors. *Proc Natl Acad Sci USA* 1977;74:5463–5467.
18. Church GM, Gilbert W: Genomic sequencing. *Proc Natl Acad Sci USA* 1984;81:1991–1995.
19. Saiki RK, Arnheim N, Erlich HA: A novel method for the detection of polymorphic restriction sites by cleavage of oligonucleotide probes: Application to sickle cell anemia. *Biotechnology* 1985;3:1008–1012.

20. Saiki RK, Scharf S, Faloona F, Erlich HA, et al: Enzymatic amplification of beta-globin genomic sequences and restriction site analysis for diagnosis of sickle cell anemia. *Science* 1985;230:1350–1354.
21. Smith LM, Sanders JZ, Kaiser RJ, et al: Fluorescence detection in automated DNA sequence analysis. *Nature* 1986; 321:674–679.
22. Botstein D, White R, Skolnick M, et al: Construction of a genetic linkage map in man using restriction fragment length polymorphisms. *Am J Hum Genet* 1980;32:314–331.
23. Southern EM: Detection of specific sequences among DNA fragments separated by electrophoresis. *J Mol Biol* 1975;98:503–517.
24. Knowlton R, Brown V, Braman J, et al: Use of highly polymorphic DNA probes for genotypic analysis following bone marrow transplantation. *Blood* 1986;68:378–385.
25. Schumm JS, Knowlton RG, Barker DF, et al: Identification of more than 500 RFLPs by random screening. *Am J Hum Genet.* In press.
26. Litt M, White R: A highly polymorphic locus in human DNA revealed by cosmid derived probes. *Proc Natl Acad Sci USA* 1985;82:6206–6210.
27. Wyman AR, White R: A highly polymorphic locus in human DNA. *Proc Natl Acad Sci USA* 1980;77:6754–6758.
28. Barker D, Schafer M, White R: Restriction sites containing CpG show a higher frequency of polymorphism in human DNA. *Cell* 1984;36:131–138.
29. Kreitman M, Aguadé M: Genetic uniformity in two populations of *Drosophila melanogaster* as revealed by four cutter hybridization. *Proc Natl Acad Sci USA* 1986;83:3562–3566.
30. Schwartz DC, Cantor CR: Separation of yeast chromosome-sized DNAs by pulse field gradient gel-electrophoresis. *Cell* 1984;67–75.
31. Carle GF, Frank M, Olson MV: Electrophoretic separations of large DNA molecules by periodic inversion of the electric field. *Science* 1986;232:65–68.
32. Myers RM, Lunelsky N, Lerman L, et al: Detection of single base substitutions in total genomic DNA. *Nature* 1985;313:495–498.
33. Studencki AB, Wallace RB: Allelespecific hybridization using oligonucleotide probes of very high specific activity: Discrimination of the human betaA and beta-Sglobin genes. *DNA* 1984;3:715.
34. Rigby PWJ, Dieckmann M, Rhodes C, et al: Labeling deoxyribonucleic acid to high specific activity *in vitro* by nick translation with DNA polymerase I. *J Mol Biol* 1977;113:237–254.
35. Melton DA, Krieg PA, Rebagliati, et al: Efficient *in vitro* synthesis of biologically active RNA and RNA hybridization probes from plasmids containing a bacteriophage SP6 promoter. *Nucl Acids Res* 1984;12:7035–7056.
36. Leary JJ, Brigati DJ, Ward DC: Rapid and sensitive colorimetric method for visualizing biotin-labeled DNA probes hybridized to DNA or RNA immobilized on nitrocellulose: Blo-blots. *Proc Natl Acad Sci USA* 1983;80:4045–4049.
37. Morton NE: Sequential tests for the detection of linkage. *Am J Hum Genet* 1955;7:277–318.
38. Davies KE, Pearson PL, Harper PS, et al: Linkage analysis of two cloned DNA sequences flanking the Duchenne muscular dystrophy laws on the short arm of the human x chromosome. *Nucl Acids Res* 1983;11:2303–2312.
39. Gusella JF, Wexler NS, Conneally PM, et al: A polymorphic DNA marker genetically linked to Huntington's disease. *Nature* 1983;306:234–238.
40. Reeders SP, Breuning MH, Davies KE, et al: A highly polymorphic DNA marker linked to adult polycystic kidney disease on chromosome 16. *Nature* 1985;317:542–544.
41. Tsui LC, Buchwald M, Barker DF, et al: Cystic fibrosis locus defined by a genetically linked polymorphic DNA marker. *Science* 1985;230:1054–1057.
42. Knowlton R, Cohen-Haguenauer O, Van Cong N, et al: A polymorphic DNA marker linked to cystic fibrosis is located on chromosome 7. *Nature* 1985;318:380–381.

43. Wainwright B, Scambler P, Schmidtke J, et al: Localization of cystic fibrosis locus to human chromosome 7cen-q*22*. *Nature* 1985;318:384–385.
44. White R, Woodward S, Leppert M, et al: A closely linked genetic marker for cystic fibrosis. *Nature* 1985;318:382–384.
45. Kuhn LC, McClelland A, Ruddle FH: Gene transfer, expression, and molecular cloning of the human transferrin receptor gene. *Cell* 1984;37:95–103.
46. Harper ME, Saunders GF: Localization of single-copy DNA sequences on G-banded human chromosomes by *in situ* hybridization. *Chromosoma* 1981;83:431–439.
47. Rohme D, Fox H, Herrmann B, et al: Molecular clones the mouse t complex derived from microdissected metaphase chromosomes. *Cell* 1984;36:783–788.
48. Royer-Pokora B, Kunkel LM, Monaco AP, et al: Cloning the gene for an inherited human disorder—chronic granulomatous disease—on the basis of its chromosomal location. *Nature* 1986;322:32–38.
49. Ray PN, Belfall B, Duff C, et al: Cloning of the breakpoint of an X;21 translocation associated with Duchenne muscular dystrophy. *Nature* 1985;318:672–675.
50. Kunkel LM, Monaco AP, Middlesworth W, et al: Specific cloning of DNA fragments absent from the DNA of a male patient with an X-chromosome deletion. *Proc Natl Acad Sci USA* 1985;82:4778–4782.
51. Collins FS, Weissman SM: Directional cloning of DNA fragments at a large distance from an initial probe: a circularization method. *Proc Natl Acad Sci USA* 1984;81:6812–6816.
52. Poustka A, Pohl TM, Barlow DP, et al: Construction and use of human chromosome jumping libraries from NotI-digested DNA. *Nature* 1987; 325:353–357.
53. Lathrop GM, Lalouel JM, Julier C, et al: Multilocus linkage analysis in humans: detection of linkage and estimation of recombination. *Am J Hum Genet* 1985;37:482–498.
54. Lander E, Botstein D: Mapping complex genetic traits in humans: New methods using a complete RFLP linkage map. *Proc Natl Acad Sci USA,* to be published.
55. Drayna D, White R: The genetic linkage map of the human X chromosome. *Science* 1985;230:753–758.
56. Donis-Keller H, Barker DF, Knowlton RG, et al: Highly polymorphic RFLP probes as diagnostic tools, in *Cold Spring Harbor Symposia Quantitative Biology: Molecular Biology of Homo Sapiens.* New York, Spring Harbor Press, 1987;51:317–324.
57. Barker DF, Green P, Knowlton RG, et al: A genetic linkage map of 63 chromosome 7 DNA markers. *Proc Natl Acad Sci USA* 1987. In press.
58. Lander E, Botstein D: Mapping complex genetic traits in humans: New methods using a complete RFLP linkage map, in *Cold Spring Harbor Symposia: Molecular Biology of Homo Sapiens,* New York, Cold Spring Harbor Laboratory Press, 51:49–62.
59. Lange K, Boehnke M: How many polymorphic genes will it take to span the human genome? *Am J Hum Genet* 1982;34:842–845.
60. Cavaill-Sforza LL, King M-C: Detecting linkage for genetically heterogeneous diseases and detecting heterogeneity with linkage data. *Am J Hum Genet* 1986;38:599–616.
61. McKusick VA: *Mendelian Inheritance in Man: Catalogs of Autosomal Dominant, Autosomal Recessive, and X-Linked Phenotypes* ed 6. Baltimore, Johns Hopkins University Press.

CHAPTER 3

The Varieties of Mutation

Haig H. Kazazian, Jr., MD, and
Stylianos E. Antonarakis, MD

The study of genetics relies upon the study of how each individual differs from all others. Without individual variation, geneticists would have nothing to study. The essence of variation is mutation. Mutations are the qualitative or quantitative changes in the DNA, which may be either benign or detrimental. Mutations of the former type have no known consequences, whereas those of the latter type may produce disease. Before 1978 we could observe genetic variation only at the protein level. Earlier studies led to the discovery of amino acid substitutions in normal and defective proteins. Recombinant DNA technology has now made it possible to study both the harmless and the harmful mutations at the ultimate level, that of the DNA itself. This has led to remarkable insights into how genes normally function and how mutations have arisen in various human populations.

In this chapter we will discuss the nature of mutation in structural eukaryotic genes and its consequences in gene expression. We will also discuss the question of how mutations arise in various human populations, the frequency with which particular mutations recur, and whether particular regions or sequences in the genome are relative "hotspots" for mutation.

We learned a great deal about mutation in bacteria in the 1960s, but the recent availability of recombinant DNA techniques has allowed us to discover the nature and varieties of mutation in man. In this chapter we will focus upon mutations in α-globin, β-globin, and Factor VIII.

Bacterial and viral genetics taught us that mutations were frequently single nucleotide substitutions.[1] These are either transitions in which one purine is substituted for another, for example, A for G; or one pyrimidine is substituted for another, for example, C for T; or transversions in which a purine is substituted for a pyrimidine or vice versa, for example, A for C. Deletions or additions of nucleotides numbering from one to thousands have also been described.

In human genetics prior to 1975 our knowledge of the consequences of mutation was limited to amino acid substitutions in proteins. The best examples of mutations were the many hemoglobinopathies,[2] one of which was the mutation producing sickle cell anemia.[3] This mutation, which causes a glutamic acid to valine substitution at the sixth position of the β-globin chain of hemoglobin, was described in the late 1950s.[4] But by 1965 we also knew that there were major classes of hemoglobinopathies, the thalassemias, that were not often amino acid substitutions in the globin chains.[5,6] These disorders appeared to be defects in the synthesis of either of the two globin chains (α or β) of adult hemoglobin, and they were believed to be model disorders for the study of gene expression and regulation. At the dawn of DNA analysis, we knew about mutations producing amino acid substitutions in proteins, and we surmised that most mutations of this type were the result of single nucleotide substitutions. We did not know about other types of mutations, knowledge of which has been provided for the most part through study of mutations producing the thalassemia syndromes.

LESSONS FROM THE THALASSEMIAS

The thalassemias are inherited hemolytic, hypochromic anemias secondary to defects in the synthesis of either globin chain (α or β) of adult hemoglobin.[7] For example, in homozygous defects affecting synthesis of β-globin, an excess of α chains are synthesized, these α chains precipitate within the erythroid precursor cell, and premature cell lysis results.[8,9] In addition, surviving cells have a deficiency of hemoglobin tetramers, even though some compensation occurs through production of γ-globin chains of fetal hemoglobin. Mutations affecting α-globin production lead to α-thalassemia, whereas those altering β-globin synthesis lead to β-thalassemia.

Here we wish to discuss some general points and describe the lessons learned from the now nearly complete characterization of these disorders. The reader is referred to the applicable literature for a detailed description of all the known mutations.[10–12]

Gene Deletions

The first types of mutations detected by recombinant DNA methods were deletions. Deletions were easily detected after restriction endonuclease analysis of patients' DNA by the absence or the abnormal size of various DNA fragments. In particular, gene deletions were often found in patients with α-thalassemia. In fact, the important lesson associated with α-thalassemia is the significance of gene deletion, especially deletions associated with mispairing of chromosomes at duplicated DNA sequences and unequal crossing-over.[13,14] Duplication of DNA sequences has been fairly common in evolution. This duplication is found (1) in tandem (tail to head arrangement of duplicated sequences), (2) in close proximity, and (3) at some distance, even on different chromosomes. Wherever there exists in the genome duplicated sequences of a few hundred or more base pairs that are similar and placed either in tandem or in proximity, mispairing of chromosomes may occur. If after mispairing, a crossing-over event occurs, one product will contain a deficiency of genetic material, while the other will contain an excess.

Specifically, within the α-globin gene cluster there are four highly related sequences of about four thousand base pairs (4 kb) (Fig. 3.1). These are the regions that include the $\psi\zeta$, $\psi\alpha$, α_2, and α_1 genes.[15] There are two α-globin genes, α_2 and α_1, which are roughly equal in function. If the α_2 and the α_1 genes mispair and unequal crossing over occurs between these genes, one chromosome product is left with a single fusion gene $(\alpha_2-\alpha_1)$[13] whereas the other contains three α genes $(\alpha_2, \alpha_1-\alpha_2, \alpha_1)$[16] (Fig. 3.2). Both of these chromosome products have been observed commonly in man, and the chromosome bearing the single α gene is polymorphic in blacks with an "allele frequency" of 0.3. Unequal crossing-over following mispairing in other regions of this cluster has also produced a number of chromosomes that lack functional α-globin genes.[17] Such chromosomes are commonly present in Southeast Asia, where homozygotes for chromosomes lacking α-globin

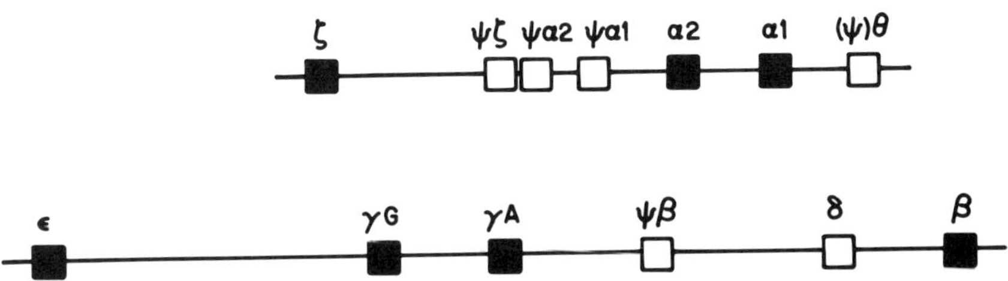

FIGURE 3.1 Structural organization of the α- and β-globin gene cluster. The α cluster at the top is spread over about 30 kilobases (kb) and contains a ζ-gene, a pseudo-ζ-gene, two pseudo-α genes, two functional α-genes, and a θ-gene. Pseudogenes are sequences that are very similar to functional genes, but they contain mutations that eliminate their ability to encode a functional product. The θ gene has been described recently,[77] and it is not yet known whether this α-like gene is functional in man. The β-globin gene cluster is spread over about 50 kb and contains one ϵ-, two γ-, and δ-, and one β-globin gene(s). In addition, there is a single pseudo-β-gene.

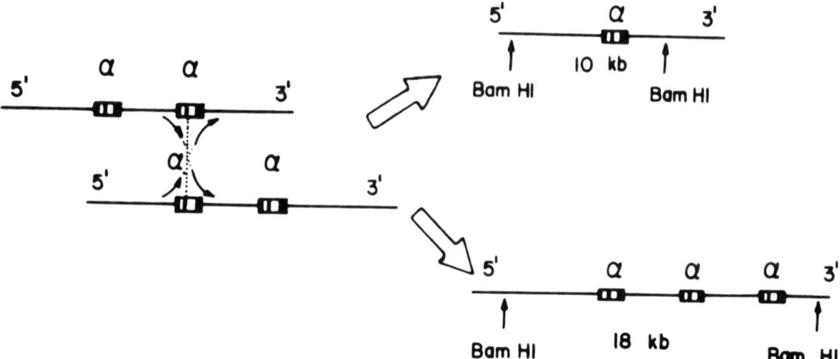

FIGURE 3.2 Mispairing and unequal crossing over produce chromosomes bearing one or three α-globin genes. Mispairing of the α_2-globin gene with an α_1-globin gene, followed by a crossing over event, produces one chromosome bearing a single α-globin gene and another chromosome containing three α-globin genes. These different chromosomes can be detected by restriction endonuclease analysis (see Chapter 2) since the Bam HI fragment of a single α-gene chromosome is 10 kb, that of a triple α-gene chromosome is 18 kb, and that of the normal chromosome with two α-genes is 14 kb.

genes are not uncommon, and these homozygotes die of hydrops fetalis either in utero or soon after delivery.

Other examples of unequal crossing over after mispairing of chromosomes have been observed. In the β-globin cluster the δ-β fusion gene, which leads to Hb Lepore, is the deletion that results after mispairing of the δ- and β-globin genes.[18] The other product of such a mispairing, an anti-Lepore chromosome, which contains a δ gene, a β-δ fusion gene, and a β gene, has also been observed.[19] Another example is the deletion of 7 kb in the growth hormone gene cluster that eliminates the normal growth hormone gene and leads to isolated growth hormone deficiency and dwarfism in the homozygous state.[20] A number of these latter deletions have been found, suggesting that mispairing and unequal crossing-over is not uncommon in the growth hormone gene cluster because approximately 500 base pair homologous segments exist 7 kb apart in the cluster.[21] Other examples of mispairing and unequal crossing-over involve the highly repeated 300 base pair sequences called Alu sequences. Examples of deletions after mispairing of Alu sequences are found in the low-density lipoprotein receptor gene and the β-globin gene cluster.[22,23]

It is clear that various deletions can occur at a low frequency for still unknown or obscure reasons.[24] However, the important lesson is that when sequences have been duplicated through evolution and are still present close to one another in a chromosome, there exists a certain likelihood of mispairing and unequal crossing-over.

In contrast to the situation in α-thalassemia, deletion as a cause of β-thalassemia is relatively uncommon. The Lepore-type deletions account for about 1% of all β-thalassemia genes in the Mediterranean basin, and a particular deletion of 619 base pairs that eliminates part of the second intron and all of the third exon of the β-globin gene accounts for about 30% of β-thalassemia genes in India.[25] Study of the molecular defects in other single genes, including Factor VIII:C,[26] HGPRT,[27] and LDL receptor,[28] suggests that, in general, deletions account for only about 1 to 5% of gene lesions.

Point Mutations

The point mutations producing β-thalassemia alleles were the first to be analyzed nearly to completion. The majority of the subjects from whom defective β-globin genes were cloned and characterized were children and young adults who were affected with β-thalassemia major. Almost all of these subjects were being transfused regularly and had a life expectancy of 20 to 30 years. Since nearly all ethnic groups residing in malaria-infested regions and affected with β-thalassemia have been studied, we now have a nearly complete picture of the types of mutations that produce this disease. From these data, we have learned much about how mutations can affect a gene encoding a protein. The great bulk of mutations producing β-thalassemia alleles are point mutations.

In order to understand the variety of types of these mutations that affect the expression of the β-globin gene, we will first discuss the structure of this gene and the steps in normal gene expression. The β-globin gene is quite small (only 1.5 kb in size) (see Fig. 3.1) and simple (it contains three exons and two introns).[29] A number of critical nucleotide sequences in the gene are demonstrated in Figure 3.3. The normal steps in expression of this and nearly all other genes encoding proteins are as follows: the gene is first transcribed into pre-mRNA, the pre-mRNA is modified at both its 5′ and 3′ ends by 5′ capping and 3′ polyadenylation, respectively. The modified pre-mRNA then undergoes splicing out of its intervening sequences or introns to form the mature mRNA; this mature mRNA is transported from nucleus to cytoplasm. In the cytoplasm, ribosomes and other machinery of protein synthesis translate the mature mRNA into protein.[30] Mutations affecting (1) transcription, (2) RNA cleavage and 3′ polyadenylation, (3) RNA splicing, and (4) translation have all been observed.[11,12]

Transcription Mutations

Transcription mutations have been found 5′ to the cap, or start, site of transcription in regions known to be important in transcription (promoter elements). Promoter regions have been determined from studies in which

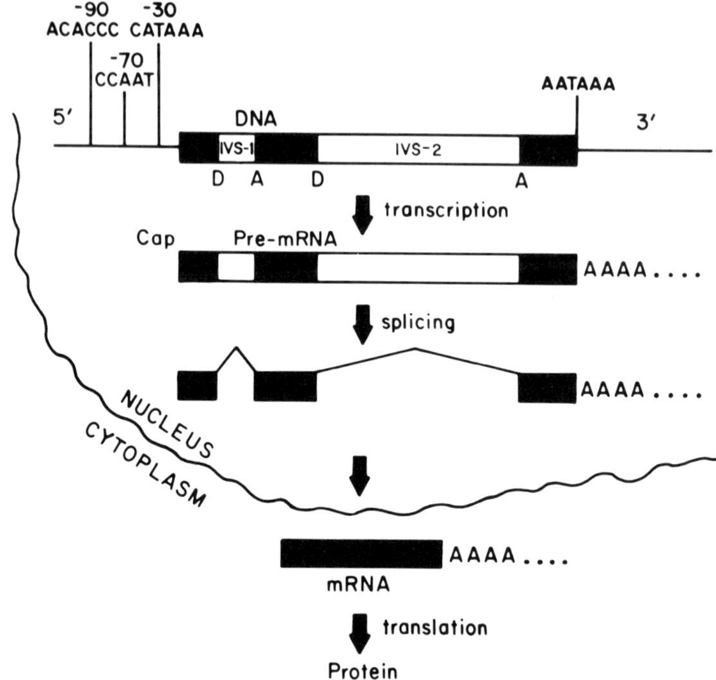

FIGURE 3.3 *β*-Globin gene structure and expression. *β*-globin gene sequences important in gene expression are shown at the top. Three promoter sequences required for transcription of the gene DNA into pre-mRNA are shown at the 5′ end of the gene at −90, −70, and −30 nucleotides. D and A at splice junctions refer to donor and acceptor splice site sequences. The RNA cleavage-polyadenylation signal AATAAA is present at the 3′ end of the gene. The gene is transcribed into RNA, its 5′ end is modified (cap) and its 3′ end is polyadenylated (AAAA). The modified pre-mRNA then has intron sequences spliced out, and the mRNA is transported to the cytoplasm, where it is translated into *β*-globin.

cloned genes were subjected to mutagenesis and inserted into cells in vitro, and expression of the mutated gene was measured. Other evidence of promoter elements has come from sequence homologies 5′ to other genes encoding proteins.[31] Four different mutations have been found in the TATA box, a region located about 30 nucleotides upstream or 5′ to the cap site, which is thought to be important for the normal transcription of those genes that are overexpressed, such as *β*-globin[11,12] (CATAAA on the *β*-globin gene —Fig. 3.4). (The cap site is designated +1, so the TATA box is present at −30 nucleotides upstream of the *β*-globin gene.) Another region thought to be important in transcription of genes such as *β*-globin is the CCAAT homology at −70 nucleotides. No mutation in this region has yet been found in *β*-thalassemia. At −85 to −90 is a six-base sequence, ACACCC, which has

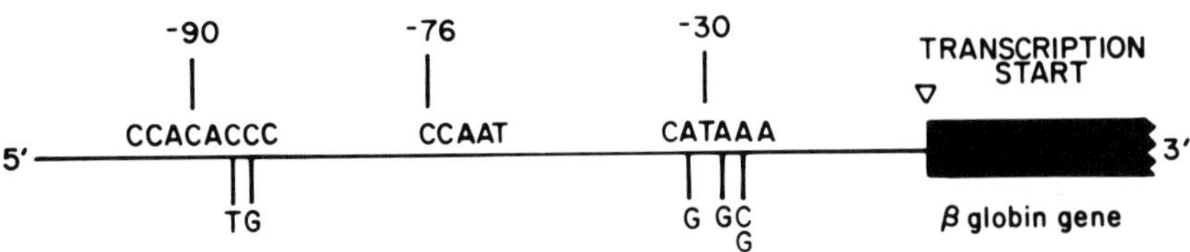

FIGURE 3.4 Transcription mutations in the β-globin gene. Mutations in different β-thalassemia genes in promoter regions are shown. These mutations are found at positions −88, −87, −31, −29, and −28. Two different mutations have been found at position −28, and none have been seen in the CCAAT sequence.

also been implicated through site-specific mutagenesis experiments as a crucial promoter element for transcription of β-globin genes.[32] Two mutations have been observed in this distal promoter element in β-thalassemia genes. They are in the two C residues near the 3′ end of the sequence, at positions −87 and −88.[33,34] The effects of all six mutations in this region, the two at −87 and −88 and the four in the TATA box homology, are relatively mild. They reduce the RNA output of the mutant gene by 75 to 80%, but do not eliminate it.[11,35,36] These mutations are termed β^+-thalassemia alleles because reduced numbers of β-chains result from these mutant genes. β^0-thalassemia genes, of which many examples are discussed below, contain mutations that completely eliminate β-globin production.

RNA Cleavage and 3′-Polyadenylation Mutation

A single mutation has been observed that greatly affects cleavage of the β-globin RNA transcript.[37] Nearly all genes encoding proteins have the six-nucleotide sequence, AATAAA, about 15 nucleotides 5′ to the RNA cleavage site. These nucleotides appear to act as a signal for cleavage of the growing RNA chain.[38] Once the endonuclease-cleavage is made, the resulting RNA has a polyadenylic acid (poly A) tail of 100 to 150 residues added to it. The poly A tail is thought to increase the stability of the mRNA. The β-thalassemia mutation is a single nucleotide substitution, C for T, in the AATAAA signal sequence[37] (Fig. 3.5). This substitution greatly inhibits endonuclease cleavage of the growing RNA. Indeed, another RNA species containing 900 additional nucleotides is found in vivo. This abnormal RNA is the product of failed cleavage at the mutated AACAAA sequence. RNA cleavage does occur when the transcription machinery encounters the next AATAAA sequence 3′ to the β-globin gene, which occurs 900 nucleotides downstream from the normal cleavage sequence at the 3′ end of the β-globin gene.

How this mutation actually produces β-thalassemia is not clear. Theoretically, the enlongated mRNA should be translated normally. However, its

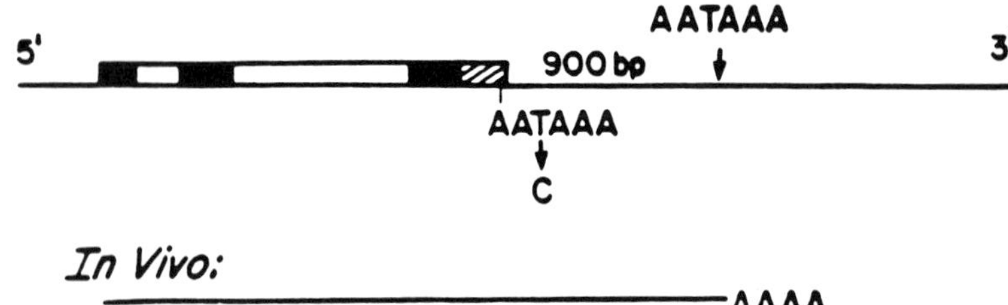

FIGURE 3.5 RNA cleavage-polyadenylation mutation in the β-globin gene. The T-C mutation in the AATAAA signal sequence leads to poor cleavage of the RNA transcript. Transcription proceeds to the next AATAAA signal 900 bp 3′ to the gene. A discrete RNA transcript 900 bp longer than the normal β-globin mRNA is found in vivo.

low concentration in reticulocytes in vivo would suggest that it is unstable and that β-thalassemia is the result of greatly reduced concentrations of the elongated β-mRNA.

RNA Splicing

Of the total of 38 different point mutations known that produce β-thalassemia, 18 are mutations affecting RNA splicing.[11,12] RNA splicing is critical to normal gene expression because the introns must be precisely removed to produce authentic mRNA for translation into protein. Mutations may alter RNA splicing either by changing normal splice sites at intron-exon junctions or by creating new splice sites in introns or exons. These mutations may occur at so-called cryptic sites, which do not undergo splicing under normal circumstances but do so when mutation affects the normal site. To enhance the reader's understanding of the following discussion, a few definitions of terms are appropriate. The 5′ exon-intron junction is called the *donor splice site* and the 3′ intron-exon junction is the *acceptor splice site* (see Fig. 3.3). Comparison of the nucleotide composition in these regions from sequenced genes of many kinds has shown that the 5′ end of the intron invariably begins with the nucleotides GT and the 3′ end of the intron is always AG.[31,39] Nucleotides residing at both sides of the splice junction at either end of the intron have been implicated as important for the splicing mechanism because certain nucleotide sequences are often present in these positions. These often seen nucleotides are called consensus sequences. For example, the three nucleotides prior to the 5′ splice site and the six nucleotides after the site are included in the consensus sequence of the donor splice site. This consensus sequence is $^{\mathrm{C}}_{\mathrm{A}}AG/GT^{\mathrm{A}}_{\mathrm{G}}$AGT, and the consensus sequence of the acceptor splice site is (Py$_{11}$ N$^{\mathrm{C}}_{\mathrm{A}}$AG/G (the vertical line refers to the splice junction itself, and Py sequences are pyrimidines, C or T).

Mutations that alter the GT or AG at the splice junctions lead to complete elimination of normal splicing and are β^{O}-thalassemia genes (see Table 3.1 and Fig. 3.6 for examples).[11,12] Mutations in consensus sequences at positions 5 and 6 of the donor site of intron-1 and at position −3 in the acceptor site of intron-2[40] do not eliminate use of the normal splice site and are β^{+}-thalassemia genes.[11] These mutations greatly slow normal splicing and often splicing occurs at cryptic splice sites. The mutation at intron-1 position 6 is noteworthy because it is fairly common in the Mediterranean basin and does not have a major effect on normal splicing.[34,35] Persons heterozygous for this mutation and a more severe β^{O}-thalassemia mutation do not usually require blood transfusions, whereas homozygotes for this mutation may be difficult to distinguish from the usual heterozygotes who contain one normal and one severe β-thalassemia gene. The mutation at the position −3 of the acceptor site of intron-2 is interesting in that it is the first consensus acceptor site mutation, and it causes a moderate slowing of normal splicing in vitro.[40]

A cryptic acceptor site (nucleotide sequences that are very similar to the normal acceptor splice site) is found at position 579 of the 850 nucleotide intron-2. Although not normally used, this site can be utilized as a result of mutation in the normal acceptor site (see Fig. 3.6). Single nucleotide substitutions that produce new donor sites in IVS-2 at positions 654, 705, and 745[34,41,42] alter normal splicing by causing aberrant splices from the site of the mutation to the normal acceptor site. When this occurs, the normal acceptor site has been used, and the normal donor site splices with the cryptic acceptor at intron-2 nucleotide 579.[35,41]

Mutations at intron-1 nucleotide 110 and intron-1 nucleotide 116 alter sequences that are similar to those of normal acceptor sites and turn them into excellent acceptor sites.[11,43] These mutations then result in small segments of intron-1 remaining in many of the β-mRNA molecules, and these molecules cannot be properly translated into β-globin.

One cryptic donor site in exon-1 has been subject to three different β-thalassemia mutations. These mutations have merely altered the sequence in this region of the gene to make it conform more closely to the consensus sequence for donor splice sites. These mutations then lead to use of the cryptic donor site, which is either never used or used very rarely in the normal gene compared to the normal donor IVS-1 site. This leads to a β-globin mRNA that is missing a portion of exon-1 and to reduced production of normally spliced β-mRNA. Two of the mutations of this type also change the amino acid inserted in mRNAs that are the product of splicing at the normal sites.[10,11] One of these genes, that for β^{E}-globin, is one of the most common variant hemoglobin genes in the world, and it produces both the variant globin and a β-thalassemia state. Splicing of β^{E} precursor mRNA occurs at the normal sites and also at the site of the β^{E} mutation. Normal

TABLE 3-1 Mutations in β-Thalassemia

Mutant Class	Type ($0 = \beta^{0}$, $+ = \beta^{+}$)	Origin	Direct Detection
Nonfunctional mRNA			
Nonsense mutants			
1) codon 17 (A-T)	0	Chinese	Oligonucleotide
2) codon 39 (C-T)	0	Mediterranean	Oligonucleotide
3) codon 15 (G-A)	0	Asian Indian	Oligonucleotide
4) codon 121 (A-T)	0	Polish	Eco RI
5) codon 37 (G-A)	0	Saudi Arabian	Ava II
Frameshift mutants			
6) −2 codon 8	0	Turkish	Oligonucleotide
7) −1 codon 16	0	Asian Indian	Oligonucleotide
8) −1 codon 44	0	Kurdish	Oligonucleotide
9) +1 codons 8/9	0	Asian Indian	Oligonucleotide
10) −4 codons 41/42	0	Asian Indian	Oligonucleotide
11) −1 codon 6	0	Mediterranean	Mst II
12) +1 codons 71/72	0	Chinese	Oligonucleotide
RNA Processing mutants			
Splice junction changes			
1) IVS-1 position 1 (G-A)	0	Mediterranean	Oligonucleotide
2) IVS-1 position 1 (G-T)	0	Asian Indian	Oligonucleotide
3) IVS-2 position 1 (G-A)	0	Mediterranean	Hph I
4) IVS-1 3′-end −17 bp	0	Kuwaiti	Fnu 4H
5) IVS-1 3′-end −25 bp	0	Asian Indian	Fnu 4H
6) IVS-2 3′-end (A-G)	0	American black	Oligonucleotide
7) IVS-2 3′-end (A-C)	0	American black	Oligonucleotide
Consensus changes			
8) IVS-1 position 5 (G-C)	+	Indian	Oligonucleotide
9) IVS-1 position 5 (G-T)	+	Mediterranean	Oligonucleotide
10) IVS-1 position 6 (T-C)	+	Mediterranean	Oligonucleotide
11) IVS-2 3′-end CAG-AAG	+	Iranian	Oligonucleotide
Internal IVS changes			
12) IVS-1 position 110 (G-A)	+	Mediterranean	Oligonucleotide
13) IVS-1 position 116 (T-G)	?	Mediterranean	Mae I
14) IVS-2 position 705 (T-G)	+	Mediterranean	Oligonucleotide
15) IVS-2 position 745 (C-G)	+	Mediterranean	Rsa I
16) IVS-2 position 654 (C-T)	0	Chinese	Oligonucleotide
Coding regions substitutions affecting processing			
17) codon 26 (G-A)	E	Southeast Asian	HbE
18) codon 24 (T-A)	+	American black	Oligonucleotide
19) codon 27 (G-T)	Knossos	Mediterranean	Hb Knossos
Transcriptional mutants			
1) −88 C-T	+	American black	Oligonucleotide
2) −87 C-G	+	Mediterranean	Avr II
3) −31 A-G	+	Japanese	Oligonucleotide
4) −29 A-G	+	American black	Oligonucleotide
5) −28 A-C	+	Kurdish	Oligonucleotide
6) −28 A-G	+	Chinese	Oligonucleotide
RNA cleavage + polyadenylation mutants			
1) AATAAA − AACAAA	+	American black	Oligonucleotide

(Total number = 38, June 1986)

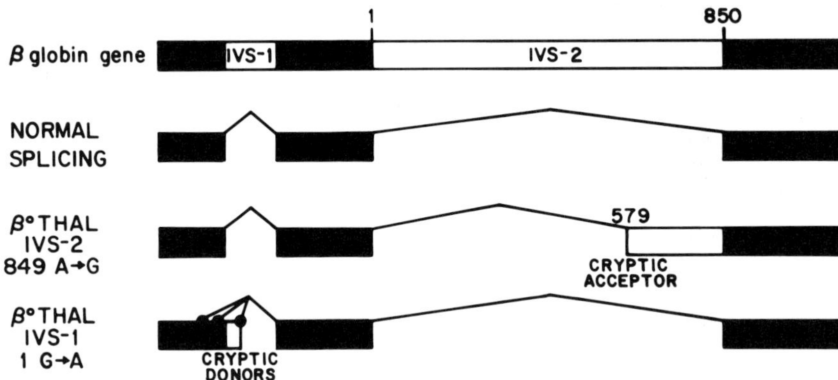

FIGURE 3.6 Examples of mutations affecting RNA splicing. The β-globin gene and the normal splicing pattern of its pre-mRNA are shown at the top. The numbers 1 and 850 above the β-globin gene denote the first and last nucleotides of the 850-nucleotide IVS (intron)-2. The third entry depicts the RNA splicing pattern observed when the β-globin gene contains an A-G mutation in the AG acceptor splice site of IVS (intron)-2. No RNA splicing occurs to the normal acceptor site and all the RNA molecules undergo splicing between the normal donor site of intron-2 and the cryptic acceptor site at position 579 of intron-2. The last entry demonstrates the RNA splicing patterns that occur when the β-globin gene contains a G-A mutation in the GT donor site of IVS (intron)-1. No RNA splicing occurs between the normal donor site and the normal acceptor site of intron-1. Each RNA transcript chooses one of three cryptic donor sites, two in exon-1 and one in intron-1, for splicing with the normal acceptor site of intron-1.

splicing produces β^E globin, whereas abnormal splicing produces a nonfunctional β-globin mRNA.[44]

Mutations Affecting Translation

These mutations are of two types, chain-terminator nonsense mutations and frameshift mutations. Five different nonsense mutations are known, all of which are single nucleotide substitutions that alter triplet codons for an amino acid to produce one of the termination codons in mRNA, that is, UAG, UAA, or UGA.[10,11] Although some 29 single nucleotide substitutions could produce nonsense codons in the coding region of the β-globin gene, only these five nonsense mutations have been observed. Since most affected population groups have been sampled, it appears that the occurrence of certain mutations to nonsense codons is unlikely.

Frameshift mutations are deletions or additions of one, two, or four nucleotides in the coding region of the gene. Because these mutations change the sense of all the codons that follow them, they alter completely the sequence of amino acids or, in some cases, terminate the protein chain prematurely. Seven frameshift mutations have been found in β-thalassemia genes.[10,11]

Other Mutations that Reduce β-Globin Gene Expression

Deletions that eliminate the β-globin gene in addition to other genes in the β-globin gene cluster reduce β-globin gene expression as a matter of course. These deletions are interesting for the variable effects they have in increasing γ-globin gene expression. The reader is referred to the excellent review on this subject by Bunn and Forget.[10]

Of greater interest are the deletions that leave the β-globin gene intact but extinguish its expression. Two deletions of this variety have been reported. In one, about 100 kb of DNA is deleted from the β-globin gene cluster and upstream to it. However, the β-globin gene and 2.5 kb upstream to it are left intact (Fig. 3.7).[45] This β-globin gene is very poorly expressed, even though it is normal by DNA sequence and by expression upon gene transfer into HeLa cells in vitro.[46] A second deletion ends further upstream, leaving intact the β-globin gene and about 30 kb 5′ to it.[47] The β-globin gene in this second case is also poorly functional in the heterogyzous person. These deletions are thought to be examples of *position effect.*

This term refers to the fact that expression of a gene depends upon its location in the genome. This effect was first observed by Drosophila geneticists who showed that a particular expressed gene could be extinguished by its translocation to another location in the genome.[48] The mechanism by which position effect occurs is thought to be a change in the chromatin configuration in which the gene resides. If the gene resides in chromatin that has an "open" configuration, the gene will be active. If the gene of interest is in chromatin with a "closed" configuration, the gene will be inactive. It has been shown that the normal chromatin configuration surrounding the β-globin gene in adult erythroid cells is "open."[46] On the other hand, the chromatin surrounding the β-globin gene in the chromosome with the 100-kb deletion that leaves the β-globin gene and 2.5 kb upstream to it intact is

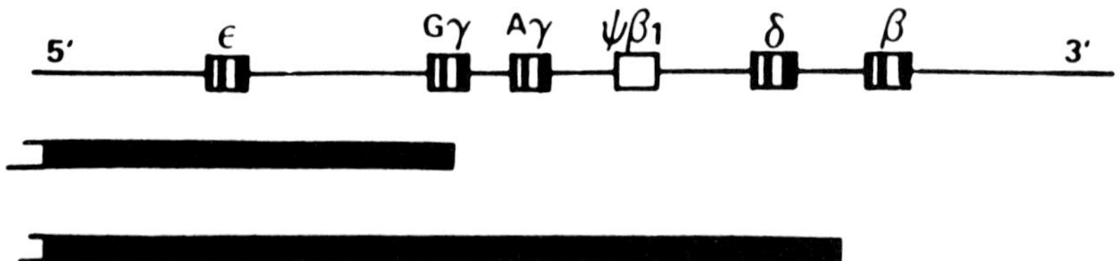

FIGURE 3.7 Deletions that produce position effects on expression of the β-globin gene. The black bars represent the extents of two deletions in the β-globin gene cluster. The 5′ end of the top deletion is unknown, whereas that of the bottom deletion is about 50 kb 5′ to the globin genes. Individuals heterozygous for either of these deletions and a normal β-globin gene cluster produce little or no β-globin from the chromosome bearing the deletion even though the deletion leaves the β-globin gene intact.

"closed."[46] Thus, the chromatin configuration in which any gene is present has a profound effect on the expression of that gene.

Point Mutations that Increase γ-Globin Gene Expression

Another set of interesting mutations that reduce β-globin gene expression are the *up-promoter mutations* of the γ-globin genes that cause one form of the hereditary persistence of fetal hemoglobin syndrome. These mutations are single nucleotide substitutions at either ~117 or ~200 nucleotides upstream of the cap site of the $^{G}\gamma$ or the $^{A}\gamma$-globin gene.[49-51] The effects of a mutation of this type are (1) to increase specifically the production of the γ-globin gene preceded by the mutation and (2) to decrease proportionately the β-globin gene expression from the chromosome bearing the mutation. Thus, the relative output of globin chains from a chromosome bearing a nondeletion $^{A}\gamma$ hereditary persistence of fetal hemoglobin mutation is estimated to be 20 $^{A}\gamma$: 80 β-chains instead of the <1 $^{A}\gamma$: >99 β-chains from a normal chromosome.

Four mutations of this type have been described. The $^{G}\gamma$-globin mutation is located 202 nucleotides upstream of the cap site, while the $^{A}\gamma$-globin mutations are located 198, 196, and 117 nucleotides 5′ to the cap site. It has been speculated that these sites are binding regions for a normal transacting repressor that turns off γ-globin gene expression at the time of γ- to β-globin switching in late fetal life. Mutation at these sites may lead to reduced binding of repressor and continued γ-globin gene expression into adult life.

A single β-thalassemia mutation has been described that is located at some distance from the β-globin gene and is associated with a mild clinical phenotype.[52] The nature of this mutation is unknown, but it may represent alteration of a positive transacting factor important in the normal stimulation of β-globin gene expression.

Origins and Spread of β-Thalassemia Genes

Since each ethnic or racial group carries its own battery of different mutations producing β-thalassemia alleles, it is apparent that the mutant alleles observed in modern times have arisen and expanded in frequency after the racial divergence of man. Among the major population groups affected, 13 different alleles have been observed in all populations of the Mediterranean basin, 8 in Asiatic Indians, 7 in Chinese, and 6 in American blacks. Analysis of the normal polymorphisms (both those determined by restriction endonuclease analysis and by DNA sequencing) in the β-globin gene suggests that a small number of normal β-globin gene types was present in man well before the divergence of the races. Since four normal types of β-globin genes are commonly present in all racial groups, the population size at the time of racial divergence was probably in the range of thousands, rather than hundreds or tens. Thus, β-thalassemia mutations present prior to racial divergence should have survived the moderate population bottleneck attendant upon racial separation. In that case, ancient mutations under positive selection should be observed in all racial groups. This is not so. Because mutational events to genes affecting β-globin expression must have occurred since the dawn of man, the ethnic distribution of mutant alleles seen today should reflect a time of onset after racial divergence and the occurrence of the positive selection pressure for heterozygous individuals, which is thought to have been falciparum malaria.

On the other hand, a growing number of β-thalassemia genes (eight at last count) have been found in more than one ethnic group. The best explanation for these alleles is separate independent origins of the same mutation. For example, the −29 A-G allele is present in blacks and Chinese (52), and the −88 A-G allele is present in blacks and Asiatic Indians (53). The chromosomal background in the β-globin gene cluster has been determined by restriction site polymorphisms in the DNA. The pattern of restriction site polymorphisms in a chromosome has been termed a *haplotype.*[34,55] The −29 and −88 mutations have occurred in these groups on different β-globin gene haplotypes which are different even in the β-globin gene itself. These data make mutant gene migration highly improbable. Interestingly, the common Mediterranean β-thalassemia allele, nonsense codon 39, has been observed as a new mutation in a European person.[56] Examples of independent origins of β-thalassemia alleles are shown in Table 3.2.

A number of β-thalassemia alleles have spread from one haplotype to another within the same ethnic group. The majority of these observations can be explained by crossing-over events in meiosis within a region of 9 kb 5′ to the β-globin gene. This region has been suggested from these observations and other data to be a hotspot for meiotic recombination.[11,55]

TABLE 3-2 Examples of Recurrent Mutation in β-Thalassemia

Mutant Allele	Ethnic Groups in Which Allele Is Observed
β^{E}	Southeast Asians and Europeans
$\beta^{IVS\text{-}1,nt\ 5}$	Indians and Chinese
$\beta^{IVS\text{-}1,nt\ 5}$	Mediterraneans and Europeans
$\beta^{Frameshift\ 41-42}$	Indians and Chinese
β^{-88}	Blacks and Indians
$\beta^{IVS\text{-}2,nt\ 1}$	Mediterraneans and blacks
β^{-29}	Blacks and Chinese
$\beta^{Nonsense\ 39}$	Mediterraneans and Europeans

In a handful of instances the same mutation is observed within an ethnic group on different β-globin genes as determined by polymorphisms within the β-globin gene.[11] These observations are difficult to explain by independent origins of the mutation since these mutations have only been found in one ethnic group. The best explanation for this type of spread of a mutation from one genetic background to another is interallelic gene conversion. This is the process, observed in yeast and *Drosophila*, by which short stretches of DNA sequence are passed from one allele at a locus to another.[57,58] If such events have occurred in the β-globin gene to produce the observations cited, the data indicate that the converted regions would have to be 500 nucleotides or less. Another curious observation is that, even though a large number of known β-globin mutations are present in introns, none of these have participated in a presumed interallelic gene conversion event. In contrast, there are five examples of such events affecting mutations in exons or coding regions.

Mutations of the Factor VIII Gene: New Lessons from a Giant Gene

Although it is the most thoroughly characterized, the β-globin gene is one of the smallest of genes. The study of larger genes may give other kinds of information. One such large gene is that which codes for Factor VIII.

Hemophilia A (classic hemophilia) is the most common inherited disease of blood coagulation. This disorder, which is caused by a deficiency or abnormality of Factor VIII, is inherited as an X-linked trait. The locus for Factor VIII has been assigned to the long arm of the human X chromosome at Xq28.[59] About 50% of patients have Factor VIII levels that are less than 5% of normal, and the remainder have levels that are between 5 and 20% of normal. Among those with levels below 5%, some produce an inactive Factor VIII-like material that reacts with appropriate antibodies, and others fail to do so. Specific antibodies against Factor VIII, called Factor VIII inhibitors, develop after transfusion in approximately 6% of patients with hemophilia A.[60] Patients with the lowest Factor VIII levels (<1 unit/dl) are the most severely affected and the most prone to the development of circulating Factor VIII inhibitors.

Over the past year we at Johns Hopkins and Gitschier et al at Genentech, Inc. have made an effort to determine the molecular basis of classic hemophilia (hemophilia A). In 1984, Gitschier et al and Toole et al reported the cloning of the Factor VIII gene, the gene that specifies the clotting factor that, when deficient or defective, produces hemophilia A.[61,62] In contrast to the tiny β-globin gene (1.5 kb), the Factor VIII gene is a giant gene (186 kb). It is composed of 9 kb of exon sequences in 26 separate exons and 177 kb of introns (Fig. 3.8).

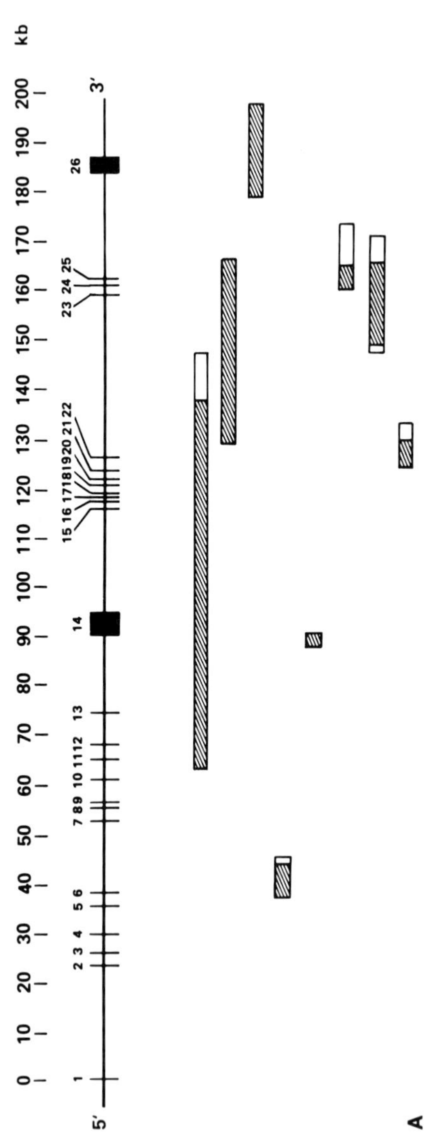

5'
3'
kb
0
10
20
30
40
50
60
70
80
90
100
110
120
130
140
150
160
170
180
190
200
1
2 3 4
5 6
7 8 9 10 11 12
13
14
15 16 17 18 19 20 21 22
23 24 25
26
1
2
3
4
5
6
7
8
A

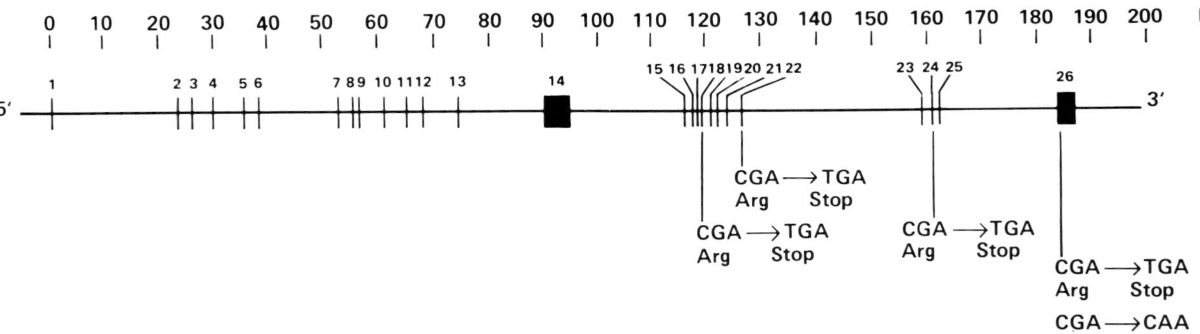

FIGURE 3.8 Deletions (**A**) and point mutations (**B**) in the Factor VIII:C gene producing hemophilia A. (**A**) Factor VIII:C gene structure with its 26 exons spread over 186 kb is shown at the top. Eight different deletions are shown below the gene. Blackened areas represent known deleted sequences; open areas at ends represent sequences within which the deletion must end. (**B**) Point mutations affecting CGA sequences in exons 18, 22, 24, and 26 are shown.

In a study of 120 males with hemophilia A, Gitschier et al found five different mutant alleles, two deletions and three point mutations.[63,64] The deletions were all present toward the 3′ end of the gene, and the point mutations were CGA-TGA mutations producing nonsense codons in exons 24 and 26, and at the same triplet codon in exon 26 a CGA-CAA missense mutation in a mildly affected male.

Antonarakis et al studied 10 patients with hemophilia A initially and discovered a large 70-kb deletion in the middle of the factor VIII:C gene and a CGA-TGA nonsense mutation in exon 18.[65] Later, Youssoufian et al studied another 70 hemophilia A males and discovered five deletions and seven point mutations[66,67] (see Fig. 3.8). Thus, it appears that of every 100 patients studied the precise mutant allele producing hemophilia can be characterized in 10 to 15 of them. This is possible using a relatively simple screening of the Factor VIII gene structure in such patients.

A number of generalizations can be derived from the study of mutations in the Factor VIII gene. First, as expected for an X-linked disorder with reduced reproductive fitness, the majority of affected families carry their own private mutant allele.

Second, about 6% of the mutant alleles are deletions, in contrast to the small number of deletions in β-thalassemia genes. This finding is probably related to (1) the large size of exon sequences (>9000 bp) in Factor VIII as compared to β-globin (450 bp), (2) the spreading of the exon sequences in Factor VIII over 186 kb, and (3) the possibility of unequal crossing over because of the similarity of DNA sequences in the introns.

Third, a large number of point mutations have been found in CG dinucleotides of the type CG-TG and CG-CA. These substitutions have produced both nonsense and missense mutations. The mechanism underlying the susceptibility to mutation of CG dinucleotides is presumably methylation of C residues at the 5-position in the pyrimidine ring (^{m}C)[68] when C is located 5′ to G. Such a ^{m}C can then become spontaneously (nonenzymatically) deaminated directly to T. This accounts for CG-TG mutations and, when the ^{m}C is on the non-coding strand, a CG-CA change. Four instances of recurrent origin of hemophilia A mutations have now been observed.[65,66] Two of these are single nucleotide substitutions CGA-TGA in exon 18, codon 1960, and two are CGA-TGA substitution in exon 22, codon 2135. Since recurrences of these mutations were observed in less than 100 hemophilia A genes, it can be calculated that up to 10,000 recurrences of these changes may have occurred in man. Thus, these CG dinucleotides may represent mutation hotspots in man. None of these data was predicted by the experience with β-globin because in this small-gene CG dinucleotides do not appear in first and second or second and third nucleotides of codons.

There are other reasons why our view of mutation events producing disease may have been skewed by attempts to generalize from the studies of β-globin. Mutations affecting heterozygous expression of the small β-globin gene are under positive selection in malarial endemic regions. Thus, any mutation occurring in malarial regions that produces a deficiency of β-globin gene expression in heterozygotes will attain a high frequency. This means that some mutant alleles presently observed at high frequency may be the product of low-probability events and that the present frequency of any particular β-thalassemia allele does not necessarily reflect the frequency with which mutation to that allele occurs. In addition, the β-globin gene is very small, leading to underrepresentation of mutations of uncommon sequences, such as CG dinucleotides.

In contrast, hemophilia is not under favorable selection and the disorder has been genetically lethal with little reproduction by affected individuals. Because the Factor VIII gene is X-linked, nearly all mutations that produce hemophilia in the male will be observed. In contrast, in autosomal recessive disorders the mutant allele is not observed unless it is in the homozygous state. Thus, only a minority of autosomal recessive mutant alleles are observed at any time. Even an allele with the very high gene frequency of 0.10 is observed in only about 2.5% of people who carry it. A large proportion of males with hemophilia A have new mutations within two generations, and the average life of any particular mutation in a stationary population has been estimated by Haldane to be two to four generations.[69] Thus, the mutations of hemophilia A observed today are all relatively recent. Since (1) no apparent selection exists for hemophilia A genes, (2) mutant alleles turn over relatively rapidly in the population, and (3) the gene involved is very large, a calculation of the frequency of the occurrence of various deleterious mutations should be relatively unbiased. The observation of a high frequency of (1) CG-TG or CG-CA changes and (2) deletions of various sizes is quite striking.

GENERALIZATIONS ABOUT MUTATIONS AND THE FREQUENCY OF SINGLE-GENE DISEASES

A number of mutant alleles have been characterized for (1) the LDL receptor gene defects that are responsible for familial hypercholesterolemia,[70] (2) the HPRT gene, an X-linked gene, which is defective in Lesch-Nyhan syndrome,[27,71] (3) the ornithine transcarbamylase (OTC) gene, an X-linked gene, which is defective in urea cycle disorders,[72] and (4) the growth hormone gene,[20] among others. The data from all these mutant alleles, as well as those of the hemoglobins and clotting factors, can be sorted out, and some general principles and hypotheses can be formulated with regard to gene defects.

The frequency of deletions among deleterious mutations at a locus may be proportional to the exon size and the number of kilobases over which parts of exons are spread. It will also be higher in regions of the genome in which homologous repeating sequences are present. In these regions, for example, the α-globin gene region, the growth hormone gene cluster, the β-globin gene cluster, mispairing in meiosis and unequal crossing over will be a common and frequent cause of deletion. In general, deletion of sequences leading to loss of gene function is no worse than a nucleotide substitution that also leads to loss of gene function as long as the deletion does not affect more than one gene locus.

CG residues in exons appear to be significant hotspots for deleterious mutation to TG or CA because of methylation of cytosines in this position. We estimate that such dinucleotides may be 10 to 20 times more prone to mutation than other dinucleotides, and therefore recurrent mutation should be observed frequently at these dinucleotides. In addition to the hemophilia A mutations cited above, Nussbaum and colleagues have reported the same Taq I site mutation in two unrelated males with OTC deficiency.[72] The Taq I recognition sequence is TCGA, so both of these mutations in the OTC gene could well be CGA-TGA nonsense mutation. Barker et al had previously suggested that CG-TG and CA changes could be mutation hotspots because changes of this type appeared more frequently as polymorphisms in intron and flanking DNA in man.[73] In addition, CG dinucleotides are observed at a rate that is about 35% of expected in exon sequences, suggesting that these sequences may have been subject to negative selection during evolution.[74]

The frequency of CG dinucleotides in exons does not appear to vary more than 30 to 50%. In addition, the size of individual exons is relatively constant, being 150 ± 50 nucleotides. This means that the number of splice junctions will vary directly with the total exon length. If a large fraction of deficiency alleles at a locus are due to mutation in CG dinucleotides or splice junctions, one could predict that for X-linked lethal disorders, disorders in which a relatively unbiased view of the frequency of various types of mutation is possible, the frequency of the disease in males may be roughly proportional to the total exon size of the affected gene. This rule seems to be approximately accurate for HPRT deficiency (exon size = 658 bp;[71] frequency of disease ≅ 1 in 100,000 males), OTC deficiency (exon size = 1070 bp;[75] frequency of disease ≅ 1 in 50,000 males), Factor IX deficiency (exon size = 1386 bp;[76] frequency of disease ≅ 1 in 50,000 males) and Factor VIII:C deficiency (exon size 7050 bp;[61] frequency of disease ≅ 1 in 10,000 males). The hypothesis would suggest that since Duchenne muscular dystrophy has a frequency of ≅ 1 in 5,000 males, the affected gene has an exon size of about 14,000 bp. This would make the coding region of this gene the largest yet described in man.

Autosomal recessive disorders that have a frequency of greater than 1 in

50,000 live births in a widespread population have probably attained this frequency by selection or by founder effect and genetic drift. In these disorders one would predict that the number of mutant alleles is one if founder effect is operative and is more than one but finite in number (perhaps 5 to 10 per involved ethnic group) if positive selection exists for individuals who are heterozygous for a mutant allele. This latter situation is the case in β-thalassemia and α-thalassemia. It may well be the case in phenylketonuria (PKU). In this autosomal recessive disorder, DiLella et al have developed evidence that the mutant genes are associated with a small number of haplotypes or DNA polymorphism patterns[4] at the phenylalanine hydroxylase locus in Danes.[77] They have characterized the mutation in two PKU genes associated with common haplotypes and found that one mutant allele is exclusively seen on one haplotype and the second alleles is exclusively associated with the second haplotype. These data are reminiscent of the situation with β-thalassemia alleles and suggest that a small number of mutant alleles, perhaps 5 to 10, exist in high frequency in Northern Europe, and they suggest the existence of positive selection of an unknown nature for PKU alleles. It will be interesting to see how many mutant alleles will be found for cystic fibrosis in Northern Europeans. This autosomal recessive disease has a carrier frequency of 1 in 20 in that population. We predict that a situation similar to that observed in β-thalassemia and PKU will be observed in cystic fibrosis, that is, a limited number of mutant alleles at a single locus in each ethnic group.

The reciprocal is true of rare recessive disorders. If a recessive disease has a frequency of 1 in 90,000 in the population, 1 in every 150 in the population is a carrier of a mutant allele, and the gene frequency of such alleles is 1 in 300. It is quite likely that a large number of alleles exist in these circumstances and that nearly all affected individuals who are not the products of consanguineous matings are "genetic compounds" (carriers of two different mutant alleles) as opposed to "true" homozygotes.

Our knowledge of the molecular genetics of autosomal dominant disorders is too limited to make broad assessments of the type outlined above. Why some disorders often occur as new mutations or with highly variable clinical pictures, for example, neurofibromatosis, and others are nearly always associated with a positive family history, for example, Huntington's disease, is not clear at this time. Answers in this area should be forthcoming soon.

REFERENCES

1. Drake JW: *The Molecular Basis of Mutation.* San Francisco, Holden-Day, 1970.
2. Bunn HF, Forget BG (eds): *Hemoglobin: Molecular, Genetic and Clinical Aspects.* Philadelphia, WB Saunders Co., 1986, pp 381–399.

3. Pauling L, Itano H, Singer SJ, et al: Sickle cell anemia: A molecular disease. *Science* 1949;110:543.
4. Ingram VM: A specific chemical difference between the globins of normal human and sickle cell anemia hemoglobin. *Nature* 1956;178:792.
5. Heywood JD, Karon M, Weissman S: Amino acids: Incorporation into α and β chains of hemoglobin by normal and thalassemic reticulocytes. *Science* 1964;146:530.
6. Weatherall DJ, Clegg JB, Naughton MA: Globin synthesis in thalassemia: An in vivo study. *Nature* 1965;208:1061.
7. Weatherall DJ, Clegg JB (eds): The *Thalassemia Syndromes*. London, Blackwell Scientific Publications, 1981.
8. Fessas P: Inclusions of hemoglobin in erythroblasts and erythrocytes of thalassemia. *Blood* 1963;21:21.
9. Nathan DG, Stossel TB, Gunn RB, et al: Influence of hemoglobin precipitation on erythrocyte metabolism and α and β thalassemia. *J Clin Invest* 1969;48:33.
10. Bunn HF, Forget BG (eds): *Hemoglobin: Molecular, Genetic and Clinical Aspects*. Philadelphia, WB Saunders Co., 1986, pp 223–321.
11. Orkin SH, Kazazian HH Jr: The mutation and polymorphism of the human β-globin gene and its surrounding DNA. *Ann Rev Genet* 1984;18:131–171.
12. Antonarakis SE, Kazazian HH Jr, Orkin SH: DNA polymorphism and molecular pathology of the human globin gene clusters. *Hum Genet* 1985;60:1–14.
13. Embury SH, Miller JA, Dozy AM, et al: Two different molecular organizations account for a single α-globin gene of the thal 2 genotype. *J Clin Invest* 1980;66:1319.
14. Phillips JA, Vik TA, Scott AF, et al: Unequal crossing-over: A common basis of single α-globin genes in Asians and American Blacks with hemoglobin H disease. *Blood* 1980;55:1066.
15. Lauer J, Shen CK, Maniatis T: The chromosomal arrangement of human α-like globin genes: Sequence homology and α-globin gene deletions. *Cell* 1980;20:119.
16. Goossens M, Dozy AM, Embury SH, et al: Triplicated α-globin loci in humans. *Proc Natl Acad Sci USA* 1980;77:518.
17. Winichagoon P, Higgs DR, Goodbourn SE, et al: The molecular basis of α-thalassemia in Thailand. *EMBO J* 1984;3:1813.
18. Flavell RA, Kooter JM, DeBoer E, et al: Analysis of the $\delta\beta$ globin gene loci in normal and Hb Lepore DNA: Direct determination of gene linkage and intragene distance. *Cell* 1978;15:25.
19. Ohta Y, Yamoaka K, Sumida I, et al: Hemoglobin Miyada, a β-δ fusion peptide (anti-Lepore type) discovered in a Japanese family. *Nature* 1977;234:218.
20. Phillips JA, Hjelle BL, Seeburg PH, et al: Molecular basis for familial isolated growth hormone deficiency. *Proc Natl Acad Sci USA* 1981;78:6372–6375.
21. Chakravarti A, Phillips JA, Mellits KH, et al: Patterns of polymorphisms and linkage disequilibrium suggest independent origins of the human growth hormone cluster. *Proc Natl Acad Sci USA* 1984;81:6085–6089.
22. Lehrman MA, Schneider WJ, Sudhof TC, et al: Mutation in LDL receptor: Alu-Alu recombination deletes exons encoding transmembrane and cytoplasmic domains. *Science* 1985;227:140–146.
23. Jagadeeswaran P, Tuan D, Forget BG, et al: A gene deletion ending at the midpoint of a repetitive DNA sequence in one form of hereditary persistence of fetal hemoglobin. *Nature* 1982;296:460–470.
24. Vanin EF, Hanthorn PS, Kioussis D, et al: Unexpected relationships between four large deletions in the human β-globulin gene cluster. *Cell* 1983; 35:701.
25. Orkin SH, Old JM, Weatherall DJ, et al: Partial deletion of β-globin gene DNA in certain patients with β^{0} thalassemia. *Proc Natl Acad Sci USA* 1979;76:2400.

26. Antonarakis SE: The molecular genetics of hemophilia A. *Adv Hum Genet.* To be published, 1987.
27. Stout JT, Caskey CT: HPRT: Gene structure, expression and mutation. *Ann Rev Genet* 1985;19:127–148.
28. Brown MS, Goldstein JL: A receptor-mediated pathway for cholesterol metabolism. *Science* 1986;232:34–47.
29. Lawn RM, Efstratiadis A, O'Connell C, et al: The nucleotide sequence of the human β-globin gene. *Cell* 1980;21:638.
30. Bunn HF, Forget BG (eds): *Hemoglobin: Molecular, Genetic and Clinical Aspects.* Philadelphia, WB Saunders Co., 1986, pp 169–222.
31. Breathnach R, Chambon P: Organization and expression of eukariotic split genes coding for proteins. *Ann Rev Biochem* 1981;50:349.
32. Dierks P, van Ooyen A, Cochran MD, et al: Three regions upstream from the cap site are required for efficient and accurate transcription of the rabbit β globin gene in mouse 3T6 cells. *Cell* 1983;32:695–706.
33. Orkin SH, Antonarakis SE, Kazazian HH Jr: Base substitution at position −88 in a β-thalassemic globin gene: Further evidence for the role of distal promoter element ACACCC. *J Biol Chem* 1984;259:8679.
34. Orkin SH, Kazazian HH, Jr, Antonarakis SE, et al: Linkage of β-thalassemia mutations and β-globin gene polymorphisms with DNA polymorphisms in human β-globin gene clusters. *Nature* 1982;296:627.
35. Triesman R, Orkin SH, Maniatis T: Specific transcription of RNA defects in five cloned β-thalassemia genes. *Nature* 1983;302:591.
36. Antonarakis SE, Orkin SH, Cheng TC, et al: β-thalassemia in American blacks: Novel mutations in the TATA box and an acceptor splice site. *Proc Natl Acad Sci USA* 1984;81:1154.
37. Orkin SH, Cheng TC, Antonarakis SE, et al: Thalassemia due to a mutation in the cleavage-polyadenylation signal of the human β-globin gene. *EMBO J* 1985;4:453.
38. Proudfoot NJ, Brownlee GG: 3′ noncoding region sequences in eukariotic messenger RNA. *Nature* 1976;263:211.
39. Mount SM: A catalogue of splice junction sequences. *Nucl Acids Res* 1982;10:459.
40. Wong C, Antonarakis SE, Goff SC, et al: β-thalassemia due to a single base substitution in a consensus acceptor splice sequence of the β-globin gene. To be published.
41. Dobkin P, Pergolizzi RG, Bahre P, et al: Abnormal splice in a mutant human β-globin gene not at the site of a mutation. *Proc Natl Acad Sci USA* 1983;80:1184.
42. Cheng TC, Orkin SH, Antonarakis SE, et al: β-thalassemia in Chinese: Use of in vivo RNA analysis and oligonucleotide hybridization in systematic characterization of molecular defects. *Proc Natl Acad Sci USA* 1984;81:2821.
43. Meatherall JE, Collins FS, Pan J, et al: β^{O} thalassemia caused by base substitution that creates an alternative splice acceptor site in an intron. To be published.
44. Orkin SH, Kazazian HH Jr, Antonarakis SE, et al: Abnormal RNA processing due to the exon mutation of β^{E} globin gene. *Nature* 1982;300:768.
45. Van der Ploeg LHT, Konings A, Oort M, et al: Gamma beta-thalassemia studies showing that detection of the gamma and delta genes influences beta-globin gene expression in man. *Nature* 1980;283:637–642.
46. Kioussis D, Vanin E, deLange T, et al: Beta globin gene inactivation by DNA translocation in gamma beta-thalassemia. *Nature* 1983;306:662–666.
47. Pirastu M, Curtin P, Kan YW: Gene deletion distant from the β-globin locus inactivates the β-globin gene. *Clin Res* 1984;32:439A.
48. Lewis EB: in Demerec M (ed): *Advances in Genetics.* New York, Academic Press, 1950, vol 3, p 73.

49. Collins FS, Metherall JE, Yamakawa M, et al: A point mutation in the A gamma globin gene promoter in Greek HPFH. *Nature* 1985;313:325–326.
50. Collins FS, Stoeckert CJ, Serjeant GR, et al: G gamma beta HPFH: Cosmid cloning and identification of a specific mutation 5′ to the G gamma gene. *Proc Natl Acad Sci USA* 1984;81:4894–4998.
51. Gelinas R, Endlich B, Pfeiffer C, et al: G to A substitution in the distal CCAAT box of the A gamma globin gene in Greek HPFH. *Nature* 1985;313:323–325.
52. Semenza GL, Delgrosso K, Poncz M, et al: The silent carrier allele: β-thalassemia without a mutation in the β-globin gene or its immediate flanking regions. *Cell* 1984;39:123–128.
53. Huang SZ, Wong C, Antonarakis SE, et al: The same TATA box β-thalassemia mutation in Chinese and U.S. blacks: Another example of independent origins of mutation. *Hum Genet*, to be published.
54. Wong C, Antonarakis SE, Goff SC, et al: On the origin and spread of β-thalassemia: Recurrent observation of four mutations in different ethnic groups. *Proc Natl Acad Sci USA*, 1986;83:6523–6532.
55. Antonarakis SE, Boehm CD, Giardina PJV, et al: Nonrandom association of polymorphic restriction sites in the β-globin gene clusters. *Proc Natl Acad Sci USA* 1982;79:137–141.
56. Chehab FF, Honig GR, Kan YW: Spontaneous mutation in β-thalassemia producing the same nucleotide substitution as that in a common hereditary form. *Lancet* 1986;1:3–5.
57. Baltimore C: Gene conversion: Some implications for immunoglobulin genes. *Cell* 1981;24:592–594.
58. Jackson JA, Fink GR: Gene conversion between duplicated genetic elements in yeast. *Nature* 1981;292:306–311.
59. Filipi G, Rinaldi A, Archidiacono N, et al: Linkage between G6PD and fragile X syndrome. *Am J Hum Genet* 1983;15:113.
60. Brinkhouse KM, Roberts HR, Weiss AE: Prevalence of inhibitors in hemophilia A and B. Thomb Diath Haemorrh (Suppl) 1982;41:315.
61. Gitschier J, Wood WI, Goralka TM, et al: Characterization of the human Factor VIII gene. *Nature* 1984;312:326–330.
62. Toole JJ, Knoph JL, Wozney JL, et al: Molecular cloning of a cDNA encoding human antihemophilic factor. *Nature* 1984;312:342–347.
63. Gitschier J, Wood WI, Tuddenham EGD, et al: Detection and sequence of mutations in the Factor VIII gene of hemophiliacs. *Nature* 1985;315:427–430.
64. Gitschier J, Wood WI, Shuman MA, et al: Identification of a missense mutation in the Factor VIII gene of a mild hemophiliac. *Science* 1986;232:1415–1416.
65. Antonarakis SE, Waber PG, Kittur SD, et al: Hemophilia A: Detection of molecular defects and of carriers by DNA analysis. *N Eng J Med* 1985;313:842–848.
66. Youssoufian H, Kazazian HH, Phillips DG, et al: Recurrent mutations in hemophilia A: Evidence for CpG dinucleotides as mutation hotspots. *Nature* 1986;324:380–382.
67. Youssoufian H, Antonarakis SE, Phillips DG, et al: The molecular genetics of hemophilia A: Five different parital deletions of Factor VIII:C gene. *Proc Natl Acad Sci USA*, 1987;84:3772–3776.
68. Coulondre C, Miller JH, Farabaugh PJ, et al: Molecular basis of base substitution hotspots in *Escherichia coli. Nature* 1978;274:775–780.
69. Haldane JBS: The rate of spontaneous mutation of a human gene. *J Genet* 1935;31:317–326.
70. Brown MS, Goldstein JL: A receptor-mediated pathway for cholesterol homeostasis. *Science* 1986;232:34–37.
71. Melton DW, Konecki DS, Breunard J, et al: Structure, expression and mutation of HPRT gene. *Proc Natl Acad Sci USA* 1984;81:2147–2151.

72. Nussbaum RL, Boggs BA, Beaudet AL, et al: New mutation and prenatal diagnosis in ornithine transcarbamylase deficiency. *Am J Hum Genet* 1986;38:149–159.
73. Barker D, Schafer M, White R: Restriction sites containing CpG show a higher frequency of polymorphism in human DNA. *Cell* 1984;36:131–138.
74. Nussinov R: Eukaryotic dinucleotide preference rules and their implications for degenerate codon usage. *J Mol Biol* 1981;149:125–131.
75. Horwich A, Fenton WA, Williams K, et al: Structure and expression of a cDNA for the nuclear precursor of human mitochondrial ornithine transcarbamylase. *Science* 1984;224:1068–1074.
76. Yoshitake S, Schadi BG, Foster DC, et al: Nucleotide sequence of the gene for human Factor IX. *Biochem* 1985;24:3736–3748.
77. DeLella AG, Marvit J, Lidsky AS, et al: A splicing mutation in PKU is linked to a specific RFLP haplotype of the human phenylalanine hydroxylase gene. *Nature,* 1986; 322:799–803.
78. Marks J, Shaw J-P, Shen C-KJ: Sequence organization and genomic complexity of primate $\theta 1$ globin gene, a novel α-globin-like gene. *Nature* 1986;321:785–788.

CHAPTER 4

Clinical Applications of Gene Mapping and Diagnosis

John A. Phillips, III, MD

Recombinant DNA technology has provided the tools necessary to study the genetic bases of various inherited human disorders by direct examination of the DNA blueprint. These techniques are highly sensitive and specific and they can be applied to the analysis of the genetic complement contained in somatic cells from various tissues. Thus, while the expression of most genes occurs only in certain select locations in the body, any tissue can be used as a source of DNA for the study of any gene. For example, by examining DNA from the leukocytes of peripheral blood, information about the molecular defects causing growth hormone deficiency, hemophilia, sickle cell anemia, thalassemia and a variety of other genetic disorders was gained without the need for biopsies or complex biochemical assays. Recently these techniques have been applied to find the location of genes responsible for adult-onset polycystic kidney disease, cystic fibrosis, Duchenne's muscular dystrophy, and Huntington's disease. While the gene mapping approaches used have provided tools for the detection of these disorders in families at risk, more importantly, they served as models for investigating the bulk of inherited human diseases for which the biochemical defects are unknown. In this chapter I will discuss present and future applications of the techniques presented in earlier chapters to the detection of a variety of clinical disorders.

GENE DIAGNOSIS—GENERAL REMARKS

The human genetic endowment or genome consists of about 6×10^9 base pairs (bp) of DNA per diploid cell. This complement of DNA resides in 25 chromosomes, including the 22 pairs of autosomes (chromosomes 1 through 22), the 2 sex chromosomes (XX or XY, depending on the sex), and the mitochondrial chromosome. Assuming a typical human gene is 40×10^3 bp or 40 kilobases (kb) in length, it follows that a given gene comprises about 1/10,000 of the genetic information contained in a cell. Recombinant DNA techniques provide the sensitivity needed to detect alterations in the DNA sequence of genes, but since extensive variation is normal, care must be taken to differentiate deleterious mutations from normal variation.

Genetic Variation

Polymorphisms

The great majority of genetic variations detected at the DNA level is the normal variation associated with DNA polymorphisms. DNA polymorphisms are extensive, and DNA sequence data suggest that about 1 in every 200 to 500 nucleotides in regions not encoding a protein is polymorphic without any clinical consequences[1,2] (see Chapter 2). This amount of variation is roughly ten times that detected through studies of proteins, suggesting that most of the polymorphic variation present in the genome must occur in non-coding sequences. Most of these DNA polymorphisms result from single nucleotide substitutions. Occasionally DNA polymorphisms are of the insertion/deletion type that occur near the α-globin, Harvey ras oncogene, insulin, and myoglobin genes.[2-4] When the DNA sequence polymorphism is a single base substitution that affects a restriction enzyme recognition site, the fragment length of the resulting DNA piece will be altered, and a restriction fragment length polymorphism (RFLP) can be detected (Fig. 4.1, *top*). The insertion/deletion type of DNA polymorphism can alter the DNA fragment size without affecting the enzyme recognition site (Fig. 4.1, *middle*). The third and probably least common type of DNA polymorphism is a variant of the insertion/deletion type. In this case, the presence or absence of a pseudogene (a nonfunctional gene whose sequence resembles that of a related but functional gene) changes the length of the DNA fragment that is bounded by two normal enzyme recognition sites (Fig. 4.1, *bottom*).[5]

Mutations

Some mutations are deletions of portions of genes or of entire genes. Other mutations result from insertion of foreign DNA sequences which, if the insertion occurs in an exon, will alter the genetic code and result in a drastically altered protein. Insertions or deletions of as few as one base in an exon will shift the triplet reading frame and can cause a completely different sequence of amino acids to be incorporated into the remainder of the protein. Single base substitutions within exons can specify the same or a differ-

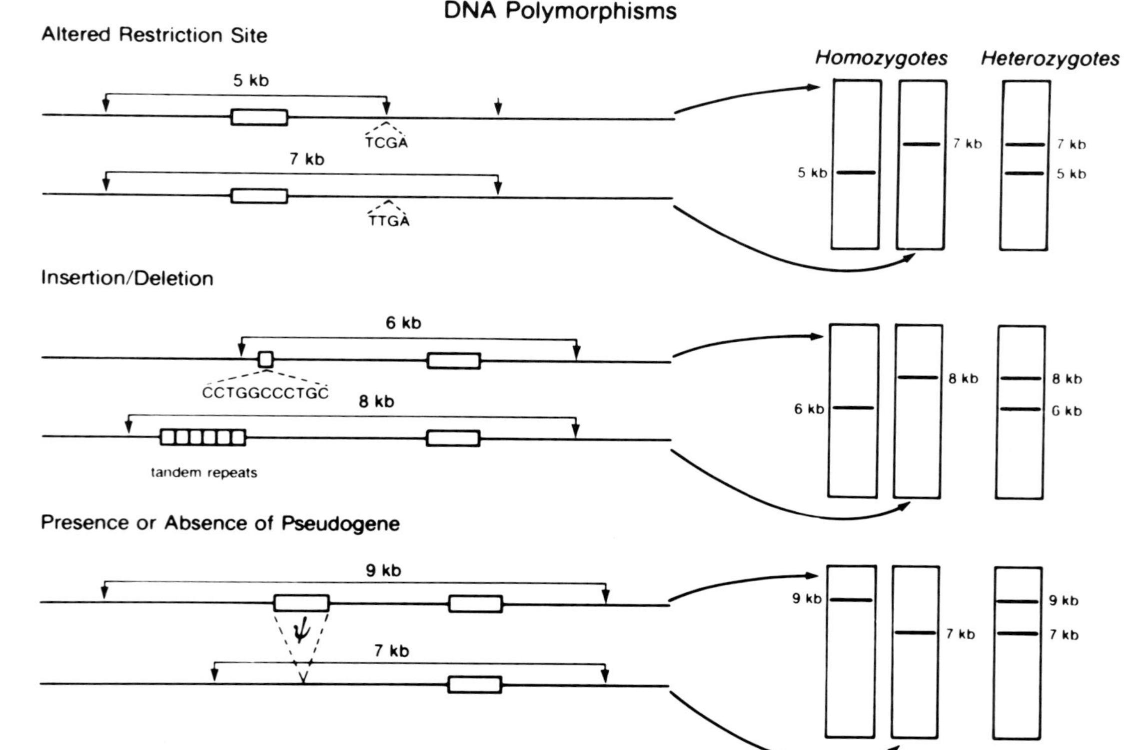

FIGURE 4.1 Types of DNA polymorphisms. *Top:* DNA polymorphism resulting from a single base substitution that eliminates a *Taq*I recognition site and yields a 7-kb rather than a 5-kb fragment (**left**) that is easily differentiated after Southern blots (**right**). **Middle:** Insertion/deletion DNA polymorphisms result from a different number of "tandem repeats" between two restriction sites, which in this case yield 6- or 8-kb fragments. **Bottom:** DNA polymorphisms due to presence or absence of a pseudogene change fragment lengths from 9 to 7 kb without affecting the recognition site.

ent amino acid and, depending on the codon involved, produce premature stop codons, or eliminate a normal stop codon to give a read-through mutation. Mutations occurring in regulatory 5′ flanking, 5′ untranslated, introns, or 3′ untranslated regions of genes do not usually alter the structure of the protein product but can result in a decreased or, rarely, an increased amount of product produced from the affected allele. Thus, some mutations within exons and most mutations in other portions of the gene may change the quantity of the gene product without altering its peptide sequence. Examples of these and other types of mutations are discussed in detail in Chapter 3. Differentiation of these various types of mutations from the normal genetic variation represented by DNA sequence polymorphisms usually requires detailed knowledge of the normal DNA sequence of the gene under study.

Heterogeneity

The great heterogeneity seen in DNA sequence alterations that can produce a single clinical phenotype such as thalassemia (see Chapter 3) complicates the detection of this and other genetic disorders by DNA analysis. The occurrence of many different defects within populations results in many affected individuals being genetic compounds (having two different abnormal alleles). Detecting the different alleles present within families and documenting their transmission to offspring often requires use of different methods of DNA analysis. A more complicated problem arises when one considers that a single phenotype, for example, familial isolated growth hormone deficiency, can be caused by genes at different loci whose alleles have patterns of expression that exhibit autosomal dominant, autosomal recessive, or X-linked modes of inheritance. Thus the same clinical phenotype can result from alleles of at least three or more different loci, and a collection of different families thought to have the same clinical disorder may actually represent a mixture of different defects. In addition to heterogeneity, the mildness of the disorder or variation in its severity seen in different affected individuals from the same family may make it difficult to determine if parents, children, or other relatives at risk are affected. This can cast doubt, in some cases, even on the mode of inheritance of the disorder being studied.

Recombination

Linkage analysis is widely applied in detecting inherited disorders through DNA analysis. When two neighboring genes (or a gene and a DNA polymorphism that is used as a marker to follow the inheritance of that gene [see Fig. 4.1]) are sufficiently close they will not segregate independently, but will be linked and transmitted together (Fig. 4.2). Once the linkage phase of the two loci is known (in coupling when the gene and marker are on the same

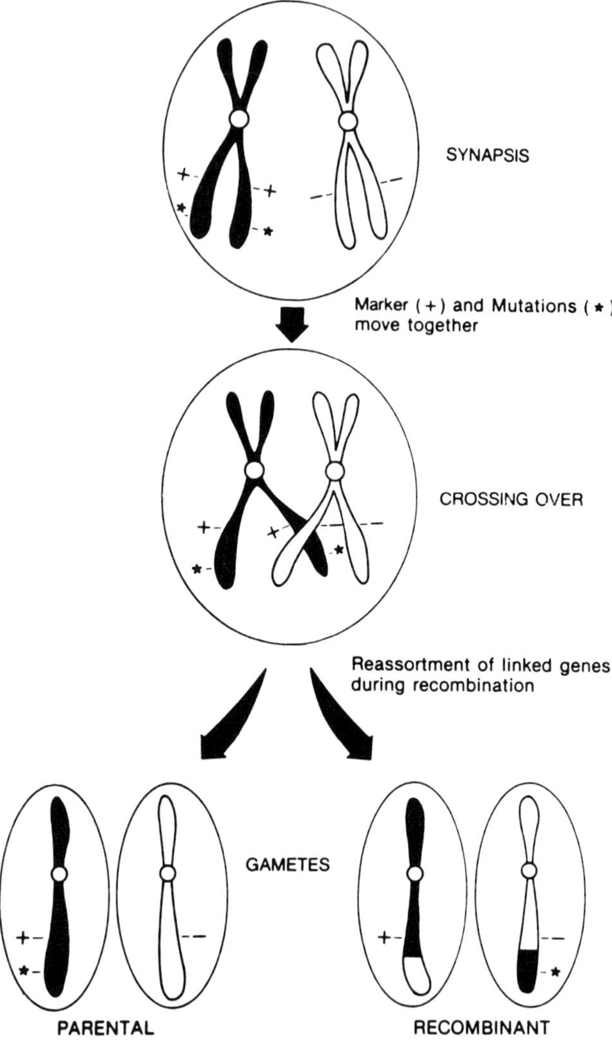

FIGURE 4.2 Crossing over and reassortment of linked genes during recombination. Note the reversed linkage phase between the marker DNA polymorphism (+ present, − absent) and the mutation (*) in parental (+ and *) compared to recombinant (− and *) chromosomes.

chromosome or in repulsion when the gene and marker are on opposite paired chromosomes), transmission of the normal or abnormal gene to offspring can be inferred from the status of the marker. However, the distance between the marker and gene locus it marks is critical. As the distance between the two increases, the probability that a recombination between them will occur also increases. A recombination, or crossing over, between the marker and gene during meiosis will cause a reversal of the parental linkage phase (see Fig. 4.2) and result in an error in the diagnosis of the genotype of offspring that is inferred from the status of the marker. One centimorgan (cM) is the genetic map distance between two loci that corresponds to a 1% chance of recombination. Given that the human genome measures about 3,300 cM and contains about 3×10^9 bp per haploid set and assuming that crossing over is evenly distributed throughout the genome, recombination between two genes that are approximately 1,000,000 bp apart should occur with a frequency of about 1% (3×10^9 bp/3.3×10^3 cM = 1×10^6 bp/cM).[6] If recombination did not occur, a single marker per chromosome would suffice to detect transmission of all of the various inherited disorders encoded on that chromosome. Because of recombination, a large number of markers of known map distance between each other will be needed to provide markers that are sufficiently close to a given gene to enable diagnosis of inherited diseases that result from alternations within the gene. How these markers are discovered and how they are used in making a complete human genetic map will be discussed following examples of more direct methods of gene diagnosis.

GENE DIAGNOSIS—APPLICATIONS

The basic tools of molecular genetics are restriction endonucleases and probes. Restriction endonucleases are necessary to produce fragments of human DNA suitable for analysis. Probes are invaluable in that they allow detection and characterization of a specific DNA sequence derived from a small portion of the 6×10^9 bp of DNA present in each somatic cell. Table 4.1 provides selected examples of cloned human sequences that are potentially useful as probes in diagnosing a variety of inherited disorders. The methods of using restriction endonucleases and probes to study genes have been discussed in Chapter 2, and I will now give examples of their application to detection of genetic disorders encountered in clinical medicine.

Chromosome-Specific Probes

Y-Chromosome-Specific Probes

Detection of Y chromosome Fragments. A clinical diagnosis of Turner's syndrome should be confirmed by cytogenetic analysis. Usually the karyotypic findings are 45,X, but occasionally additional chromosome fragments are found, or mosaicism with a mixture of chromosomal patterns in different cells (such as 45,X/46,XY) is seen. The chromosome fragments represent in some cases an X chromosome with a deletion of the "critical region" for

TABLE 4-1 Selected Probes That Are Potential Tools for Diagnosis of Various Genetic Disorders

Name	Chromosome Location	Type	Application	Genetic Disorder
Adenosine deaminase (ADA)	20q13-qter	Intragenic	Not reported	ADA deficiency
α globin	16p12-pter	Intragenic	Deletion	α thalassemia
α1 antitrypsin	14q24-q32	Intragenic	Oligonucleotide, linkage	α antitrypsin deficiency
Antithrombin III	1q23	Intragenic	Deletion, linkage	Antithrombin III deficiency
Apolipoprotein CII	19p13-q13	Paragenic	Linkage	Myotonic dystrophy
Apoprotein A-I	11q13	Intragenic	Deletion	Combined Apo AI-CIII deficiency
Arginosuccinic acid synthetase	9q34	Intragenic	Not reported	Citrullinemia
β-globin	11p12	Intragenic	Deletion, linkage, oligonucleotide, restriction site	β-thalassemia, sickle cell and other β-globin mutations
Carbamyl phosphate synthetase I (CPS)	2p	Intragenic	Linkage	CPS I deficiency
cDNA 379	Xp21	Intragenic	Deletion, linkage	Chronic granulomatous disease
Collagen α 2(I)	7q21-q22	Intragenic	Linkage	Osteogenesis imperfecta (some types)
Cystathionine β-synthetase	21q21-q22	Intragenic	Linkage	Homocystinuria
DNA Segments				
DOC R1-917	7cen-q22	Paragenic	Linkage	Cystic fibrosis
DX13	Xq28	Paragenic	Linkage	Hemophilia A
G8	4p16.1	Paragenic	Linkage	Huntington's disease

3′HVR	16p12-pter	Paragenic	Linkage	Adult-onset polycystic kidney disease
L1.28	Xp21-p22	Paragenic	Linkage	Duchenne's muscular dystrophy, some X-linked retinitis pigmentosa
met oncogene	7q21-q31	Paragenic	Linkage	Cystic fibrosis
pERT 87	Xp21	Paragenic	Deletion, linkage	Duchenne's muscular dystrophy
pJ3.11	7cen-q22	Paragenic	Linkage	Cystic fibrosis
RC8	Xp21-p22	Paragenic	Linkage	Duchenne's muscular dystrophy
ST14	Xq28	Paragenic	Linkage	Hemophilia A
Glucose-6-phosphate dehydrogenase	Xq28	Paragenic	Linkage	Adrenoleukodystrophy
Growth hormone (GH)	17q21-q22	Intragenic	Deletion	Isolated GH deficiency type 1A
Hypoxanthineguanine phosphoribosyl transferase	Xq26-q27	Intragenic	Deletion, linkage	Lesch-Nyhan's syndrome
Insulin	11p15	Intragenic	Restriction site	Diabetes mellitus (rare type)
LDL receptor	19p13	Intragenic	Deletion	Familial hypercholesterolemia
Orithine transcarbamylase (OTC)	Xp21	Intragenic	Restriction site	OTC deficiency
Phenylalanine hydroxylase	12q24	Intragenic	Linkage	Phenylketonuria
Prealbumin	18	Intragenic	Restriction site	Familial amyloid neuropathy (one type)
Steroid 21-hydroxylase	6p21	Intragenic	Deletion	Congenital adrenal hyperplasia
Y-chromosome specific	Yq	Paragenic	Deletion	Fetal sex determination

Beaudet AL: Bibliography of Cloned Human and Other Selected DNAs. *Am J Hum Genet* 1984;36:235; McKusick VA: The Human Gene Map. In *Mendelian Inheritance in Man,* Baltimore, Johns Hopkins University Press, 1986, pp xxxix–lxxxi; Willard HF, Skolnick MH, Pearson PL, et al: Report of the Committee on Human Gene Mapping by Recombinant DNA Techniques. Eighth International Conference on Human Gene Mapping. *Cytogenet Cell Genet* 1985;40:360.

Turner's syndrome or alternatively a portion of a Y chromosome.[7] Distinction between these two situations is clinically important because the presence of Y chromosome material in female gonadal tissue greatly predisposes to the development of gonadoblastomas (dysgerminomas that occur almost exclusively in abnormal gonads, frequently in those having an abnormal chromosomal complement). The utility of DNA analysis to detect the presence of Y chromosomal material in such a case is illustrated in the pedigree shown in Figure 4.3. The darkened circle represents a newborn who had apparently normal female external genitalia and clinical features of Turner's syndrome. The newborn's chromosomes included a normal appearing X and a chromosome fragment which is smaller than either an X or a Y chromosome (compare the chromosome fragment of the child to her father's Y chromosome shown on the far right). A DNA probe containing Y-chro-

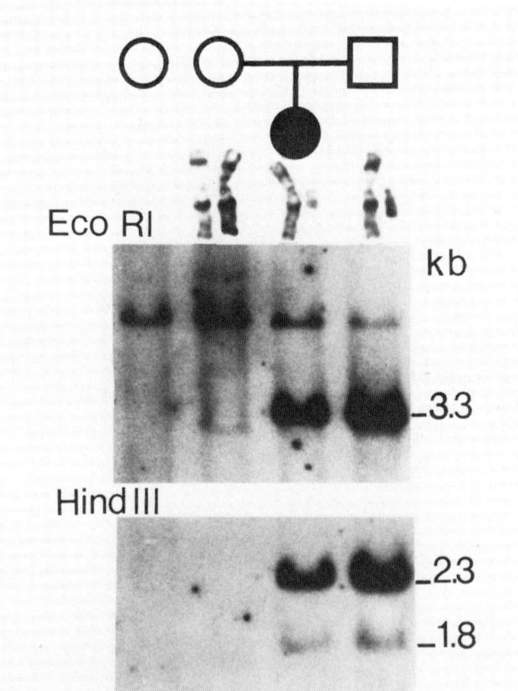

FIGURE 4.3 Chromosome and DNA analysis of Turner's syndrome with 45,X/46,X+frag karyotype. Sex chromosomes from the parents and patient are shown beneath the pedigree. Autoradiogram of DNA from female control (lane 1), mother (lane 2), child (lane 3), and father (lane 4) after digestion with *Eco*RI or *Hind*III and hybridization to a Y chromosome probe. Note the detection of Y-specific sequences in patient (lane 3), indicating that the chromosome fragment is a Y derivative.

mosome-specific sequences was used to examine restriction fragments from DNA isolated from peripheral blood leukocytes of a control female, the patient's mother, the patient, and the patient's father.[8-9] Following digestion with the restriction enzyme *Eco*RI the resulting DNA fragments were separated by size through agarose gel electrophoresis and blotted onto a nitrocellulose membrane, as described in Chapter 2. The membrane-bound fragments were then hybridized to the radiolabeled Y-specific sequences (probe) and the resulting autoradiogram is shown in Figure 4.3. Note that the Y chromosome probe shows no hybridization to the 3.3 kb *Eco*RI derived fragments in DNA samples from a normal female control or the patient's mother (lanes 1 and 2, respectively). However, DNA from the patient (lane 3) and the patient's father (lane 4) both show strong hybridization to the probe indicating they both have Y-chromosome-specific DNA sequences. Finding these Y-chromosome sequences in the patient's DNA confirms that the chromosome fragment actually represents a partially deleted Y chromosome. The decreased amount of hybridization seen in lane 3 containing the patient's DNA in comparison to that seen in lane 4 containing the father's DNA is due to the patient being a 45,X/46;X+frag mosaic (60%/40%) so that only 40% of the patient's cells had Y-chromosome fragments.

Studies of 46,XX Males. Another application of Y-chromosome-specific probes is in determining the basis of the male phenotype in individuals with a 46,XX karyotype. Such individuals (referred to as XX males) often present with postpubertal androgen deficiency associated with cryptorchidism and/or hypospadias.[10] Using Y-chromosome-specific probes Guellaen and colleagues found that DNA from such 46,XX males contained Y-chromosome-specific DNA sequences.[11] Presumably, these sequences are contained in small Y chromosome translocations that are not detected by the usual chromosome analysis techniques. Using the same DNA probe and in situ hybridization, the location of such Y chromosome translocation fragments has been demonstrated.[12] In situ hybridization involves fixing intact chromosomes to a microscopic slide followed by hybridization to the radiolabeled DNA probe. The slide is then washed and coated with a photographic emulsion that forms microscopic grains at the site of, in this case, the translocated Y chromosome sequences.

Fetal Sex Determination. A final application of the Y-specific probe is in very early fetal sex determination. The fetal DNA obtained from chorionic villi or amniocytes is denatured and blotted onto a membrane and hybridized to the probe.[13] If the fetus is a male, his DNA will anneal with the probe, producing a dot after autoradiography. This technique, called *dot blotting,* has been used to determine the sex of fetuses at risk for X-linked disorders such as hemophilia, Lesch-Nyhan syndrome, and Menkes' syndrome.

X-chromosome-Specific Probes

Hemophilia A. Hemophilia A is an X-linked recessive deficiency of clotting Factor VIII:C that occurs in 2 to 10 per 100,000 population.[14] The Factor VIII:C gene is closely linked to an X-chromosome-specific probe named DX13 that has been mapped along with the Factor VIII:C gene to chromosome band Xq28.[15] A DNA sequence polymorphism is detected by DX13/*Bgl*II, which generates two common patterns (Fig. 4.4). The larger (5.8 kb) fragment occurs when the polymorphic restriction site is absent (−), and the smaller (2.8 kb) fragment occurs when it is present (+). This difference in fragment sizes enables easy detection of both X-chromosome patterns when a female is heterozygous for the RFLP alleles (see I-2, II-2, and 3; Fig. 4.4). In the approximately one-half of females who have both the 5.8 and the 2.8 DX13/*Bgl*II alleles, the RFLP can be used as a marker from which to infer the transmission of the different tightly linked Factor VIII:C alleles to their children. The utility of this marker in linkage analysis is seen when the pedigree and autoradiogram patterns of DNA from a family at risk for hemophilia A are examined (see Fig. 4.4). The grandmother (I-2) is both a

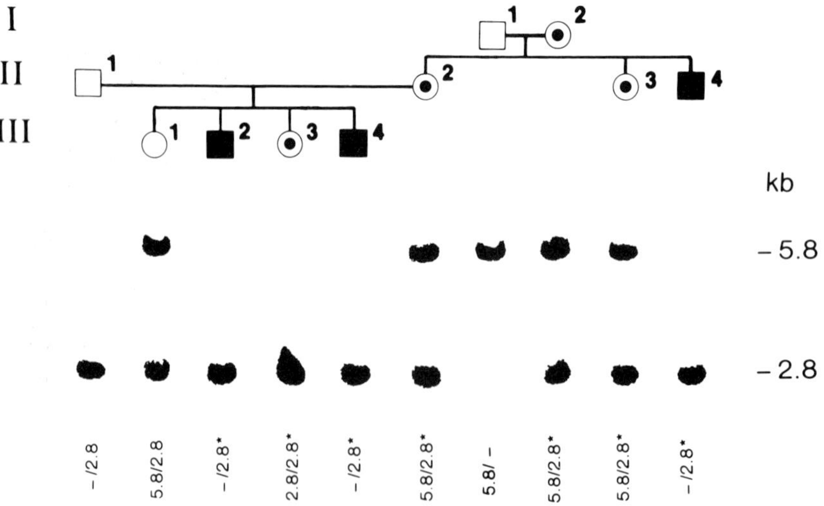

FIGURE 4.4 Autoradiogram patterns of males with hemophilia A (**solid squares**), normal males (**open squares**), carrier females (**circles with dots**) and non-carrier females (**open circles**) following digestion with *Bgl* II and hybridization with the DX13 probe.[15] Note that the + (2.8 kb) allele is in coupling with the mutant Factor VIII:C gene in this family.

carrier for hemophilia A and a heterozygote for the RFLP detected by DX13/*Bgl*II. Since her affected son inherited her 2.8 kb (+) fragment and mutant (*) Factor VIII:C allele, we can infer the coupling phase is + and * just as in the parental chromosome shown in Figure 4.2. Thus, I-2's two daughters (II-2 and 3) should both be carriers for hemophilia A because they both inherited her + RFLP allele. Similarly, the hemophilia A status of their sons and the carrier status of their daughters can also be inferred from their RFLP patterns (see Figs. 4.1, 4.2, and 4.4).

Three important points regarding diagnoses derived by linkage analysis must be considered when applying the technique to clinical situations. First, the linkage phase shown in Fig. 4.4 (mutant Factor VIII:C genes in coupling with 2.8-kb DX13/*Bgl*I-derived fragments) does not occur in all hemophilia A families. Different coupling phases between different mutant Factor VIII:C alleles and the RFLP marker, or in general between any alleles and markers, are seen in different families, and the linkage phase must be established for each family to avoid erroneous diagnoses from linkage studies. Second, although RFLPs can be used to detect the transmission of a disorder in a family without the researcher's actually knowing the precise mutation responsible, certain conditions must be met. To derive diagnoses using linkage analyses, one needs DNA samples from certain relatives (affected or normal sibs and parents or, alternatively, grandparents, aunts, and uncles) to establish the linkage phase between the given mutation and the RFLP being used as a marker. If such samples cannot be obtained to determine the linkage phase, then the study will be uninformative. A more serious problem can arise if paternity of one or more family members is incorrectly assigned, since the inferred linkage phase and diagnosis may both be incorrect. Third, as previously discussed, the distance between the paragenic DNA polymorphism being used as a marker and the defective gene is critical (see Fig. 4.2). In the case of the Factor VIII:C and DX13 loci, although both are assigned to Xq28 the physical distance separating them in kb is unknown. In the first 24 meioses studied, no recombinations between the Factor VIII:C and DX13 loci were detected, suggesting the map distance between the two should be 0-12 cM at 95% confidence limits.[15] Subsequently, 38 additional nonrecombinants were reported, further suggesting that the two loci are quite close.[16-17] Despite this, errors in diagnoses have been documented that resulted from recombinations.[18-19] To minimize such errors, paragenic RFLP markers closer to or intragenic markers actually within the Factor VIII:C gene itself are preferred. The utility and increased accuracy of such intragenic RFLPs will be discussed under gene-specific probes.

Duchenne's Muscular Dystrophy. Duchenne's muscular dystrophy (DMD) is an X-linked disease with progressive muscle wasting that leads to death in the late teens or early 20s.[20] Cytogenetic studies of certain females affected with DMD showed deletions of the Xp21 chromosome region, suggesting that Xp21 was the locus of the DMD.[21] Using this clue, X-chromosome specific probes that mapped to Xp21-22 were isolated. Two such probes, RC8 and L1.28, flank the DMD locus, and each is about 15 cM from it.[22] While diagnoses based on the RFLPs detected by either of these paragenic probes would have an error rate of about 15% due to recombination, the combination of both probes (when informative and in the absence of recombination) should have an error rate of only about 2% (15% $\times$ 15%).

To provide additional probes that are more tightly linked to the DMD locus, Kunkel and others used the phenol-enhanced reassociation technique (PERT) to selectively clone DNA sequences deleted in the male with DMD.[23] One such clone (pERT 87) was deleted in DNA from 5 of 57 unrelated males with DMD. RFLPs detected by additional probes from the same region of Xp21 showed no recombination in the first 34 meioses studied.[24] Thus, pERT 87 and flanking sequences should provide probes necessary for accurate prenatal detection of DMD in families in which a previous case is available for study to determine the linkage phase or to detect the occurrence of deletions.

Gene-Specific Probes

Gene-specific probes are DNA sequences that constitute a portion of a known gene. Such probes comprise about one-third of the reported DNA sequences compiled at the Eighth Human Gene Mapping Workshop held in 1985.[2] Gene-specific probes are increasingly used to examine the status of corresponding genes that are suspected on the basis of biochemical or other evidence to be the site of mutations that may underlie various genetic disorders. Gene-specific probes are used to detect gene deletions and certain point mutations, as well as to identify DNA polymorphisms useful in linkage analysis.

Gene Deletions: Isolated Growth Hormone Deficiency Type 1A

There are multiple types of familial isolated growth hormone deficiency, including those with autosomal recessive (type I), autosomal dominant (type II), or X-linked (type III) modes of inheritance. In turn, there is heterogeneity within IGHD type I (type 1A is associated with complete absence of and type 1B associated with deficient but detectable GH secretion). IGHD type 1A (IGHD-1A) is an example of a clinical disorder that is caused by a gene deletion. This rare disorder has an autosomal recessive mode of inheritance, and affected individuals have severe growth retardation due to complete deficiency of growth hormone (GH). Many respond only briefly to GH replacement therapy due to their tendency to develop high titers of anti-GH specific antibodies.[25-26] When the GH gene was cloned it provided a logical tool to investigate the status of GH genes in individuals with this disorder. These studies were complicated by the fact that the structural gene for GH (GH-N) is one of the five GH-related genes (5′ GH-N: CS-L″ CS-A: GH-V: CS-B 3′) contained in the GH gene cluster that is mapped to 17q22-24 (Fig. 4.5). Although these various genes share extensive homologies in their sequences, only the GH-N locus encodes GH. The CS-L gene is of unknown function and encodes a chorionic somatomammotropin-like peptide, whereas CS-A and B genes encode chorionic somatomammotropin, and GH-V is a variant growth hormone gene of unknown function that contains an internal *Bam*HI recognition site. The GH-N gene is flanked by consistent *Bam*HI recognition sites 3.8 kb apart. Although alleles of the other four related loci (CS-L, CS-A, GH-V, and CS-B) are sufficiently homologous to hybridize to the GH-N probe, they are all contained in *Bam*HI-derived fragments that differ in size from that of GH-N (Fig. 4.5). Autoradiograms of DNAs from IGHD-1A subjects lack the 3.8-kb *Bam*HI fragments that normally contain the GH-N genes (Fig. 4.6). In addition, the intensity of hybridization of the 3.8-kb fragments seen in lanes containing DNA from the heterozygous parents is intermediate between that seen in DNA samples from normal controls and their affected children. These results established that individuals affected with IGHD-1A and their parents were homozygous and heterozygous, respectively, for GH-N gene deletions. Since these deletions preclude production of any GH protein, affected individuals tend to be immunologically intolerant to exogenous GH, similarly to those hemophiliacs who develop anti-Factor VIII:C antibodies after receiving Factor VIII:C replacement.[27]

Partial or complete gene deletions have been demonstrated to be the basis of a variety of genetic disorders. Among these are some patients with α or β-thalassemia, antithrombin III deficiency, congenital adrenal hyperpla-

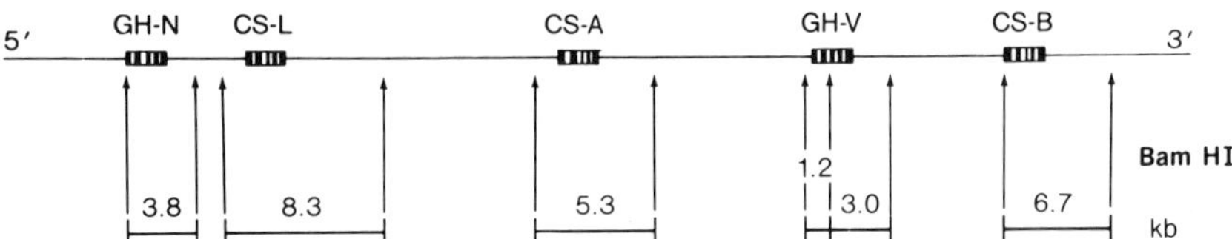

FIGURE 4.5 Partial restriction map of the human growth hormone (GH) gene cluster. The locations (**above**) and sizes (**below**) of *Bam*HI derived fragments that contain various components of the GH gene cluster (**top**) are shown. Note that the structural gene for GH (GH-N) is contained in a 3.8-kb *Bam*HI-derived fragment.

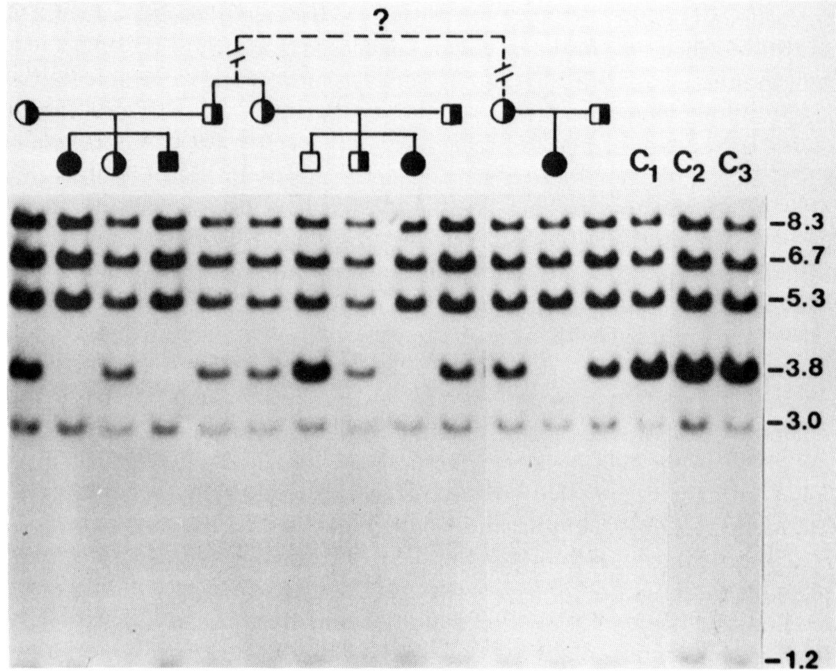

FIGURE 4.6 Autoradiogram patterns of DNAs from three families each with one or more individuals (**solid symbols**) having isolated growth hormone deficiency type 1A and three controls (C_1-C_3) following digestion with *Bam*HI and hybridization to the GH probe. Fragment sizes in kb are shown on the right (from Phillips JA, III, Hjelle BL, Seeburg PH, et al: Molecular basis for familial isolated growth hormone deficiency. *Proc Natl Acad Sci USA* 1981;78:6372).

sia due to steroid 21-hydroxylase deficiency, Duchenne's muscular dystrophy, hemophilia A and B, Lesch-Nyhan syndrome, and ornithine transcarbamylase deficiency (see Table 4.1).

Point Mutations

The point mutations causing a variety of disorders including $\alpha 1$ antitrypsin deficiency, the BO^{Arab}, and β^S globin mutations, and some forms of familial amyloidosis and hemophilia A can be directly detected by DNA analysis. These single base substitutions can be detected because they produce or eliminate a restriction endonuclease recognition site or an oligonucleotide probe can be devised that serves as a specific reagent for the detection of the mutation.

Altered Restriction Sites: Sickle Cell Anemia and Hemophilia A. Detection of the sickle cell mutation is an example of the use of restriction endonuclease analysis to detect a point mutation. This single base substitution results, in the homozygous state, in irreversible sickling of erythrocytes due to the polymerization of the abnormal hemoglobin. The deformation of the erythrocytes that results causes infarction of various tissues, hemolysis, anemia, and susceptibility to infections. Couples at risk for having children with sickle cell anemia are usually both carriers so that they have a 25% risk for having homozygous offspring. In carriers by affected matings the risk of recurrence is 50%. The mutation responsible for sickle cell anemia is an A to T substitution (transversion) in the sixth codon (GAG to GTG) of the β-globin chain (Fig. 4.7).[28] Detection of this single base substitution among the 3 billion other nucleotides present in a *haploid* genome is possible using the restriction endonuclease *Mst*II. In the normal (β^A) globin gene, CCT and GAG are the fifth and sixth codons. The A to T substitution in the sickle (β^S) gene changes the sixth codon from GAG to GTG, which substitutes valine for glutamic acid and destroys this sequence as an *Mst*II recognition site. When the β^A globin gene is cleaved with *Mst*II, a recognition site normally 5′ to the gene is cut and another cleavage occurs at codons 5 and 6, generating a 1.15-kb fragment (see Fig. 4.7).[28-30] In the case of the β^S-gene, the cleavage at codons 5 and 6 does not occur because the A–T substitution has destroyed the corresponding *Mst*II recognition, and the next intact 3′ site is cleaved,

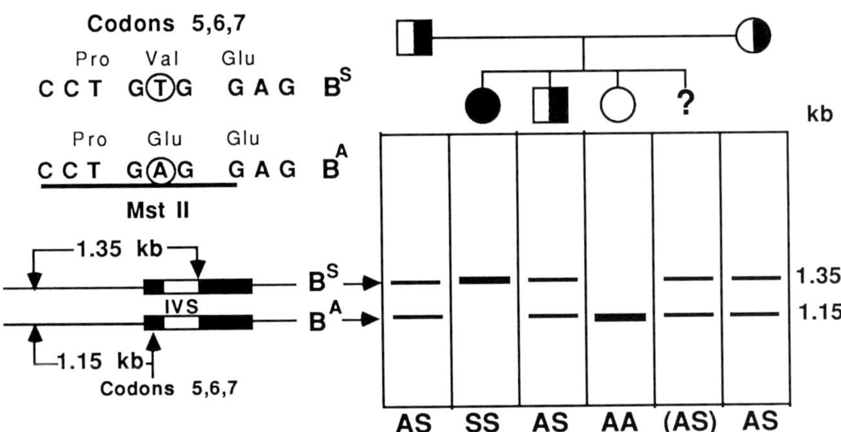

FIGURE 4.7 Detection of the sickle mutation by restriction endonuclease analysis. An A to T substitution in the sixth codon of the β^A globin gene yields the β^S allele. This change eliminates an *Mst*II recognition site, which results in the 5′ region of the β^S allele, generating a 1.35-kb fragment rather than a 1.15-kb fragment.

generating a 1.35-kb fragment. Thus, the β-globin alleles of the AS parents are recognized as 1.15-kb (β^A) and 1.35-kb (β^S) fragments (see Fig. 4.7). When DNA from these children or chorionic villi or amniotic fluid cells obtained for prenatal diagnosis are examined, the presence of only 1.15-kb fragments would predict AA. If 1.15- and 1.35-kb fragments are seen, the offspring would be predicted to be a carrier (AS) like each of the parents. Finally, if only a 1.35-kb fragment is seen, then the offspring would be diagnosed as homozygous SS, or affected.

Certain Factor VIII:C gene mutations represent examples of detection of single base substitutions by their effect on a restriction endonuclease recognition site. Gitschier et al found that the Factor VIII:C genes of some hemophiliacs yielded abnormal fragment sizes following digestion with *Taq*I.[31] These recognition site alterations have been shown to be the mutations causing Factor VIII:C deficiency.[31-32] This conclusion is drawn from the result of various substitutions that can occur within the *Taq*I recognition sequence (TCGA). Two of the three possible substitutions for the second base (C) in this sequence, T*TGA* and *TAG*A produce the underlined stop or termination codons (see Fig. 7.1, *top*). Since five of the seven *Taq*I sites that are in the Factor VIII:C gene occur in exons, introduction of stop codons at these points would result in an abbreviated Factor VIII:C protein molecule.[31-32] The mutation causing BO^{Arab} variant of β-globin and familial amyloidosis can also be detected directly by restriction enzymes because they eliminate an *Eco*RI and produce a *Pvu*II recognition site, respectively.[33-34]

Oligonucleotide-Specific Probes: α-Antitrypsin Deficiency. Point mutations that do not eliminate or produce a restriction endonuclease recognition site can be detected using mutation-specific oligonucleotide probes. These probes are short, 15- to 20-nucleotide fragments that span the point mutation being studied and the normal and mutant oligonucleotides duplicate the sequence of the corresponding portions of the normal and mutant alleles. One example of their utility is in the detection of the most common mutation responsible for α1-antitrypsin deficiency. The altered gene product (Z allele) was found to result from a G to A substitution in codon 342 (Fig. 4.8)[35-36] While the Z mutation, like the great majority of single base substitutions, does not occur within a restriction recognition site, it can be directly detected using a mutation-specific oligonucleotide. A 19-bp oligonucleotide probe specific for the M (normal) allele was synthesized and used to study DNA from normal (MM) and affected (ZZ) individuals. Under low temperature hybridization and subsequent washing conditions, the M-specific probe remains annealed to DNA from individuals with MM or ZZ genotypes. When either the hybridization or wash temperature was increased the single base mismatch lessens the amount of hybridization to the correspond-

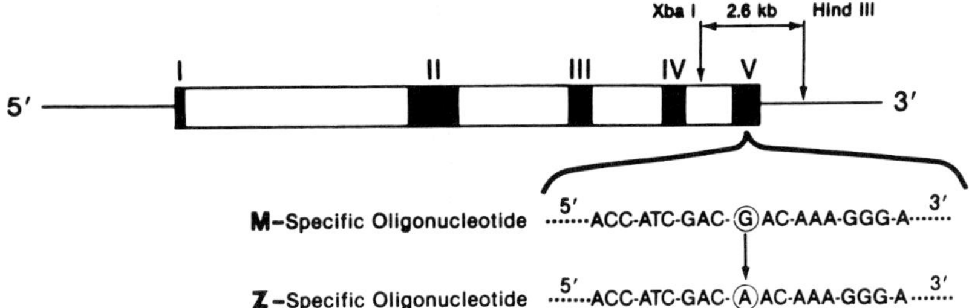

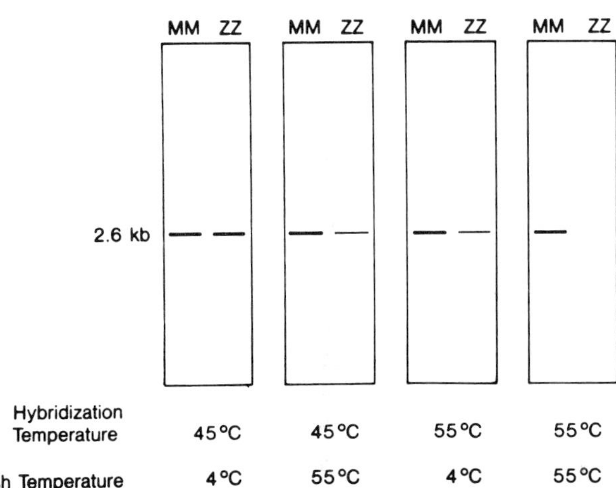

FIGURE 4.8 Detection of a single base substitution using an oligonucleotide probe. The sequences of a portion of exon V of the normal (M) and mutant (Z) alleles of α1-antitrypsin (**top**) and autoradiogram patterns of DNA from MM and ZZ individuals following digestion with *Xba* I and *Hind*III and hybridization to the M-specific oligonucleotide (**bottom**) are shown above. Note the specificity of the M-specific oligonucleotide under stringent hybridization and washing conditions for the M allele (modified from Kidd VJ, Wallace RB, Itakura K, et al: α1-Antitrypsin deficiency detection by direct analysis of the mutation in the gene. *Nature* 1983;304:320).

ing sequence of the Z alleles because the thermal stability of M-specific oligonucleotide/Z allele hybrids is less than that of the M-specific oligonucleotide/M allele hybrids (see Fig. 4.8). When both temperatures were increased, the MM and ZZ genotypes could be easily differentiated, and MZ heterozygotes could also be identified by the intensity of their hybridization to the M- and Z- specific oligonucleotide probes.

Linkage Analysis

Positive Linkage Analysis: Hemophilia A. When deletions or restriction-site-specific mutations cannot be detected by gene-specific probes, or where the affected individuals represent genetic compounds (are heterozygous for two different mutant alleles at the same locus), linkage analysis remains an alternative method to provide clinical diagnoses. The use of an X-chromosome-specific probe (DX13) as a marker in the detection of hemophilia A by linkage analysis is shown in Figure 4.4. Although DX13 is closely linked to Factor VIII:C, the two loci are sufficiently far apart to give rise to recombination and its associated errors (see Fig. 8.2). To minimize the potential for errors in diagnosis that would result from recombination, RFLP markers within the Factor VIII:C gene are preferred. An example of such an intragenic RFLP is the one detected by *Bcl*I using exons 17 and 18 of the Factor VIII:C gene as a probe (Fig. 4.9).[16-17] In this family the mother, who is an obligate carrier of hemophilia A, is heterozygous for the exon 17-18/*Bcl*I RFLP and has the 1.2- and 0.9-kb fragments associated with the − and + alleles, respectively. Her affected sons and grandsons all inherited her Factor VIII:C alleles that contains the 1.2-kb RFLP, indicating that the mutant Factor VIII:C allele is in coupling phase with the RFLP, which corresponds to the 1.2-kb fragment. Thus, her three younger daughters are all carriers because they all inherited the 1.2-kb fragment. In contrast, her

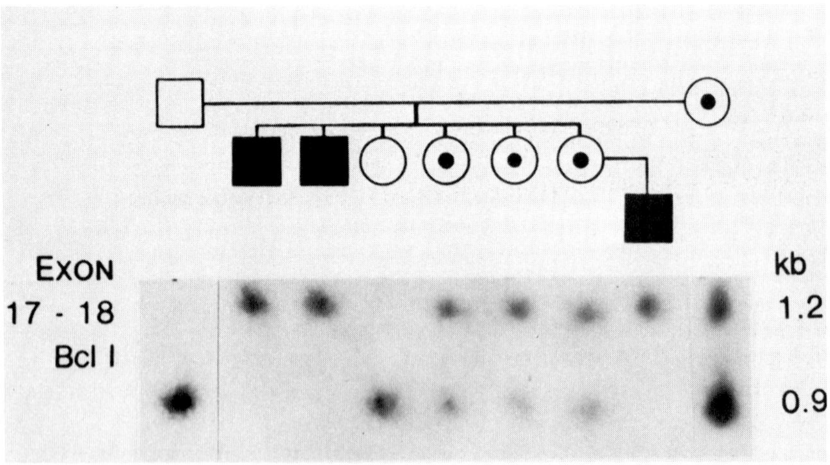

FIGURE 4.9 Autoradiogram patterns of DNAs from males with hemophilia A and their relatives following digestion with *Bcl*I and hybridization to the exon 17-18 probe derived by Gitschier and others.[17] Note that the − (1.2 kb) allele is in coupling with the mutant Factor VIII:C gene in this family. The carrier (**circles with dots**) or non-carrier (**open circles**) status of females can be inferred from the segregation of this intragenic DNA polymorphism.

oldest daughter is a non-carrier because she inherited the 0.9-kb fragment, which is in repulsion with her mothers mutant Factor VIII:C gene (see Fig. 4.9). Since the exon 17-18 probe is intragenic (within the Factor VIII:C gene), the risk for possible errors due to recombination should be negligible compared to that associated with RFLPs detected by flanking or paragenic probes such as DX13 (Fig. 4.4).

Negative Linkage Analysis: Isolated Growth Hormone Deficiency Type 1B. The putative location of mutations causing inherited disorders can be easily tested by linkage analysis. For example, isolated growth hormone deficiency type 1B (IGHD-1B) is an autosomal recessive deficiency of GH that causes pituitary dwarfism. Since the GH-N genes (see Fig. 4.5) have been shown not to be deleted in such subjects, it was hypothesized that point mutations of this gene would be found. Linkage analysis using RFLPs detected by a probe for the GH gene was used to test the validity of this hypothesis. We reasoned that if GH-N mutations were responsible for IGHD-IB, then both parents would be expected to transmit the same RFLP containing their mutant GH-N allele to both of their affected children. If they transmitted different GH-N alleles to both affected children then the mutations responsible for IGHD-1B must reside somewhere else in the genome rather than at the GH-N locus.

The autoradiogram patterns of DNAs from a family with IGHD-1B after digestion with *Hinc*II is shown in Figure 4.10. The mother is heterozygous for a GH-N/*Hinc*II RFLP, and RFLP that is tracking the growth hormone gene, and her 6.7- and 4.5-kb fragments each contain one of her GH-N alleles. Since the mother is a carrier of this autosomal recessive disorder one would expect her two affected children would both have inherited the same GH-N allele if the mutation causing IGHD-1B occurs within the GH-N gene. Interestingly, the two affected sibs did not inherit the same maternal GH-N allele (see Fig. 4.10).[37] This finding of a lack of correlation between the GH-N genes transmitted and GH deficiency indicates that, in this family, the cause of the disease is not a mutation in the GH-N gene. Thus, this study illustrates the ease with which linkage analysis can be used to *exclude* a locus, GH-N in this case, as the site of mutations that cause an inherited disorder. Furthermore, the two disorders IGHD-1A and -1B provide an excellent example of genetic heterogeneity. Whereas both disorders have a common phenotype (pituitary dwarfism) and mode of inheritance (autosomal recessive), one (IGHD-1A) shows genetic linkage to the GH-N locus while the other (IGHD-1B) does not. This demonstrates that a similar clinical phenotype can result from mutations at different locations or loci in the genome. Furthermore, these studies show that great care must be taken before combining families to be used in linkage studies, since some families may have a

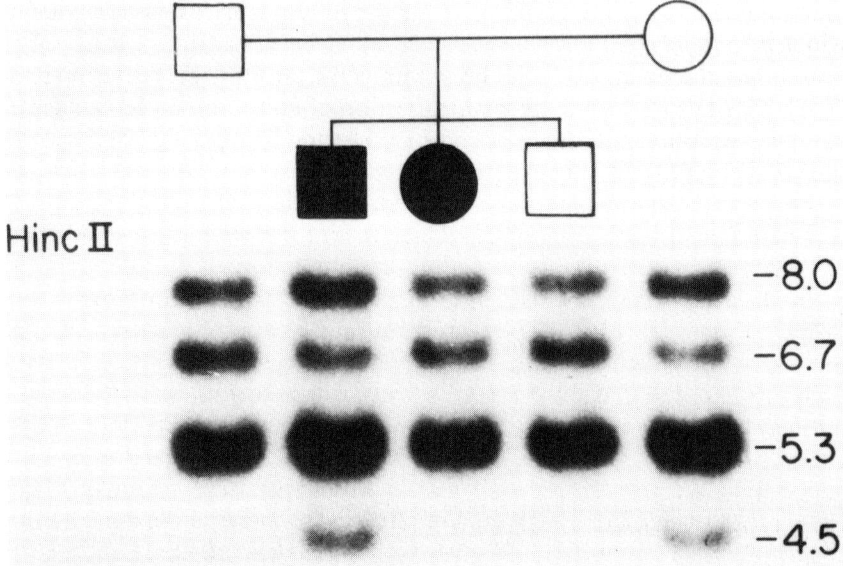

FIGURE 4.10 Autoradiogram patterns of DNAs from a family with isolated growth hormone deficiency type 1B following digestion with *Hinc*II and hybridization to the GH probe (from Phillips et al 1982).[37] Note that the two affected children (**solid symbols**) inherited different GH-N alleles (detected as 6.7-kb vs 4.5-kb RFLPs), indicating the disorder does not cosegregate with GH-N alleles.

different genetic basis for their disorder from that occurring in the other families.

Probes to Detect Disorders of Unknown Biochemical Basis

In the majority of inherited disorders the primary defect in the gene, or in fact the gene responsible for the disorder, is unknown. Examples of such disorders in which the locus responsible has not yet been identified include adult-onset polycystic kidney disease, Huntington's disease, and cystic fibrosis. Despite the lack of knowledge regarding the biochemical defects that underlie each of these diseases, DNA analysis has been used to detect the chromosomal location of the defective gene responsible for each.

Huntington's Disease

Huntington's disease (HD) has an autosomal dominant mode of inheritance and an incidence of 1 in 10,000 to 20,000. Heterozygotes are usually asymptomatic until 30 to 50 years of age.[38] Those who inherited the HD gene then develop chorea, dementia, and progressive deterioration to death within 15 years of onset of symptoms.

In an attempt to find the chromosomal location of the HD gene and devise a means of presymptomatic detection of HD, Gusella et al tested a variety of probes to determine whether any showed linkage with the disorder in two large kindreds that have many members with HD.[39] Since one family was very large (> 500 members) it seemed likely that linkage would be detected if the probes close to the HD locus were tested. Such large families are extremely useful because they provide many matings that can be examined to detect recombination, and because they avoid the possibility of heterogeneity that might arise if many smaller, unrelated families are tested. Surprisingly, one of 13 probes tested in the initial families, G8 showed tight linkage with the disorder and no recombinations were detected. Subsequent studies have also shown that G8 is linked in HD families of different ethnic and racial backgrounds but recombination between the HD and G8 loci does occur.[40] The current estimate of the map distance between G8 and the HD gene is about 4 cM. Additional studies to determine the exact risk for recombination and to verify that the probe exhibits linkage in a large number of different families are being completed. Once these results are obtained, clinical use of the probe in presymptomatic individuals, and possibly in prenatal diagnosis of HD, should follow.

Adult-Onset Polycystic Kidney Disease

Adult-onset polycystic kidney disease (APKD) has an autosomal dominant mode of inheritance and an incidence of 1 in 500 to 1,000. Heterozygotes are usually asymptomatic until adulthood, when they develop progressively enlarging cysts in the kidneys as well as in the liver, pancreas, and spleen. Without renal transplantation or dialysis, there is irreversible renal failure and death occurs at a mean age of 51 years.[41] Unfortunately, presymptomatic detection of the disorder by renal ultrasound is reported to have a high error rate, since 34% of those at risk in the second decade with normal ultrasound studies later develop the disease.[42]

Since the biochemical basis of APKD is unknown, Reeders and coworkers tested various probes in an attempt to find a clinically useful marker for the disorder.[43] In nine different families they found that a probe called 3′ HVR located near α-globin on chromosome 16 cosegregated with and showed tight linkage to the APKD locus. An example of the application of this probe to families at risk for APKD is shown in Fig. 4.11. The results shown indicate the two daughters are unlikely to have inherited APKD from their mother since they do not have the same 3′ HVR RFLP as their affected brother. Note that such studies are facilitated by the large number of RFLP (insertion/deletion) alleles that are detected by the 3′ HVR probe (see Figs.

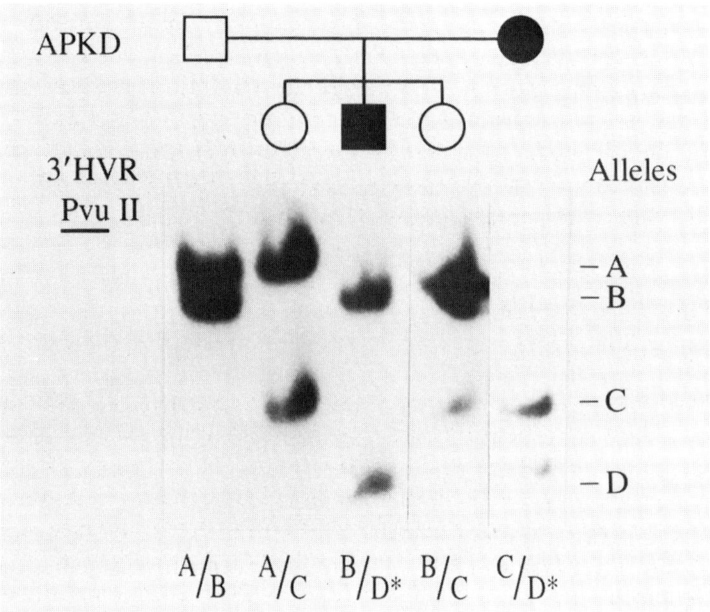

FIGURE 4.11 Autoradiogram patterns of DNAs from a family with adult-onset polycystic kidney disease following digestion with *Pvu*II and hybridization to the 3′ HVR probe described by Reeders and co-workers.[43] Note that the two daughters did not inherit the same maternal alleles as their affected brother (**solid symbol**).

4.1 and 4.11). This variety of alleles increases the probability that an individual under study will be heterozygous, and hence informative. Since the map distance between this marker and the gene causing APKD is about 5 cM, the clinical application of the marker for presymptomatic and prenatal detection of APKD is complicated by a significant risk for errors that arise through recombination. Hopefully this limitation will be overcome by identification of more tightly linked paragenic and possibly intragenic RFLPs in the future.

Cystic Fibrosis

Cystic fibrosis (CF) has an autosomal recessive mode of inheritance and an incidence of about one in 2,000 caucasian births. Affected children suffer a wide variety of severe gastrointestinal, pulmonary, and nutritional problems that result in chronic illness and shortened lifespan.

Despite years of research by many investigators the biochemical basis of CF and the location of the CF locus remains elusive. Recently, a DNA probe (DOCR1-917) that detects RFLPs following DNA digestion with *Hind*III or *Hinc*II was shown to be about 15 cM from the CF locus.[44] When the

DOCR1-917 locus was mapped to chromosome 7, other DNA markers, including the *met* oncogene and a DNA segment (pJ3.11), which were both known to be on chromosome 7, were also used in linkage studies.[45-46] Both the *met* and pJ3.11 probes were found to be very close (within 2 cM) of the CF locus, and Beaudet and others have used the *met* and pJ3.11 probes for prenatal diagnosis of cystic fibrosis by analysis of DNA isolated from either chorionic villus samples or amniotic fluid cells.[47]

HUMAN GENE MAP

Chromosomal Gene Maps

The updated human gene map as of August 1985 consisted of 1,479 human genes and markers, which included 249 cloned genes, 559 cloned arbitrary DNA segments, and 89 fragile sites.[48] Since many of the mapped loci represent diseases such as color blindness or proteins that show little variation, their utility in linkage studies is restricted to only certain families. Interestingly, the cloned genes and arbitrary segments comprise 808 of 1,479, or 55%, of assigned loci. Of these 808, 333 (88 known genes and 245 anonymous segments) detect a known RFLP.[2,48] The number of loci per chromosome varies greatly with the Y-chromosome having the fewest (7) and the X-chromosome the most (116).[48] Thus, long regions of certain chromosomes (2, 8, 10, 13, 18, 20, and Y) are devoid of mapped loci while regions of others (6, 11, 14, and X) are densely populated.[48-50] While in most cases the proportion of DNA markers to total loci per chromosome is roughly one-half, in the case of chromosomes 4, 13, 21, X, and Y there are more DNA segments mapped than known expressed loci (Fig. 4.12). Comparison of the growth rates of the number of total loci vs DNA segments from 1983 to 1985 is 170% vs 250%.[48] Thus, the number of DNA segments represents a rapidly growing majority of the total mapped loci in humans. Since over 40% of the DNA segments detect known RFLPs, the human gene map appears to be rapidly evolving into a DNA linkage map due to the number of and information content provided by DNA markers.[2,48-51]

Utility of Gene Maps to Medical Disorders

The rapid progress in determining the location of the cystic fibrosis (CF) gene was greatly helped by knowledge of the human gene map. Once the DOCR1-917 locus, which was linked to the CF locus, was assigned to chromosome 7, investigators quickly tested various probes for that chromosome.[44] Among those examined, probes for *met* and pJ3.11 exhibited tight linkage and have subsequently been proved useful in prenatal diagnosis of

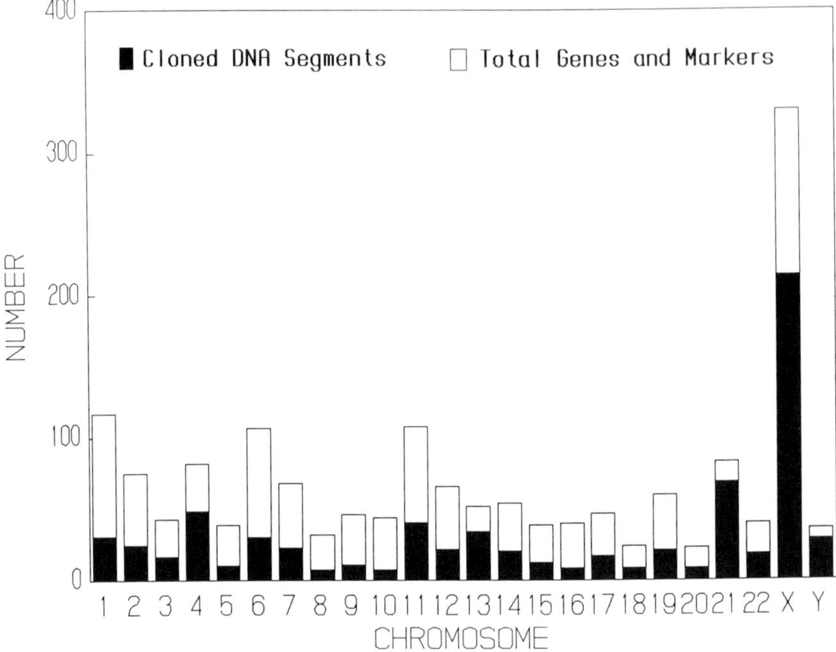

FIGURE 4.12 Genes and markers mapped to specific human chromosomes. The total number of genes and markers (including fragile sites) mapped to the various human chromosomes are depicted by **open bars** and the number of cloned DNA segments (including cloned genes and anonymous sequences) are depicted by **solid bars**.[2,48]

CF. These sequences will also be of great value in isolation of the actual CF gene because they can be used as origins for chromosome "hopping" or "walking" experiments.[45-47,52]

Determining the location of the gene responsible for any disease would be relatively easy if a complete gene map were available. A partial but functional map spanning the 3,300 cM contained in the human genome would be provided by 83 probes evenly spaced 20 cM apart.[50-51] Using these probes each could be tested for linkage to the disease gene by determining whether deletions, mutations, or RFLPs detected by the probe cosegregate with the disorder in question in a specific family (Figs. 4.3, 4.4, and 4.6 through 4.11). Since the neighboring probes that detect RFLPs would be found at 20-cM intervals, the disease locus should be ≥10 cM from the nearest marker. Once the disease gene was localized, then additional probes known to reside between the two that flank the disease gene could be tested. In this way a marker tightly linked to the disease locus could be quickly found, and this marker could be used to determine whether the disorder showed consistent linkage in a variety of families. If it did so, the possibility of genetic heterogeneity would be minimized and the probe could be used as a highly accurate tool in prenatal diagnosis or presymptomatic carrier detection.

Derivation of Linkage Maps

Obtaining a complete linkage map of the human genome is an enormous undertaking. Although 1,479 loci have been assigned to various chromosomes, most of the conventional markers represent disease phenotypes present only in rare families.[48] In addition, only about 30 represent expressed products such as blood type antigens that can serve as easily assayed and highly polymorphic markers that are practical to use in linkage analysis.[2,48] In contrast, DNA probes provide a large and rapidly growing number of informative markers. There are 333 DNA probes consisting of 88 known genes and 245 anonymous DNA segments that detect DNA polymorphisms. The great majority of the DNA polymorphisms detected are RFLPs, many of which have multiple alleles that make it likely most individuals will be heterozygous, and thus informative, for the RFLP in linkage studies. The techniques used to determine the map distances between markers and to determine the order of markers is discussed in Chapter 2.

Localization of Disease Genes

Several illustrations included in this chapter provide examples of mapping disease genes. In the family studies shown in Figures 4.4 and 4.9 the hemophilia A locus and DX13 and Factor VIII:C loci are shown to exhibit linkage, isolated growth hormone deficiency type 1A is mapped to the GH-N locus in Figure 4.6, and cosegregation of adult-onset polycystic kidney disease and the 3′ HVR probe is seen in Figure 4.11. The example of mapping of the cystic fibrosis gene was discussed under applications of probes to detect disorders of unknown biochemical cause.

FUTURE

More Disease-Specific Probes and a Better Human Gene Map

The number of reported cloned genes and anonymous DNA segments increased from 319 in 1983 to 808 in 1985.[48] Since 41% of these probes detect known RFLPs, it follows that about 100 new markers were reported in 1984 and 1985. As these and additional new probes are mapped by linkage studies and in situ hybridization the degree of saturation of human chromosomes with informative markers will increase, and the probability that a probe closely linked to a disease locus will be included should increase exponentially. When all regions of all chromosomes have been assigned markers, determining the localization of a disease locus becomes increasingly easy. In addition, as the distance between neighboring markers is determined, more and more linkage groups will be discovered, and of these groups only one or a few of the members will have to be studied to determine if the disease locus is likely to be linked to any of the genes within that linkage group.

Ultimately, geneticists and physicians will have markers that will enable the prenatal or presymptomatic detection of a tremendous number of human genetic disorders. This should lead to the discovery of heterogeneity in the causes of many disorders that are now thought to be homogenous because of their common phenotypic features. Because these disorders will fall in the purview of all the medical specialties, all physicians will need to understand this information and be able to communicate it to their patients. Finally, important factors that predispose to common diseases will, no doubt, be identified. These discoveries will result in the ability to detect heterozygotes or carriers of disorders such as phenylketonuria and cystic fibrosis as well as in possibly enabling detection of those who are heterozygotes for alleles that predispose to common disorders such as atherosclerosis, adult-onset diabetes mellitus, and hypertension. Physicians caring for these patients will find that genetic counseling and preventive medicine will become increasingly important parts of their routine care of patients.

Reverse Genetics

For the majority of human genetic disorders the biochemical basis is unknown. Several diseases discussed in this chapter such as cystic fibrosis, Duchenne's muscular dystrophy, adult-onset polycystic kidney disease and Huntington's disease have been mapped using recombinant DNA and cytogenetic techniques.[21-24,39-40,43-47] Once the chromosomal location has been established by these studies, cloning strategies can be devised to isolate the actual gene involved.[52] A good example of this approach, referred to as *reverse genetics,* is the isolation of the gene responsible for chronic granulomatous disease (CGD).[53] The CGD locus was mapped to Xp21 by the occurrence of the disease in patients with Xp21 deletions and linkage of CGD to Xp21 specific clones.[53-54] Using this knowledge, Royer-Pokora and colleagues isolated messenger RNA from granulocytic cells and used it to synthesize complementary DNA (cDNA). This cDNA was then annealed to mRNA from β-cells of CGD patients, resulting in an enrichment for cDNAs encoding the transcript which is deficient in CGD. This enriched cDNA was then used to screen a genomic library of Xp21 clones. The result was discovery of a specific cDNA clone (379 cDNA) whose product was abnormal or not transcribed in four different CGD patients, thus proving that mutations at this locus were responsible for CGD in the patients studied.[53] Similar approaches using linkage analysis, chromosome walking, and cDNA enrichment should be applicable to other diseases (adult-onset polycystic kidney disease, cystic fibrosis, and Huntington's disease) where the localization of the gene has been established.[52-53]

Forensic Applications

The use of recombinant DNA techniques in forensic medicine also has great promise. Certain sequences called *minisatellite regions* detect a tremendous number of alleles in the normal population.[4] The potential utility of these in paternity testing, documentation of transplant engraftment, and the analysis of tissue samples for forensic purposes rests on the high probability for heterozygosity and individual specific patterns.

Detection of Neoplasias

Over 90% of chronic myelogenous leukemia (CML) cases are associated with a characteristic chromosome translocation.[55] In this reciprocal translocation a portion of the q arm of chromosome 22 is translocated to 9q to form a $9q^+$ chromosome, and a small portion of 9q containing the *c-abl* oncogene is translocated to chromosome 22 to form the Philadelphia chromosome (Ph^1).[55,56] Using portions of 9q and 22q as probes, the Ph^1 breakpoints of the translocation have been found to be clustered within a small (<5 kb) region on chromosome 22 referred to as the *breakpoint cluster region (bcr)*.[57-58] Since the great majority of CML cases studied could be detected by alternations in restriction patterns using the *brc* probe, DNA analysis of bone marrow and peripheral blood samples should be useful in diagnosis, monitoring responsc to treatment, and detecting early relapses as well as differences in translocations.

Other neoplasias associated with consistent deletions include retinoblastoma (Rb) (13q14) and aniridia, or Wilms' tumor (11p13).[52] In the case of retinoblastoma, many autosomal dominant kindreds exist. If DNA markers tightly linked to the Rb locus or showing deletion in affected individuals were available, more accurate counseling and detection of carriers would be feasible.

Technical Improvements

New Methods of Labeling Probes

Currently, most DNA probes are radiolabeled with ^{32}P. The resulting probes have a relatively short half-life, which is awkward for diagnostic laboratories where consistency and long reagent shelf-life are needed. The use of biotinylated nucleotides to label probes by enzymatic reaction should provide an attractive alternative in clinical applications.[59]

Ribonuclease A Analysis

Ribonuclease A analysis provides an improved method of detecting single base substitutions.[60] This technique uses the specificity of ribonuclease A to cleave gene-specific RNA probes at the single base mismatches between them and the DNA strands with which they have formed RNA/DNA hybrids. This specific cleavage enables detection of single base differences between the normal probe sequence and DNA from a putative mutant gene without requiring DNA sequencing. Potential drawbacks include the high probability that many such differences represent DNA polymorphisms and the different efficiencies of ribonuclease A to detect different mismatches.

Denaturing Gradient Electrophoresis

Although agarose and polycrylamide gels are currently used to separate DNA fragments, the mobilities of molecules with single base substitutions are not significantly different. Using denaturing gradient gels mutants with one or two base substitutions can give distinctively different mobility profiles from corresponding normal alleles.[61] This methodology has the potential to identify mutations that do not alter restriction sites.

Perspective

It has been 9 years since the first diagnosis using DNA analysis was done for sickle cell anemia.[62] Since that time, accurate tests using DNA analysis have been developed for a number of inherited diseases (see Table 4.1). In the next several years the number of such applications will predictably increase manyfold. During the same time, advances in gene mapping should provide markers that will effectively span the genome and provide tools to detect mutations underlying many inherited disorders caused by unknown biochemical derangements.

ACKNOWLEDGMENTS

The author thanks Mrs. Judy Copeland for expert preparation of the manuscript. This work was supported in part by National Institutes of Health grant number AM35592 and Research Career Development Award grant number AM01434.

REFERENCES

1. Cooper DN, Smith BA, Cooke HJ, et al: An estimate of unique DNA sequence heterozygosity in the human genome. *Hum Genet* 1985;69:201.
2. Gusella JF: Recombinant DNA techniques in the diagnosis of inherited disorders. *J Clin Invest* 1986;77:1723.
3. Bell GI, Selby MJ, Rutter WJ: The highly polymorphic region near the human insulin gene is composed of simple tandemly repeated sequences. *Nature* 1982;295:31.
4. Jeffreys AJ, Wilson V, Thein SL: Hypervariable minisatellite regions in human DNA. *Nature* 1985;314:67.
5. Anagnon NP, O'Brien SJ, Shimara T, et al: Chromosomal organization of the human DHFR genes: Dispersion, selective amplication and a novel form of polymorphism. *Proc Natl Acad Sci USA* 1984;81:5170.
6. Kurnit DM, Hoehn H: Prenatal diagnosis of human genome variation. *Ann Rev Genet* 1979;13:235.
7. Gantt PA, Byrd JR, Greenblatt RB, et al: A clinical and cytogenetic study of fifteen patients with 45,X/46,XY gonadal dysgenesis. *Fertil Steril* 1979;34:216.
8. Butler MG, Dev VG, Phillips JA, III, et al: A child with 45,X/46,Xdel(Y)(q12) identified with a Y specific probe. *Fertil Steril* 1986;46:718.
9. Burk RD, Patrick MA, Smith KD: Characterization and evaluation of a single-copy sequence from the human Y chromosome. *Molec Cell Biol* 1985;5:576.
10. de la Chapelle A: The etiology of maleness in XX men. *Hum Genet* 1981;58:105.
11. Guellaen G, Casanova M, Bishop C, et al: Human XX males with Y single-copy DNA fragments. *Nature* 1984;307:172.
12. Andersson M, Page DC, de la Chapelle A: Chromosome Y-specific DNA is transferred to the short arm of X chromosome in human XX males. *Science* 1986;233:786.
13. Lau YF, Dozy AM, Huang JC, et al: A rapid screening test for antenatal sex determination. *Lancet* 1984;1:14.
14. Biggs R: Defects in coagulation, in Emery AEH, Rimoin DL (eds): *Principles and Practice of Medical Genetics.* Edinburgh, Churchill Livingstone, 1983, pp 1068–1072.
15. Harper K, Pembrey ME, Davies KE, et al: A clinically useful DNA probe closely linked to haemophilia A. *Lancet* 1984;2:6.
16. Janco RL, Phillips JA, III, Orlando P, et al: Carrier testing strategy in haemophilia A. *Lancet* 1986;1:148.
17. Gitschier J, Drayna D, Tuddenham EGD, et al: Genetic mapping and diagnosis of haemophilia A achieved through a *Bcl*I polymorphism in the Factor VIII gene. *Nature* 1985;314:738.
18. Winter RM, Harper K, Goldsmith E: First trimester prenatal diagnosis and detection of carriers of haemophilia A using the linked DNA probe DX13. *Br Med J* 1985;291: 765.
19. Peake IR, Lillicrap DP, Liddell MD, et al: Linked and intragenic probes for haemophilia A. *Lancet* 1985;2:1003.
20. Emery AEH: The muscular dystrophies, in Emery AEH, Rimoin DL (eds). *Principles and Practice of Medical Genetics.* Edinburgh, Churchill Livingstone, 1983, p 396.
21. Lindenbaum RH, Clarke G, Patel C, et al: Muscular dystrophy in an X:1 translocation female suggests that Duchenne locus is on X chromosome short arm. *J Med Genet* 1979;16:389.
22. Davies KE, Pearson PL, Harper PS, et al: Linkage analysis of two cloned DNA sequences flanking Duchenne muscular dystrophy locus on the short arm of the human X chromosome. *Nucl Acid Res* 1983;11:2303.
23. Kunkel LM, Monaco AP, Middlesworth W, et al: Specific cloning of DNA fragments

absent from the DNA of a male patient with an X chromosome deletion. *Proc Natl Acad Sci USA* 1985;82:4778.
24. Monaco AP, Bertelson CJ, Middlesworth W, et al: Detection of deletions spanning the Duchenne muscular dystrophy locus using a tightly linked DNA segment. *Nature* 1985;316:842.
25. Phillips JA, III, Hjelle BL, Seeburg PH, et al: Molecular basis for familial isolated growth hormone deficiency. *Proc Natl Acad Sci USA* 1981;78:6372.
26. Phillips JA, III, Ferrandez A, Frisch H, et al: Defects of growth hormone genes: Clinical syndromes, in Raiti S, Tolman RA (eds): *Human Growth Hormone.* Plenum Medical Book Company, 1986, pp 211–226.
27. Shapiro SS: Genetic predisposition to inhibitor formation, in Hoyer LW (ed): *Factor VIII Inhibitors.* New York, Alan R. Liss, 1984, pp 45–55.
28. Wilson JT, Milner PF, Summer ME, et al: Use of restriction endonucleases for mapping the allele for β^S-globin. *Proc Natl Acad Sci USA* 1982;79:3628.
29. Chang JC, Kan YW: A sensitive new prenatal test for sickle-cell anemia. *N Engl J Med* 1982;307:30.
30. Orkin SH, Little PFR, Kazazian HH Jr, et al: Improved detection of the sickle mutation by DNA analysis: Application to prenatal diagnosis. *N Engl J Med* 1982;307:32.
31. Gitschier J, Wood WI, Tuddenham EGD, et al: Detection and sequence of mutations in the Factor VIII gene of haemophiliacs. *Nature* 1985;315:427.
32. Gitschier J, Wood WI, Shuman MA, et al: Identification of a missense mutation in the Factor VIII gene of a mild hemophiliac. *Science* 1986;232:1415.
33. Phillips JA, III, Scott AF, Kazazian HH Jr., et al: Prenatal diagnosis of hemoglobinopathies by restriction endonuclease analysis: Pregnancies at risk for sickle cell anemia and SO^{Arab} disease. *Johns Hopk Med J* 1979;145:57.
34. Wallace MR, Dwulet FE, Conneally PM, et al: Biochemical and molecular genetic characterization of a new variant prealbumin associated with hereditary amyloidosis. *J Clin Invest* 1986;78:6.
35. Kidd VJ, Wallace RB, Itakura K, et al: α1-Antitrypsin deficiency detection by direct analysis of the mutation in the gene. *Nature* 1983;304:230.
36. Kidd VJ, Woo SLC: Recombinant DNA probes used to detect genetic disorders of the liver. *Hepatology* 1984;4:731.
37. Phillips JA, III, Parks JS, Hjelle BL, et al: Genetic basis of familial isolated growth hormone deficiency type 1. *J Clin Invest* 1982;70:489.
38. Tyler A, Harper PS: Attitudes of subjects at risk and their relatives towards genetic counselling in Huntington's chorea. *J Med Genet* 1983;20:179.
39. Gusella JF, Wexler NS, Conneally PM, et al: A polymorphic DNA marker genetically linked to Huntington's disease. *Nature* 1983;306:234.
40. Folstein SE, Phillips JA, III, Meyers DA, et al: Huntington's disease: Two families with differing clinical features show linkage to the G8 probe. *Science* 1985;209:776.
41. Dalgaard OZ: Bilateral polycystic disease of the kidneys. A follow-up of 284 patients and their families. *Acta Med Scand* 1957;328(suppl):1.
42. Bear JC, McManamon P, Morgan J, et al: Age at clinical onset and at ultrasonographic detection of adult polycystic kidney disease: Data for genetic counseling. *Am J Med Genet* 1984;18:45.
43. Reeders ST, Breuning MH, Davies KE, et al: A highly polymorphic DNA marker linked to adult polycystic kidney disease on chromosome 16. *Nature* 1985;317:542.
44. Tsui LC, Buchwald M, Barker D, et al: Cystic fibrosis locus defined by a genetically linked polymorphic DNA marker. *Science* 1985;230:1054.
45. White R, Woodward S, Leppert M, et al: A closely linked genetic marker for cystic fibrosis. *Nature* 1985;318:382.

46. Wainwright BJ, Scambler PJ, Schmidtke J, et al: Localization of cystic fibrosis locus to human chromosome 7cenq22. *Nature* 1985;318:384.
47. Beaudet AL, Rosenbloom C, Spence JE, et al: Linkage of cystic fibrosis (CF) and the met oncogene. *Ped Res* 1986;20:470A.
48. Willard HF, Skolnick MH, Pearson PL, et al: Report on the committee on human gene mapping by recombinant DNA techniques. Eighth International Conference on Human Gene Mapping. *Cytogenet Cell Genet* 1985;40:360.
49. Drayna D, Davies K, Hartley D, et al: Genetic mapping of the human X chromosome by using restriction fragment length polymorphisms. *Proc Natl Acad Sci USA* 1984;81:2836.
50. White R, Leppert M, Bishop DT, et al: Construction of linkage maps with DNA markers for human chromosomes. *Nature* 1985;313:101.
51. Botstein D, White RL, Skolnick M, et al: Construction of a genetic linkage map in man using restriction fragment length polymorphisms. *Am J Hum Genet* 1980;32:314.
52. Schmickel RD: Contiguous gene syndromes: A component of recognizable syndromes. *J Peds* 1986;109:231.
53. Royer-Pokora B, Kunkel LM, Monaco AP, et al: Cloning the gene for an inherited human disorder—chronic granulomatous disease—on the basis of its chromosomal location. *Nature* 1986;322:32.
54. Baehner RL, Kunkel LM, Monaco AP, et al: DNA linkage analysis of X chromosome-linked chronic granulomatous disease. *Proc Natl Acad Sci USA* 1986;83:3398.
55. Rowley JD: A new consistent chromosomal abnormality in chronic myelogenous leukemia identified by quinacrine fluorescence and Giemsa straining. *Nature* 1973;243:290.
56. deKlein AA, Geurts van Kessel A, Grosweld G, et al: A cellular oncogene is translocated to the Philadelphia chromosome in chronic myelocytic leukemia. *Nature* 1982;300:765.
57. Groffen J, Stephenson JR, Heisterkamp N, et al: Philadelphia chromosomal breakpoints are clustered within a limited region, *bcr* on chromosome 22. *Cell* 1984;36:93.
58. Collins SJ: Breakpoints on chromosomes 9 and 22 in Philadelphia chromosome-positive chronic myelogenous leukemia (CML). *J Clin Invest* 1986;78:1392.
59. Leary JJ, Brigati DJ, Ward D: Rapid and sensitive colorimetric method for visualizing biotin-labeled DNA probes hybridized to DNA or RNA immobilized on nitrocellulose: Bio blots. *Proc Natl Acad Sci USA* 1983;80:4045.
60. Myers RM, Larin Z, Maniatis T: Detection of single base substitutions by ribonuclease cleavage at mismatches in RNA:DNA duplexes. *Science* 1985;230:1242.
61. Myers RM, Lumelsky N, Lerman LS, et al: Detection of single base substitutions in total genomic DNA. *Nature* 1985;313:495.
62. Kan YW, Dozy AM: Antenatal diagnosis of sickle cell anemia by DNA analysis of amniotic fluid cells. *Lancet* 1978;2:910.

CHAPTER 5

Inborn Errors of Metabolism in the Molecular Age

David L. Valle, MD, and
Grant A. Mitchell, MD

The study of inborn errors of metabolism began at the turn of the century with Sir Archibald Garrod, Regius Professor of Medicine at Oxford.[1] Working in a time when mendelism was being rediscovered, Garrod studied four disorders: cystinuria, albinism, pentosuria, and most productively, alkaptonuria, a disorder caused by a defect in tyrosine degradation. Garrod proposed that each of these disorders resulted from inherited, life-long defects in the ordered processes of metabolism. He also suggested that rare disorders such as these were but the most easily recognized characteristics of an individual's genetic makeup. He reasoned that just as each of us has a characteristic physical appearance, we each have genetically determined metabolic and physiologic strengths and weaknesses—what Garrod termed our "chemical individuality."[2]

From Garrod's time onward, inborn errors of metabolism have been useful models of genetic disease and have contributed to our understanding of chemical individuality. The rate of progress was slow at first and, over the years, has been markedly influenced by the development of new technologies. The pace increased dramatically in the 1950s and 1960s with the advent of chromatographic methods, quantitative amino acid analysis, electrophoretic techniques for the separation of proteins, radioisotopic methods for enzyme measurements, cell culture techniques, and the development of gas chromatography and mass spectrometry. Each of these methods improved our capability to detect new inborn errors, analyze their metabolic consequences, and predict their genetic basis. Today the powerful techniques of molecular biology provide the first opportunity to determine directly the nature of the genetic defects responsible for these diverse disorders and to understand how these mutations disrupt the synthesis, posttranslational modification, processing, and localization of these interesting and clinically relevant gene products. In this chapter we will review the contributions of molecular technology to our knowledge of inborn errors, and emphasize the continued role of these disorders as model systems for genetic analysis. Finally, we will project future directions of study for this field.

SOME GENERAL FEATURES OF INBORN ERRORS

Definition

Garrod coined the phrase *inborn error of metabolism* to describe a group of lifelong disorders of metabolism that he supposed to be caused by inherited deficiency of an enzyme.[1] More recently, Rosenberg has expanded the definition of inborn errors of metabolism to include all biochemical disorders due to genetically determined, specific defects in the structure and/or function of protein molecules.[3] Both definitions emphasize the specific, monogenic nature of these disorders. The latter definition enlarges the scope of Garrod's definition from enzymes to all proteins. The biologic basis for this expansion is the realization that enzymes are members of but one of many classes of proteins (others include structural proteins, plasma transport proteins, membrane transport proteins, receptors, etc.) and the understanding that genetic defects in the structure and/or function of any protein will result in biochemical perturbations. In general, physicians continue to limit the definition of inborn errors of metabolism to monogenic disorders whose phenotype includes recognizable disturbances in the complex systems of biochemical interconversions known as intermediary metabolism. Many of the examples we will cite in this chapter fit easily under this heading. However, we favor the broader definition because of its basis in biology and because, as our understanding of the nature and consequence of mutations becomes more molecular, the lessons learned from one gene are easily transposable to others regardless of whether the protein product is an enzyme, a receptor, or a structural component of a cell membrane.

Features of Inborn Errors

In general, inborn errors of metabolism are rare disorders. The incidence of a particular inborn error may vary in different ethnic groups, but almost always is much lower than the common maladies of adult life such as hypertension, atherosclerosis, cancer, arthritis, and the like. For many inborn errors, the age at onset is early in postnatal life, at a time when the individual no longer has access to maternal homeostatic systems to compensate for his or her endogenous defect. Exceptions to this generalization include some inborn errors whose symptoms clearly begin in utero (eg, certain disorders of energy utilization,[4] and defects of genes whose protein products have a major functional role in utero, such as the α-thalassemias and the monogenic malformation syndromes). Exceptions at the other end of the spectrum include disorders whose expression is accentuated by the postpubescent internal milieu (eg, acute intermittent porphyria) or those that require time for the accumulation of some toxin or undigestable metabolic byproduct (eg, the late onset varieties of the lysosomal storage diseases[5] and the LDL receptor defects[6]) or for death of sufficient number of cells to limit the function of a particular organ or tissue (eg, possibly Huntington's disease).[7]

Inborn errors are possible for nearly all loci. All genes are susceptible to mutation and, particularly as our molecular knowledge increases, we can expect to identify an ever-increasing number of inborn errors. Already, many metabolic pathways are nearly or completely saturated (Fig. 5.1). Genes underrepresented in the lists of inborn errors will include those whose products are so vital or so rigidly dependent on their normal configuration that mutation results in a drastic reduction in function and lethality early in development. Possible examples of this class include DNA- and RNA-synthesizing enzymes, tRNA-charging enzymes, and enzymes catalyzing certain critical steps in metabolism, such as ornithine decarboxylase, which catalyzes the first step in polyamine biosynthesis. Even for these vital gene products, we can expect to find clinical phenotypes associated with mutations that only modestly impair the function of the gene products. At the other extreme, gene products that are redundant, little used, or highly tolerant to structural change are also infrequently associated with inborn errors. For example, the ribosomal RNA genes are so abundant that deletion of many, which occurs when one of the acrocentric chromosomes on which they are found lacks a satellite, has no discernible phenotypic effect and is known only as a benign chromosomal heteromorphism.[8]

An important lesson learned from the study of inborn errors is that gene products interact with one another in the form of developmental and homeostatic systems. These interactions may be very intimate, such as those between subunits of a heteromeric protein, or they may be of a more physiologic type at organellar, cellular or organ levels mediated by shared metabolites, hormones, and other regulatory factors. This systematic interaction of gene products is easily overlooked as investigators focus on molecular topics. However, realization of this arrangement is vital to understanding the relationship between genes and phenotypes. The phenotype of a particular genetic defect mainly reflects failure of the entire homeostatic system. Hence, defects of any of several components of the system may result in similar, if

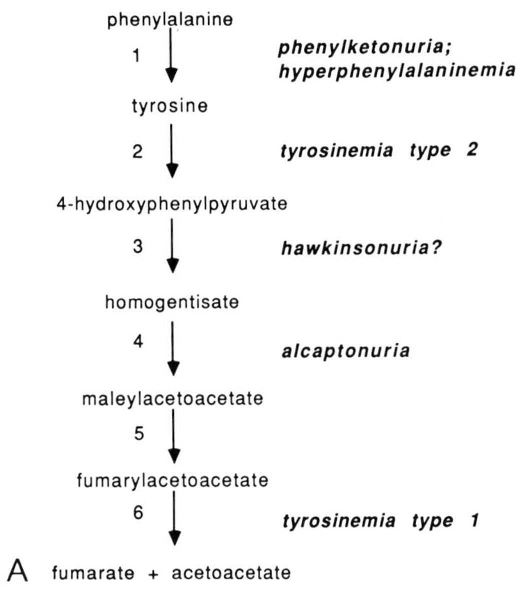

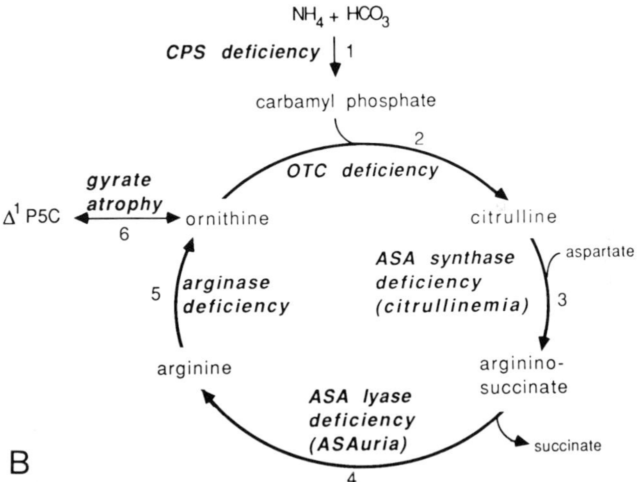

FIGURE 5.1 Some metabolic pathways are nearly saturated with inborn errors. **A**: The inherited disorders of aromatic amino acid catabolism. The enzymes indicated are (1) phenylalanine hydroxylase; (2) tyrosine aminotransferase; (3) 4-hydroxy-phenylpyruvic dioxygenase; (4) homogentisic acid 1,2-dioxygenase; (5) maleylacetoacetic acid isomerase; and (6) fumarylacetoacetase. **B**: The inherited disorders of the urea cycle. The enzymes indicated are: (1) carbamyl phosphate synthase (CPS); (2) ornithine transcarbamylase (OTC); (3) argininosuccinic acid synthase (ASA); (4) ASA lyase; (5) arginase; and (6) Ornithine-δ-aminotransferase (OAT). Other abbreviation: Δ^1P5C, Δ^1-pyrroline-5-carboxylate.

The names of the corresponding inborn errors appear in boldface italics.

not identical, phenotypes. The concept of genetic heterogeneity, or mutations at two or more loci resulting in the same or similar phenotypes, is accounted for by this interaction among gene products.

The genes involved in blood glucose are a good example of a homeostatic system. The products of these genes interact in a complex system capable of maintaining blood glucose concentrations within the narrow range of 3 to 6 mM despite intermittent input of variable amounts of glucose precursors and constantly changing rates of glucose utilization depending on the level of activity and the state of nutrition. At least 30 gene products are involved in the system (intestinal dissacharidases, transmembrane glucose transporters, enzymes of glycogen synthesis and degradation and glycolysis). Defects at several of the genes result in episodic hypoglycemia—a failure of the glucose homeostatic system. This elaborate interaction of gene products also predicts the existence of regulatory mechanisms controlling the expression of genes whose products are all part of a particular homeostatic system. We are beginning to understand these regulatory mechanisms on a molecular level, but much remains to be learned.

MOLECULAR STUDIES OF GENES INVOLVED IN INBORN ERRORS OF METABOLISM

The initial step in a molecular study of a gene almost always is the isolation of a cDNA, a DNA molecule complementary to its messenger RNA or mRNA. Using the cDNA, a wide variety of molecular investigations of the corresponding gene are possible. In this section we will discuss methods of cDNA cloning; mRNA structure and nucleotide sequence; gene structure, function, and location; the detection of and consequences of mutations responsible for inborn errors; and the possibilities for treatment of patients with these defects.

cDNA Cloning

The first step in cDNA cloning is the isolation of mRNA from a particular cell or tissue, which is usually chosen because it is a rich source of the desired mRNA. The retroviral enzyme, reverse transcriptase, is used to synthesize cDNA from the mRNA. Because the cell or tissue mRNA will contain transcripts of many genes, the resultant pool of cDNAs will be heterogeneous and the investigator must sort through this pool to find the cDNA of interest. To this end, the cDNAs contained in this mixture are inserted into some replicable carrier DNA molecule (vector), one cDNA per vector, to form a cDNA library. Typical vectors include various derivatives of bacteriophage λ or one of several varieties of autonomous, self-replicating, circular DNA molecules found in bacteria known as *plasmids*. Standard vectors have been engineered so as to be convenient for insertion of the cDNA and so that the recombinant molecules (insert plus vector) can be separated by a variety of methods to identify and isolate the desired, cloned cDNA.

Initiating the cloning procedure with mRNA is advantageous because the mRNA pool, although heterogeneous, is not nearly so complex as would be a pool of genomic DNA fragments cut into mRNA-sized pieces. In addition to the expressed genes, the genomic DNA pool would contain sequences of nonexpressed genes and a great deal of DNA from the spaces between genes. Expressed genes make up less than 10% of genomic DNA. Converting the mRNA to cDNA is advantageous because the double-stranded cDNA is much more stable, can be cut at specific sites and spliced and, most importantly, the cDNA, when inserted into vector, is easily stored, screened, replicated, and isolated in large quantities from the bacterial host (see Chapter 2).

Table 5.1 lists a variety of strategies to enrich cellular mRNA with the desired mRNA as well as methods for finding a particular cDNA in a library. Before the development of these methods, progress in isolating cDNA clones for genes involved in inborn errors of metabolism was slow because in most tissues the relevant mRNA molecules were low in abundance ($<0.01\%$ of the total mRNA). This is due to the large number of genes (approximately 10^4/liver cell) which, in most tissues, are expressed in roughly equivalent amounts. Regardless of the approach, there are always two particularly important aspects of cDNA cloning: (1) isolation of putative positive clones from some sort of heterogenous pool and (2) verification of the identity of the clone(s). The two methods of cDNA cloning most widely used currently are (1) screening a suitable cDNA library with synthetic oligonucleotide probes,

TABLE 5-1 Methods of cDNA Cloning

Enrichment for a specific mRNA
Tissue selection[49]
Overproducing cell line[13,16]
Size fractionation[74]
Polysome immunoprecipitation[75-77]
Subtraction hybridization[78]
Detection of positive clones
Differential hybridization to cDNA prepared from tissue induced and noninduced for mRNA of interest (+/− hybridization)[79]
Hybrid selection[74]
Probe with homologus region of another gene or same gene from another species[80-81]
Oligonucleotide probes predicted from amino acid sequence[9-10]
Antibody screening of expression libraries[11-12]
Genomic probes identified by chromosome deletion[82-83]

and (2) screening a cDNA expression library constructed in phage λgt11 with antibodies to the protein of interest.

Screening with Oliogonucleotide Probes

A set of oligonucleotides (usually with lengths in the range of 18–26 mers) is constructed with sequences complementary to that predicted for the mRNA from the corresponding amino acid sequence of the protein product. The redundancy of the genetic code prevents precise prediction of the nucleotide sequence. However, most of the uncertainty is in the third base position of the codon and can be minimized by choosing a stretch of sequence that contains amino acids with low codon redundancy; depending on the amino acid, there are one to six codons. Pools of all possible oligonucleotides (typically comprised of 8–256 members, depending on the amount of redundancy) are radiolabeled and used to probe a cDNA library, which is usually arrayed on a nitrocellulose membrane at high density (200–500 bacterial colonies or phage plaques per cm^2). Hybridization conditions are selected according to the length and nucleotide composition of the oligonucleotides. Positive clones are then isolated by picking an area containing a positive signal and using serial dilution and repeated screening to isolate the positive clone. The cloning of the β subunit of human hexosaminidase A by Gravel and colleagues[9] and of human adenosine deaminase by Orkin and others[10] are good examples of this approach.

Screening Expression Libraries with Antibodies

A second widely used method of cDNA cloning utilizes antibodies against the protein product to detect cDNAs that have been inserted into the expression vector phage λgt11. The site of cDNA insertion (cloning site) in this vector is an EcoRI restriction site located within the inducible β-galactosidase gene (Fig. 5.2). When this gene is induced in recombinant phage, a hybrid or fusion protein is produced in which the first few residues are β-galactosidase and the remaining residues are those directed by the cDNA sequence. If the inserted cDNA is in the proper orientation and correct reading frame (which will occur one-sixth of the time for randomly inserted cDNAs), a portion of the fusion protein will correspond to the normal protein product of the mRNA complementary to the cDNA. After induction, the library is screened with a specific antibody directed to the protein of interest. Immunoadsorbed, polyclonal antibodies with high affinity for a variety of epitopes are the best choice. Positive clones are then isolated by dilution and repeated screening. The cloning of the urea cycle enzyme argininosuccinate lyase by O'Brien and colleagues[11] and α-galactosidase, the enzyme deficient in Fabry's disease, by Desnick and co-workers[12] are good examples of this approach.

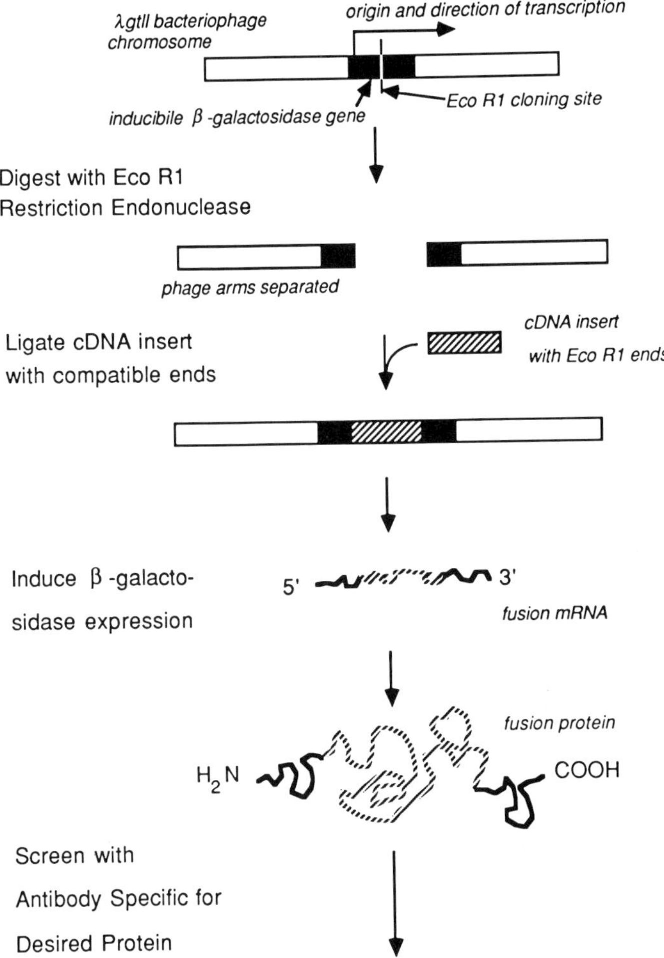

FIGURE 5.2 Creation and screening of a λgt11 expression library.

Both of these methods have a variable but significant false-positive rate. Therefore, the identity of putative positive clones must be verified by some alternative method. Most typically this is achieved by comparing the amino acid sequence predicted from the nucleotide sequence of the cDNA with that observed by direct sequencing of the protein of interest. Current protein microsequencing technology provides considerable sequence from as little as 100 to 200 picomoles of protein.

The first molecular cloning of a cDNA for a gene involved in a classical inborn error of metabolism was reported by Beaudet and colleagues, who cloned the human urea cycle enzyme, argininosuccinic acid synthetase, in 1981.[13] In the ensuing 6 years, cDNAs for scores of genes have been cloned.[14] In addition to providing nucleotide and amino acid sequence information, these cDNAs have been used as hybridization probes to characterize and quantitate the corresponding mRNA in cells and tissues from normals and patients with a variety of IEMs; and to isolate, characterize, and map the corresponding genes. What follows is an account of the experimental approaches frequently used and the information we have gained from these studies and the impact this knowledge has had on our understanding of the inborn errors of metabolism.

mRNA Structure

Sequencing

Nucleotide sequencing is typically the first step in the analysis of a cDNA and often provides the information necessary for verification of its identity. In practice, any of several readily available programs for personal computers are used to store and analyze the sequence data as it accumulates. The programs enable one to identify sites of restriction endonuclease cleavage, to translate the sequence in all reading frames in both orientations, and to search for the deduced amino acid sequence for sites of potential posttranslational modification (phosphorylation, glycosylation, cleavage) and for regions of homology with other proteins.

Structure

With the full-length sequence of a particular cDNA in hand, the structure of its mature mRNA can be determined (Fig. 5.3). At the 5′ end (which is the first to be transcribed and the first to enter the ribosome, and corresponds to the amino-terminus of the protein) following a posttranscriptionally added 7-methyl guanosine residue (the cap), there is usually a short, 50 to 100-nucleotide nontranslated region. A few mRNAs (<5%), often encoding key regulatory proteins, have long 5′-nontranslated regions of several hundred nucleotides in length, which may play a role in regulating the translation of the message.[15] The genes for ornithine decarboxylase, the first enzyme in the polyamine biosynthetic pathway;[16] 3-hydroxy-3-methyl glutaryl coenzyme A reductase, the rate limiting enzyme in cholesterol synthesis;[17] and the nuclear-acting oncogene c-myc[18] all specify mRNAs with long 5′-nontranslated regions. Exactly how this long nontranslated region influences translation is not known, but when it is removed experimentally, the rate of translation of these messages increases dramatically.[19]

mRNA Structure

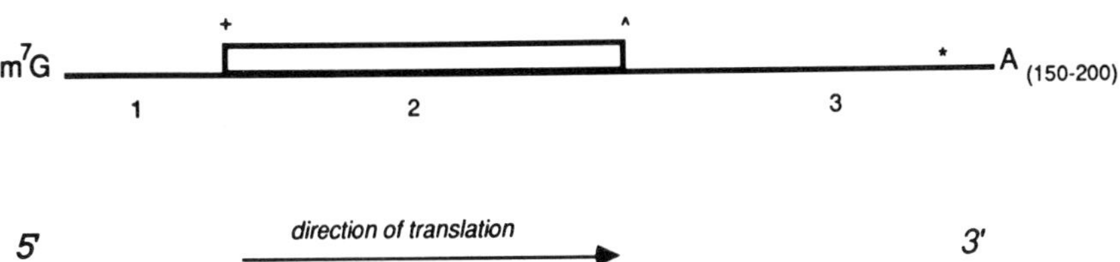

FIGURE 5.3 The features of eukaryotic messenger RNAs: (1) 5′ nontranslated region starting with a 7-methylguanosine cap (m^7G); (2) translated portion, denoted by the rectangle, beginning with an initiation AUG codon (+), and ending at a stop codon (^); and (3) 3′ nontranslated region, with poly A tail 15 to 20 nucleotides downstream from the polyadenosine addition signal (*).

The translated, or open reading frame, region of an mRNA invariably starts with a methionine codon (AUG) and continues for the entire length of the polypeptide. The open reading frame is terminated by one of three possible stop codons (UAA, UAG, UGA) and is followed by a 3′-nontranslated region of variable length ranging from a few to a few thousand nucleotides in length. Finally, at the extreme, 3′ end of the mRNA there are 100 to 200 nucleotides of posttranscriptionally added adenosine residues (poly-A tail). The consequence, if any, of the great variation in length of 3′-nontranslated region between mRNAs is not known. However, certain sequences within the 3′-nontranslated region clearly are important. Shaw and Kamen have shown that one or more copies of the sequence AUUUA in this region is a characteristic of very short lived mRNAs ($t_{1/2} < 30$ minutes) and confers this characteristic on otherwise stable mRNAs when molecularly inserted into their 3′-nontranslated region.[20] A second important sequence in the 3′-nontranslated region is the hexanucleotide AAUAAA which is found 15 to 20 nucleotides 5′ (or upstream) from the poly A addition site. It is thought to function as a recognition signal for an endonuclease, which cleaves the elongating transcript at the site of subsequent addition of the adenosine residues.

Predicted Amino Acid Sequences

cDNA cloning and sequencing has replaced in large part direct chemical analysis as the most commonly used method for determining amino acid composition and sequence of proteins. As might be expected, this nucleotide sequence data has proved extremely useful. Readily available personal computer software can be used to search the deduced amino acid sequence for consensus sequences for endoproteolytic cleavage,[21] phosphorylation,[22] glycosylation,[23] and cofactor binding,[24] and for regions suitable for spanning membranes.[23] Predictions of post-translational processing and subcellular localizations can be tested by direct immunologic and biochemical experiments and frequently lead to considerable new information about the protein. For example, in their studies of familial hypercholesterolemia, Brown and colleagues isolated and sequenced a cDNA for the low-density lipoprotein receptor (LDL).[23] The deduced amino acid sequence predicted a single transmembrane spanning region separating the receptor into large extracellular and small cytoplasmic domains.[23] The extracellular domain contained a cluster of 18 serine and threonine residues suitable for o-glycosylation. These results verified and extended previous biochemical studies showing the receptor was membrane bound and contained o-linked sugars. Similarly, Woo and his colleagues in their molecular analysis of human phenylalanine hydroxylase found information relevant to earlier biochemical studies that had indicated that phenylalanine hydroxylase could be phosphorylated and that partial proteolysis of the intact 50-kD monomer released a 15-kD phosphorylated peptide that inhibited the catalytic activity of the remaining 35-kD peptide.[22] In the deduced amino acid sequence they found a consensus sequence for a cAMP-dependent protein phosphorylation. By comparing the phenylalanine hydroxylase amino acid sequence with that of other hydroxylases, they assigned its active site to the middle and carboxy-terminal thirds of the protein and the phosphorylatable, auto-inhibitory activity to the amino-terminal third.[22]

Homology comparisons have also provided considerable information on the evolutionary relatedness of a variety of proteins. By comparing the sequences of rat tyrosine hydroxylase with human phenylalanine hydroxylase, Ledley and co-workers estimated that tyrosine and phenylalanine hydroxylase began to diverge from some common precursor about 700 to 800 million years ago.[22] Even more remarkable is the not infrequent discovery of unexpected homology between two proteins whose functions were not known to be related. For example, human clotting Factor VIII has two domains homologous to regions of the Cu^{2+}-binding protein ceruloplasmin,[25] and LDL receptor has three domains homologous with a portion of epidermal growth factor and another region in the ligand-binding area comprised of a 40-amino-acid sequence repeated 7 times that is homologous to a single 40-amino-acid segment of complement factor C9.[26] Such information suggests previously unknown functions for particular proteins and also provides information about the evolutionary origins of these molecules.

In summary, cDNA cloning and sequencing of genes involved in inborn errors have increased our knowledge of the normal structure, posttranslational modification, regulation, and evolutionary history of these important proteins. This information provides an increasingly detailed and sophisticated framework for understanding the consequences of the mutations found in patients with these disorders.

Gene Structure and Regulation

The structure and organization of several genes well known to physicians by the diseases with which they are associated is now beginning to unfold. Some examples are presented in Table 5.2 and compared with β-globin, one of the first gene structures to be determined. In each case, investigators utilized the corresponding cDNA clones as a radiolabeled hybridization probe to isolate portions of these genes from libraries of total genomic DNA. Because these genes may be 100 kb or more in length, the libraries used for this purpose are often constructed in special plasmid-like vectors (cosmids) that have been engineered to accommodate large inserts (20–50 kb) of genomic DNA; even so, several overlapping clones are often required to cover the entire gene.

Gene Structure

In comparison to the β-globin gene, which is about 1.5 kb long and has three exons, most of these genes are larger (50–100 kb or greater) and more complex. The number of exons is greater and is roughly predicted by the number of amino acid residues in the protein.[27] This reflects the fact that exon lengths are not random and are clustered about means of 52, 140, 223, and 299 nucleotides.[28] The 3′-most exon, which often is larger and encodes the entire 3′-nontranslated portion of the mRNA, is an exception to this rule. Intron lengths have no periodicity and range from as few as 50 nucleotides to as long as 30 to 40 kb. How the mechanisms that splice out introns to assemble the mature mRNA can function so precisely over such long distances is a fascinating question yet to be answered. The information will be important to the study of inborn errors since, as pointed out in Chapter 3, mutations that prevent normal splicing are particularly disruptive to mRNA stability and function.

Transcriptional Regulation

For many genes associated with inborn errors there is an existing body of biochemical data regarding induction, turnover, and tissue distribution of the protein product. Study of transcriptional regulation of these same genes will confirm, extend, and explain much of these biochemical data. We can expect to learn why certain genes are expressed in only one or a few tissues (eg, ornithine transcarbamylase and phenylalanine hydroxylase in liver, globins in erythroid cells), whereas others, whose products often perform essen-

TABLE 5-2 Features of Some Genes Associated with Inborn Errors

Gene	Size (kb)	mRNA (kb)	Protein Molec Wt (kD)	No. of Exons	Promoters	Regions Homologous to	Pseudogenes	Inborn Error
β-globin[45]	1.5	0.7	16	3	TATA	α-globin	2	Many, including sickle cell disease
Argininosuccinic acid synthetase[36]	63	1.6	46	14	TATA and GC rich	—	14	Citrullinemia
Ornithine transcarbamylase[84-85]	50	—	40	9	—	—	0	Ornithine transcarbamylase deficiency
Phenylalanine hydroxylase[57]	90	2.4	50	13	—	Tyrosine hydroxylase	0	Phenylketonuria, benign hyperphenylalaninemia
HPRT[49]	44	1.6	25	9	GC rich	—	4	Lesch-Nyhan syndrome, HPRT-deficient gout
Adenosine deaminase[86]	32	1.6	41	12	GC rich	—	0	Adenosine deaminase deficiency
LDL receptor[26]	>45	5.5	120	18	—	EGF	0	Familial hypercholesterolemia
Collagen α1(I)[87-88]	18	6	150	51	TATA and GC rich	Other collagens	0	Osteogenesis imperfecta
Factor VIII[89]	186	9	330	26	GATA	Ceruloplasmin	0	Classical hemophilia
DMD[82]	1000	14	—	—	—	—	—	Duchenne's muscular dystrophy

EGF, epidermal growth factor; C9, the ninth component of complement; –, information not available tial metabolic functions, are expressed in nearly all tissues. This latter group of genes is often referred to as *"housekeeping" genes* or proteins, and examples include HPRT, glucose-6-phosphate dehydrogenase, adenosine deaminase, and many others. Experiments with transgenic animals indicate that the sequences contained in the 200 to 300-nucleotide 5′ flanking region of several tissue specific genes are necessary and sufficient to confer both tissue-specific expression and proper developmental regulation.[30] Sequences in this region have also been shown to be necessary for glucocorticoid induction of gene activity.[31] Other experiments comparing the promotors in the region of the gene just 5′ to the first exon have shown that several housekeeping genes lack classic TATA sequences (the "TATA box"), which is located 25 to 30 nucleotides 5′ to the first exon of tissue-specific genes (eg, globins and immunoglobins). Instead, housekeeping genes so far examined have CG-rich sequence motifs 40 to 50 nucleotides or more 5′ to exon 1. These sequences are potential binding sites for a transcriptional factor (Spl) and appear to represent a new class of promotors characteristic of housekeeping genes.[32] Bird has pointed out that the dinucleotide CG occurs relatively uncommonly in vertebrate genomes that 60 to 90% of the existing CG dinucleotide sequences are methylated at the 5′ position of cytosine ring, and that the remaining nonmethylated CG nucleotides are clustered in "islands" associated with housekeeping genes.[33] In most instances these are located in the 5′ flanking region as described above; in one instance (G6PD) they are at the 3′ end of the gene. Bird argues that these CG islands play a role in the broad-tissue expression of housekeeping genes; however, he also points out that some genes have both CG clusters and TATA boxes, so that interactions and permutations of these two regulatory sequences are possible.

Pseudogenes

For many of the inborn error–associated genes thus far studied, more than one copy of the gene is present in the genome. Usually only one of these multiple copies is the active structural gene, while the others, called *pseudogenes,* have one or more mutations that make them defective.[34] Nonprocessed pseudogenes have a normal intron-exon arrangement and are almost always contiguous to the active gene. Presumably they arise by duplication of the active gene followed by the accumulation of mutations that render them nonfunctional. The human β-globin gene cluster contains two nonprocessed β-globin pseudogenes. A more common type of pseudogene has an mRNA-like structure, lacking introns and having a poly A stretch at the 3′ end. The origin of these processed pseudogenes is thought to involve in vivo formation of cDNA transcripts of mature mRNA molecules by reverse transcriptase produced following retroviral infection.[34] These cDNAs insert with unknown frequency at random sites in the genome, and if this happens in a germ line cell, they will be transmitted to future generations. Because this mechanism of pseudogene formation requires expression in a germ line cell, processed pseudogenes will be most commonly observed for housekeeping genes.

Many of the inborn error–associated genes examined to date have been found to have processed pseudogenes.[34] The most notable example is argininosuccinic acid synthetase.[35] The structural gene is located on the long arm of chromosome 9, and there are 14 processed pseudogenes scattered throughout the genome including sites on both the X and Y chromosome.[36] Sequence analysis of three of these showed 89 to 93% homology with the exons of the active gene, suggesting they all arose some 10 to 20 million years ago. These sequences account for the large number of hybridizing fragments on a genomic Southern blot probed with argininosuccinic acid cDNA and complicate the search for mutations affecting those few fragments that actually represent the structural gene. Once structural gene clones are obtained, probes can be developed from intronic regions that will not hybridize to processed pseudogenes and therefore will simplify the Southern blot pattern.

Mapping

Chromosomal localization of the genes involved in inborn errors has proceeded at a rapid pace, and these genes account for a significant fraction of mapped sequences. McKusick has emphasized this point by assembling a map of the morbid anatomy of the human genome.[37] Molecular mapping methods have largely replaced earlier somatic cell hybrid techniques that depended on detection of electrophoretic migration differences between analogous rodent and human proteins. For genes that have processed pseudogenes, mapping has been helpful in structural studies. Once its chromosome assignment can be made, genomic libraries prepared from the relevant chromosome can be used to obtain structural gene clones which are not contaminated by pseudogene sequences.

Summary

Many of the genes which have contributed to our current knowledge of gene structure, gene families, pseudogenes and transcriptional regulation are those that were initially selected for investigation because of their association with a particular human inborn error. This emphasizes lessons previously learned from biochemical study of inborn errors: many genes are likely to be identified by mutations causing clinically relevant phenotypes; the genes so far identified exemplify an array of interesting genetic and regulatory mechanisms; and the lessons learned from their study will be applicable to all genes.

Mutations

Characterization of mutations is a high priority for many investigators working with genes associated with inborn errors. The stimuli for this go beyond the desire to know the precise defect in each patient. Comparisons among patients uncover heterogeneity in the mutations causing defective function of a particular gene, which can be related to clinical variability. Delineation of mutations also provides insight into the regulation of the gene and the cell biology and function of its protein product. Finally, this information may be used to develop improved methods of screening and diagnosis.

Methods of Detection

A variety of approaches have been used to detect mutations. Table 5.3 lists several. Optimally, determination of cDNA structure and sequence and elucidation of gene structure and organization are completed prior to beginning a search for specific defects. Although the numbers vary for each gene examined, in general, only about 5 to 10% of clinically significant mutations are due to gross alterations in gene structure detectable by simple Southern blot analysis of genomic DNA. An additional few percent of mutations are detected by this method because the mutation alters the recognition site of a specific restriction endonuclease resulting in a DNA fragment(s) of abnormal size. Mutations altering the recognition site for the TaqI endonuclease are a special example of this and are described in greater detail in Chapter 3. Elucidation of the remaining 90% or so of mutations is a formidable undertaking. The magnitude of this problem is emphasized by the realization that many of the mutations are due to single nucleotide substitutions in genes that are 50 to 100 kb or even 1,000 kb in length and that encode mature mRNA molecules ranging from several hundred to several thousand nucleotides in length (see Table 5.2). The problem is compounded by normal variation in the nucleotide sequence. When alterations from the normal sequence are found, additional analysis is required before these changes can be identified as the disease-causing mutation.

TABLE 5-3 Some Methods for Detecting Mutations

Restriction site change in genomic DNA[48]
Haplotype analysis and sequencing[45]
Oligonucleotide probes[38–45]
Sequencing cloned mRNA from patients with inborn errors[54–55]
S1 nuclease A cleavage of RNA : DNA duplexes[36,39]
Ribonuclease A cleavage of RNA : DNA or RNA : RNA duplexes[90–91]
Denaturing gradient electrophoresis[92–93]

Northern Blots. Examination of the size and amount of mRNA transcript is a useful initial step to detect mutations of genes that are expressed in accessible cells or tissues. Cultured skin fibroblasts and/or lymphoblasts are good sources of mRNA for many genes. For most messages enough RNA to perform several preliminary analyses (50 – 100 μg of whole-cell RNA, 1 – 2% of which is mRNA, whereas the remainder is mainly ribosomal and transfer RNA) can be obtained from 10^7 fibroblasts or from 10^8 lymphoblasts. Once isolated, the RNA is denatured, separated by size in agarose gels, transferred to a nitrocellulose or nylon membrane solid support (or "filter"), and detected by hybridization to a specific radiolabeled nucleotide probe (usually the corresponding cDNA). The sensitivity of this "Northern" blot procedure is adequate to detect quantitative alterations of roughly 30% or more and size alterations of 10 to 20% or more, depending on the size of the normal mRNA transcript.

Nuclease Degradation. Methods to detect subtle alterations in mRNA often involve the use of nucleases that degrade single-stranded but not double-stranded RNA. These methods take advantage of the fact that in certain nonaqueous solutions (eg, formamide) single-stranded mRNA molecules will form double-stranded duplex molecules with complementary RNA (RNA : RNA duplexes) or with complementary single-stranded DNA (RNA : DNA heteroduplexes). If one strand is a radiolabeled normal RNA (or DNA) probe and the other is the mutant mRNA, the mutated nucleotide(s) will not find a complement in the normal strand, and this mismatched region will be susceptible to digestion with single-strand specific nucleases such as RNase A or S_1 nuclease. Following nuclease digestion, the duplexes are denatured and the single-stranded molecules are separated by size in agarose gels. Cleavage into smaller fragments indicates a mismatch, and the size of the fragments can be used to determine its location. Cloning and sequencing of the corresponding genomic fragments are then required to delineate the mutation. Not all mismatches will be cut by S_1 or RNase A in these assays. The sensitivity depends upon several factors: the specific bases involved (RNase A cleaves only C and U residues): the type of mismatch (substitution, insertion, deletion) and its length; the neighboring sequences (GC pairing is stronger than AT pairing and allows less spreading of the helix); and experimental conditions (eg, temperature and salt concentration). Results to date indicate that simple point mutations can be detected by RNase A protection analysis.

Once a particular mutation has been delineated, oligonucleotide probes of about 20 nucleotides in length can be synthesized complementary to either the mutant or to the normal sequence. These can then be used as hybridization probes. At certain temperatures and salt concentrations, only probes with a perfect complete match to the target sequence will hybridize, permitting discrimination of the normal from the mutant sequence.[38] These probes can be used to follow the segregation of the mutant gene in families and may eventually be useful to screen populations for particular mutant alleles.

The Nature of Mutations

Investigators studying inborn errors of metabolism are accustomed to describing the phenotype of mutation at the protein level by the presence or absence of an immunologically detectable protein (CRM^+, CRM^-), by molecular size and charge (electrophoretic migration variants), and by specific amino acid abnormalities. As shown in Table 5.4, a similar classification is possible with mRNA. Although the patterns are different for each disorder, the overall picture is one of considerable molecular heterogeneity. For many disorders about 5 to 10% of unrelated patients have no detectable mRNA ($mRNA^o$); 10 to 20% have reduced but detectable amounts of mRNA ($mRNA^-$); and about 5% have some alteration in mRNA size ($mRNA^{\Delta sz}$). The remaining 50% or so have normal amounts of normally sized mRNA ($mRNA^+$). Patients with $mRNA^o$ phenotypes may have regulatory mutations blocking transcription or mutations that so disrupt mRNA splicing or stability that no detectable mRNA (<5% of normal) is present. Patients with an abnormally sized mRNA may have a deletion or addition within an exon or an alteration in splicing that does not affect message stability. Patients with $mRNA^+$ phenotype are likely to have alterations of one or a few nucleotides in the coding region that result in nonsense, missense or frame shift mutations.

The extent of heterogeneity in the mutations causing a rare inborn error is exemplified by the studies of Beaudet and colleagues, who used both Northern blotting and S_1 nuclease assays to examine argininosuccinic acid synthetase mRNA in citrullinemia.[36,39,40] They found at least seven different mutant alleles, including those that produced no ASA mRNA, six different $mRNA^+$, S_1 nuclease-sensitive mutant alleles, and $mRNA^+$ allele(s) that remain intact in the S_1 nuclease assay. When the precise nucleotide abnormalities are determined in each of these classes, the number of different mutations is certain to increase. A consequence of this high level of mutational heterogeneity is that most patients with rare inborn errors will, in fact, be genetic compounds rather than true homozygotes. The unlimited variety of possible interaction between different mutant molecules contributes to the variability among patients with a particular inborn error.

Conversely, in a few inborn errors that have reached a relatively high frequency ($\pm 10^4$) in a particular population, there are indications that one or a few mutant alleles account for most of the mutant genes in the population. Examples are given below. Thus, most patients with these disorders are

TABLE 5-4 mRNA Phenotype of Selected Inborn Errors as Seen by Northern Blot Analysis

Disease	Protein	Subtype	No. of Pts	Normal	$mRNA^{\Delta sz*}$	mRNA	$mRNA^{-}$	$mRNA^{o}$
Lesch-Nyhan syndrome[94]	HPRT		15	11	1			3
HPRT-deficient gout[94]	HPRT		9	8				1
Adenosine deaminase deficiency[95-97]	ADA	Partial deficiency	4	3		1		
		Severe deficiency	5	4		1		
Tay-Sachs disease[42,43]	β-Hexosaminidase α-subunit	Ashkenazi Jewish	5					5
		French Canadian	2					2
		Other	1	1				
Sandhoff's disease[98]	β-Hexosaminidase β-subunit	Juvenile	5	4			1	
		Infantile	11	3			4	4
Gaucher's disease[44]	β-Glucosaminidase	CRM^{+}	5	5				
		CRM^{-}	1	1				
Phenylketonuria[99]	Phenylalanine hydroxylase		2	1			1	
Propionic acidemia[100]	Propionyl Co-enzyme A carboxylase	Group A (α subunit)	6	2				4
		Group B (β subunit)	3	3				
		Group C	3	3				
		Group BC	3	3				
Citrullinemia[39]	Argininosuccinate synthase			4				
McArdle's disease[101]	Muscle phosphorylase		8				3	5
Hepatoerythropoetic porphyria[102]	Uroporphyrinogen decarboxylase		2	2				
Chronic granulomatous disease[78]	Unknown		4	1				3

homozygotes rather than compounds. Possible explanations for the high frequency of one or a few alleles in these disorders include founder effects and/or positive selection for heterozygotes. The latter has been shown to occur for sickle hemoglobin heterozygotes and certain thalassemia heterozygotes in regions of the world where malaria is endemic. Aeterozygotes for the sickle cell allele or for certain thalassemia alleles are more resistant to malaria than homozygous normals. Inborn errors that appear to fit this model include phenylketonuria (PKU), Tay Sachs disease, and type I, or nonneuronopathic, Gaucher's disease. PKU has a frequency of about 10^{-4}, and DiLella and associates have shown with haplotype analysis and oligonucleotide probes that two to three mutant phenylalanine hydroxylase alleles account for the majority of PKU cases in certain regions of Europe.[41] In Tay Sachs disease and type I Gaucher's disease, the evidence is not as complete. Both have frequencies of about 5×10^{-4} in the Ashkenazi Jewish population, and Northern blot analysis of a large number of patients has failed to yield evidence for heterogeneity of mutation.[42–44] The same reasoning would predict that cystic fibrosis, with a frequency of 5×10^{-4}, is also likely to be caused by one or a few mutant alleles. It is interesting to speculate on how these mutant genes, so harmful in the homozygous state, have reached such a high frequency.

The number of inborn error–causing mutations that have been specified at the nucleotide level is small and, in general, the mutations are similar to those characterized in the globin gene.[45] TaqI site changes and some gross structural mutations have been delineated in several X-linked genes, including ornithine transcarbamylase, Factor VIII and HPRT.[46–49] Several mutations including gross rearrangements and point mutations have been described in type I collagen genes in patients with osteogenesis imperfecta.[50–51] DiLella and co-workers have reported a single nucleotide change (G → A transition in the donor splice site of intron 12) in phenylalanine hydroxylase, which results in abnormal mRNA processing.[41] Brown and colleagues, in their study of LDL receptor defects in familial hypercholesterolemia, have shown that a large deletion involving exons 13, 14, and 15 accounts for an $mRNA^{o}$ allele,[52] and that two smaller changes (one a single nucleotide substitution, the other a four-nucleotide duplication) in the region of the cytoplasmic domain of the LDL receptor result in $mRNA^{+}$ mutant alleles that encode faulty receptors which fail to cluster in coated pits and therefore cannot transport LDL into cells.[53] Two point mutations have been identified in the adenosine deaminase genes of patients with severe combined immunodeficiency.[54–55] A great many inborn error–causing mutations remain to be identified and related to the large collection of data on the functional phenotype of these mutant proteins. In particular, elucidation of the mutation-causing aberrations in the regulation of expression of these genes, alterations in protein stability (CRM^+ and CRM^- mutations), changes in cofactor binding (the vitamin-responsive inborn errors), and alterations of subcellular localization of these proteins all promise to be extremely interesting.

Diagnosis

Before the advent of molecular methods, diagnosis of inborn errors was accomplished by measurement of abnormal levels of metabolites or alterations of protein function. The precision of these techniques accounts, in part, for the favored position of inborn errors as model genetic diseases. However, these methods are not completely specific because the biochemical phenotypes are distant from the gene and are influenced by other members of the homeostatic system (other proteins, hormones, diet, general state of health, etc.). Imprecision in diagnosis leads to problems in understanding variation between patients and consequently with prognostication, treatment, and counseling of patients and their families.

The diagnostic precision possible with molecular methods represents a substantial improvement. The methods used include direct identification of mutant genes in cases in which a restriction site has been introduced or removed. Alternatively, sets of oligonucleotide probes complementary to the wild type and the mutant sequences are particularly useful when the mutation does not alter restriction fragment size. Mutational heterogeneity prevents application of the oligonucleotide method to populations, unless special characteristics of either the population or the disorder indicate that one mutant allele is predominant. Less direct but still reliable methods of diagnosis involve establishment of linkage of the mutant gene to a nearby polymorphic restriction site or to a set of neighboring polymorphic restriction sites (a haplotype). An added advantage of the molecular methods of diagnosis is that they do not require acquisition of tissue that expresses the protein of interest. Thus, diagnosis of disorders caused by genes whose expression is limited to liver or other specialized tissues can be accomplished by examining DNA from any source (leukocyte, fibroblast, amniocyte, chorionic villi) in the individual's body.

The benefits and opportunities afforded by molecular methods of diagnosis are exemplified by recent progress on PKU. Because phenylalanine hydroxylase is expressed only in liver, diagnosis of this common inborn error is usually made at the substrate level by documenting plasma phenylalanine levels in excess of 1.2 mM, or about 25 times normal.[56] Other individuals, similar in number to PKU patients, have phenylalanine levels in excess of normal but below 1.2 mM and are said to have benign hyperphenylalaninemia. Metabolic tests for PKU heterozygotes are cumbersome and often yield ambiguous results. Phenylalanine hydroxylase is not expressed in amniocytes, and prenatal diagnosis by enzyme analysis is not possible. Equipped with the knowledge from their studies of phenylalanine hydroxylase cDNA and the structural gene, Woo and others have applied molecular methods to the problems of diagnosis of PKU and related disorders. Following the model of studies on β-thalassemia,[45] these investigators have described a series of polymorphic restriction sites in and about the phenylalanine hydroxylase gene and have organized them into 12 haplotypes.[57] Linkage studies with these phenylalanine hydroxylase associated RFLPs showed that the mutations causing PKU and benign hyperphenylalaninemia are allelic.[58] Prenatal diagnosis of PKU by RFLP linkage analysis is possible.[59] Haplotypic analysis of controls and PKU patients in a Danish population showed that 89% of the mutant phenylalanine hydroxylase genes were confined to four common haplotypes.[60] The previously described phenylalanine hydroxylase splicing mutation accounted for 38% of all the mutant alleles and was always associated with a particular haplotype that was rare in the normal gene pool.[41] Oligonucleotide probes could distinguish this mutant gene from normal and were used to correctly identify heterozygotes. The other PKU alleles in the Danish population have not been defined at a molecular level but are known by their association with other haplotypes. The severity of the metabolic phenotype is predicted, in part, by the particular combination of mutant alleles in the patient.[60] Thus, variation at the phenylalanine locus is responsible for a major fraction of the phenotypic variability. Because a small number of mutant alleles account for most of the patients, a pool of the appropriate oligonucleotides could be used for heterozygote screening in the general population. This rapid progress in the diagnosis of PKU and related disorders highlights the power of these molecular methods and is likely to continue as other inborn error–associated loci are studied.

Treatment

The many successes of molecular biology in solving fundamental problems in biology have led to considerable optimism for direct treatment of genetic disorders by gene therapy. This subject is well covered in Chapter 6. Suffice it to say here that inborn errors will be the models for these experiments. Most of the work to date has focused on defects in purine metabolism, including the Lesch-Nyhan syndrome, nucleoside phosphorylase deficiency, and adenosine deaminase deficiency. Serial measurements of the specific biochemical abnormalities associated with these inborn errors provides the obvious advantage of allowing investigators to follow the progress of these experiments. An appreciation for the difficulties encountered in trying to circumvent these mutations is less obvious, but is certainly apparent to those responsible for the care of these patients.

ONCOGENES

Throughout this chapter we have emphasized that mutations of virtually all genes will result in biochemical and metabolic consequences resembling those of inborn errors of metabolism. Investigations into the mechanisms of oncogenesis, particularly the study of the role of oncogenes in this process, are beginning to yield information on the biochemical and metabolic processes involved in the development of the malignant state. Oncogenes are viral or cellular genes that, when altered genetically, have the potential to cause or contribute to the malignant phenotype. About 40 have been described and extensively reviewed.[61–65] Many have been identified by using malignant tissue as a source of DNA in a gene transfer assay to find a gene in the tumor cells that transfers the malignant phenotype to nontransformed recipient cells.[63] Oncogenes identified in this manner are mutant alleles of normal cellular genes that are called *proto-oncogenes* or *c-oncogenes.* Other c-oncogenes have been identified by homology of their nucleotide sequence to *retroviral oncogenes (v-oncogenes).* The latter are sequences in certain retroviral genomes that are responsible for the ability of these viruses to cause tumors and elicit neoplastic transformation of cultured cells. V-oncogenes arise by recombination between retroviral and cellular genomes so that c-oncogenes are transferred to the retroviral genome in a process called transduction. Aberrant regulation of these transduced oncogenes or acquisition of mutations results in the conversion of a normal cellular gene to one capable of causing cancer.

The protein products of oncogenes function either in the cytoplasm or nucleus (or in some cases in both) by one of four general mechanisms: protein phosphorylation at either tyrosine or serine residues,[64] metabolic alterations in binding or hydrolysis of GTP,[64] control of gene expression by activation of transcription of certain genes,[65] and participation in DNA replication.[64]

Mutations of c-oncogenes and resultant aberration in the function of their products lead to malignancy. In this regard, the malignant phenotype fits within the definition of an inborn error of metabolism as a biochemical disorder due to a specific genetically determined defect in the structure or function of a protein molecule. Like other inborn errors, the malignant phenotype is the result of some biochemically definable perturbation of a homeostatic system, and study of the aberrant phenotype is yielding information about both the normal and abnormal functions of the gene product within the system. However, there are several differences between the disorders commonly recognized as inborn errors and the malignancies that result from oncogene mutations. The malignant phenotype almost always results from exuberant or unregulated function of an oncogene product, whereas the converse is true for inborn errors. Furthermore, and most notably, the mutant genes causing inborn errors are inherited and usually have major phenotypic consequences only when both alleles are defective; they are recessive traits. In contrast, the oncogene mutations are not inherited and in most instances act as dominants. As a consequence of transmission in the germline, the familial inborn errors affect all tissues that express the particular gene; the oncogene abnormalities are clonal, affecting only the progeny of the cell that suffered the somatic mutation. As far as we know, there are no examples of inherited disorders due to mutations in the genes now recognized as oncogenes. Perhaps inheritance of such a mutant allele would be lethal in utero.

A second class of genes, less well understood, has also been associated with oncogenesis. The identity of these genes has been inferred from the study of familial tumors, such as retinoblastoma and Wilms tumor, in which the malignant cell line is hemizygous or homozygous for a chromosomal deletion.[63] Thus, in contrast to the oncogenes mentioned above, these genes result in tumors when they are nonfunctional. Some have emphasized this contrast by calling the latter genes *antioncogenes.*[66] The recessive nature of this second type of cancer-associated gene, the transmission of defective copies in the germline, the fact that several tissues can be involved (eg, inheriting the retinoblastoma gene or allele predisposes one to both retinoblastoma and osteosarcoma)[66] and the fact that the phenotype results from a reduced activity of the gene product are all features reminiscent of inborn errors. It will be interesting to see how this comparison holds up as we learn more about these genes and their products.[83]

FUTURE DIRECTIONS

We can anticipate that the number of cloned genes will continue to increase at a rapid rate and that study of their structure, function, and regulation will expand our understanding of inborn errors. The number of recognized inborn errors will increase as new defects are discovered and as the biochemical bases of disorders already known unfold. The potential for making precise molecular diagnoses will increase dramatically and, accordingly, our ability to decipher genetic heterogeneity will improve. Recognition of this source of clinical variability may enable us to bring the roles played by other genetic variables and the environment into better perspective.

What of our understanding of the pathophysiology of inborn errors? How do these mutations now seen with elegant clarity result in the complicated clinical problems that have challenged physicians since Garrod's time? One area of investigation into pathophysiology likely to be active in the near future will involve the expression and isolation of large quantities of cloned mutant proteins in bacterial or cell culture systems so that amounts sufficient for biochemical and crystallographic analysis can be obtained.[67] These experiments should provide a better understanding of the consequences of mutations on the structure and function of proteins.

Other experiments relevant to pathophysiology will involve the expression of cloned mutant genes in transgenic animals.[30] Here the aim will be to delineate the effect of the aberrant protein on the whole organism. For some genes, for example, those encoding structural proteins, expression of the mutant protein in an otherwise normal animal may be a sufficient model of the disease. For other genes, it may be necessary to markedly decrease the expression of the endogenous genes in order to obtain pathologic effects. The large number of well-characterized mutations in mice will be useful in this regard. The recent preliminary reports of expression of the Pi-Z allele of α-1-antitrypsin and of human sickle cell β-globin are examples of this approach.[67-70] In the former, liver abnormalities characteristic of α-1-antitrypsin deficiency could be observed, whereas in the latter, reduction of the endogenous mouse β-globin gene function will be necessary to have any hope of actually studying the sickling phenomenon. Breeding the sickle transgene into a mouse strain carrying murine β-thalassemia may result in a sufficiently high fraction of circulating sickle hemoglobin to mimic sickle cell disease.[68]

A more direct approach to making animal models of inborn errors will utilize molecular methods to mutagenize or otherwise specifically inhibit the products of endogenous genes. Experiments utilizing transgenic animals expressing high levels of a specific antisense RNA[71-72] or possibly techniques involving production of mutations in target genes by injecting the corresponding cDNA into viable cells (heteroduplex mutagenesis[73]) may succeed in creating specific animal models that will be of great value in studies of pathophysiology and experimental therapy.

ACKNOWLEDGMENTS

The authors gratefully acknowledge the help of Ms. Sandra Muscelli with the preparation of this manuscript. Part of the work that led to ideas expressed in this chapter was supported by National Eye Institute grant number 5R01EY02948 and by grant 5M01RR-00052 to the Pediatric Clinical Research Unit. Dr. Mitchell is a bursar of the Fonds de la Recherche en Sante du Quebec. Dr. Valle is an investigator in the Howard Hughes Medical Institute.

REFERENCES

1. Garrod AE: The Croonian lectures. *Lancet* 1908;2:1–7,73–79,142–148,214–220.
2. Childs B: Sir Archibald Garrod's conception of chemical individuality: A modern appreciation. *N Engl J Med* 1970;282:71–77.
3. Rosenberg LE: Inborn errors of metabolism, in *Metabolic Control and Disease,* Philadelphia, WB Saunders, 1980, pp 73–102.
4. Goodman SI, Lenich AC: Glutaric acidemia, medium- and long-chain acyl CoA dehydrogenase deficiencies and multiple acyl-CoA dehydrogenation deficiency (glutaric acidemia type II), in, *Inherited Diseases of Amino Acid Metabolism,* Bickel H, Wachtel U (eds): New York, Springer-Verlag, 1985, pp 383–387.
5. O'Brien JS: The gangliosidoses, in Stanbury JB, Wyngaarden JB, Fredrickson DS, et al (eds): *Metabolic Basis of Inherited Disease,* New York, McGraw-Hill, 1983, pp 945–969.
6. Brown MS, Goldstein JL: How LDL receptors influence cholesterol and artherosclerosis. *Sci Am* 1984;251:58–66.
7. Farrer LA, Conneally M: Predictability of phenotype in Huntington disease. *Arch Neurol* 1987;44:109–113.
8. Jacobs PA: Human chromosome heteromorphisms (variants). In Steinberg AG, Bearn AG, Motulsky AG et al (eds): *Progress in Medical Genetics,* Philadelphia, WB Saunders, 1977, pp 251–274.
9. O'Dowd BF, Quan F, Willard HF, et al: Isolation of cDNA clones coding for the β subunit of human β-hexosaminidase. *Proc Natl Acad Sci USA* 1985;82:1184–1188.
10. Orkin SH, Dadonna PE, Shewach DA, et al: Molecular cloning of human adenosine deaminase gene sequences. *J Biol Chem* 1983;258:12753–12756.
11. O'Brien WE, McInnes R, Kalumuck K, et al: Cloning and sequence analysis of cDNA for human argininosuccinate lyase. *Proc Natl Acad Sci USA* 1986;83:7211–7215.
12. Calhoun DH, Bishop DF, Bernstein HS, et al: Fabry disease: Isolation of a cDNA clone encoding human α-galactosidase A. *Proc Natl Acad Sci USA* 1985;82:7364–7368.
13. Su TS, Bock HO, O'Brien WE, et al: Cloning of cDNA for argininosuccinate synthetase mRNA and study of enzyme overproduction in a human cell line. *J Biol Chem* 1981;256:11826–11831.
14. Cooper DN, Schmidtke J: Diagnosis of genetic disease using recombinant DNA. *Hum Genet* 1986;73:1–11.
15. Kozak M: Selection of initiation sites by eucaryotic ribosomes: Effect of inserting AUG triplets upstream from the coding sequence for preproinsulin. *Nucl Acids Res* 1984;12:3873–3893.
16. Kahana C, Nathans D: Nucleotide sequence of murine ornithine decarboxylase mRNA. *Proc Natl Acad Sci USA* 1985;82:1673–1677.
17. Reynolds GA, Basu SK, Osborne TF, et al: HMG CoA reductase: A negatively regulated gene with unusual promoter and 5′ untranslated regions. *Cell* 1984;38:275–285.
18. Cole MD: The myc oncogene: Its role in transformation and differentiation. *Ann Rev Genet* 1986;20:361–384.
19. Tzamarias D, Alexandraki D, Thireos G: Multiple cis-acting elements modulate the translational efficiency of GCN4 mRNA in yeast. *Proc Natl Acad Sci USA* 1986;83:4849–4853.
20. Shaw G, Kamen R: A conserved AU sequence from the 3′ untranslated region of GM-CSF mRNA mediates selective mRNA degradation. *Cell* 1986;46:659–667.
21. Bishop DF, Calhoun DH, Bernstein HS, et al: Human α-galactosidase A: Nucleotide sequence of cDNA clone encoding the mature enzyme. *Proc Natl Acad Sci USA* 1986;83:4859–4863.

22. Ledley FD, DiLella AG, Kwok SCM, et al: Homology between phenylalanine and tyrosine hydroxylases reveals common structural and functional domains. *Biochem* 1985;24:3389–3394.
23. Russell DW, Schneider WJ, Yamamoto T, et al: Domain map of the LDL receptor: Sequence homology with the epidermal growth factor precursor. *Cell* 1984;37:577–585.
24. Mueckler MM, Pitot HC: Sequence of the precursor to rat ornithine aminotransferase deduced from a cDNA clone. *J Biol Chem* 1985;260:12993–12997.
25. Lawn RM: The molecular genetics of hemophilia: Blood clotting factors VIII and IX. *Cell* 1985;42:405–406.
26. Sudhof TC, Goldstein JL, Brown MS, et al: The LDL receptor gene: A mosaic of exons shared with different proteins. *Science* 1985;228:815–822.
27. Blake C: Exons—present from the beginning? *Nature* 1983;306:535–537.
28. Naora H, Deacon NJ: Relationship between the total size of exons and introns in protein-coding genes of higher eukaryotes. *Proc Natl Acad Sci USA* 1982;79:6196–6200.
29. Padgett RA, Grabowski PJ, et al: Splicing of messenger RNA precursors. *Ann Rev Biochem* 1986;55:1119–1150.
30. Palmiter RD, Brinster RL: Germ-line transformation of mice. *Ann Rev Genet* 1986;20:465–499.
31. Yamamoto KR: Steroid receptor regulated transcription of specific genes and gene networks. *Ann Rev Genet* 1985;19:209–252.
32. Dynan WS: Promoters for housekeeping genes. *TIG* 1986;2:196–197.
33. Bird AP: CpG-rich islands and the function of DNA methylation. *Nature* 1986;321:209–213.
34. Vanin EF: Processed pseudogenes: Characteristics and evolution. *Ann Rev Genet* 1985;19:253–272.
35. Freytag SO, Bock HGO, Beaudet AL, et al: Molecular structures of human argininosuccinate synthetase psuedogenes. *J Biol Chem* 1984;259:3160–3166.
36. Beaudet AL, O'Brien WE, Bock HGO, et al: The human argininosuccinate synthetase locus and citrullinemia. *Adv Hum Genet* 1986;15:161–196.
37. McKusick VA: The morbid anatomy of the human genome: A review of genetic mapping in clinical medicine. *Medicine* 1986;65:1–33.
38. Kidd VJ, Wallace RB, Itakura K, et al: α1-Antitrypsin deficiency detection by direct analysis of the mutation in the gene. *Nature* 1983;304:230–234.
39. Su TS, Bock HGO, Beaudet AL, et al: Molecular analysis of argininosuccinate synthetase deficiency in human fibroblasts. *J Clin Invest* 1982;70:1334–1339.
40. Su TS, Beaudet AL, O'Brien WE: Abnormal mRNA for argininosuccinate synthetase in citrullinaemia. *Nature* 1983;301:533–534.
41. DiLella AG, Marvit J, Lidsky AS, et al: Tight linkage between a splicing mutation and a specific DNA haplotype in phenylketonuria. *Nature* 1986;322:799–803.
42. Myerowitz R, Proia RL: cDNA clone for the α-chain of human β-hexosaminidase: Deficiency of α-chain mRNA in Ashkenazi Tay-Sachs fibroblasts. *Proc Natl Acad Sci USA* 1984;81:5394–5398.
43. Myerowitz R, Hogikyan ND: Different mutations in Ashkenazi Jewish and non-Jewish French Canadians with Tay-Sachs disease. *Science* 1986;232:1646–1648.
44. Graves PN, Grabowski GA, Ludman MD, et al: Human acid β-glucosidase: Northern blot and S1 nuclease analysis of mRNA from HeLa cells and normal and Gaucher disease fibroblasts. *Am J Hum Genet* 1986;39:763–774.
45. Antonarakis SE, Kazazian HH, Orkin SH: DNA polymorphism and molecular pathology of the human globin gene clusters. *Hum Genet* 1985;69:1–14.

46. Rozen R, Fox J, Fenton WA, et al: Gene deletion and restriction fragment length polymorphisms at the human ornithine transcarbamylase locus. *Nature* 1985;313:815–817.
47. Nussbaum RL, Boggs BA, Beaudet AL, et al: New mutation and prenatal diagnosis in ornithine transcarbamylase deficiency. *Am J Hum Genet* 1986;38:149–158.
48. Youssoufian H, Kazazian HH, Phillips DG, et al: Recurrent mutations in hemophilia A: Evidence for CpG mutation hotspots. *Nature* 1986;324:380–382.
49. Stout JT, Caskey CT: HPRT: Gene structure, expression and mutation. *Ann Rev Genet* 1985;19:127–148.
50. Prockop DJ: Mutations in collagen genes: Consequences for rare and common diseases. *J Clin Invest* 1985;75:783–787.
51. Cheah KSE: Collagen genes and inherited connective tissue disease. *Biochem J* 1985;229:287–303.
52. Lehrman MA, Schneider WJ, Sudhof TC, et al: Mutation in LDL receptor: Alu-Alu recombination deletes exons encoding transmembrane and cytoplasmic domains. *Science* 1985;227:140–146.
53. Lehrman MA, Goldstein JL, Brown MS, et al: Internalization-defective LDL receptors produced by genes with nonsense and frameshift mutations that truncate the cytoplasmic domain. *Cell* 1985;41:735–743.
54. Bonthron DT, Markham AF, Ginsburg, D, et al: Identification of a point mutation in the adenosine deaminase gene responsible for immunodeficiency. *J Clin Invest* 1985;76:894–897.
55. Valerio D, Dekker BMM, Duyvesteyn MGC, et al: One adenosine deaminase allele in a patient with severe combined immunodeficiency contains a point mutation abolishing enzyme activity. *EMBO* 1986;5:113–119.
56. Scriver CR, Clow CL: Phenylketonuria: Epitome of human biochemical genetics. *N Engl J Med* 1980;303:1336–1342;1394–1400.
57. DiLella AG, Kwok SCM, Ledley FD, et al: Molecular structure and polymorphic map of the human phenylalanine hydroxylase gene. *Biochem* 1986;25:743–749.
58. Ledley FD, Levy HL, Woo SLC: Molecular analysis of the inheritance of phenylketonuria and mild hyperphenylalaninemia in families with both disorders. *N Engl J Med* 1986;314:1276–1280.
59. Daiger SP, Lidsky AS, Chakraborty R, et al: Polymorphic DNA haplotypes at the phenylalanine hydroxylase locus in prenatal diagnosis of phenylketonuria. *Lancet* 1986; 1:229–232.
60. Guttler F, Ledley FD, Lidsky AS, et al: Correlation between polymorphic DNA haplotypes at phenylalanine hydroxylase locus and clinical phenotypes of phenylketonuria. *J Pediatr* 1987;110:68–71.
61. Varmus HE: The molecular genetics of cellular oncogenes. *Ann Rev Genet* 1984; 18:553–612.
62. Bishop JM: Viral oncogenes. *Cell* 1985;42:23–38.
63. Bishop JM: The molecular genetics of cancer. *Science* 1987;235:305–311.
64. Weinberg RA: The action of oncogenes in the cytoplasm and nucleus. *Science* 1985;230:770–776.
65. Kingston RE, Baldwin AS, Sharp PA: Transcription control by oncogenes. *Cell* 1985;41:3–5.
66. Knudson AG: Hereditary cancer, oncogenes and antioncogenes. *Cancer Res* 1985; 45:1437–1443.
67. Ledley FD, Grenett HE, McGinnis-Shelnutt M, et al: Retroviral mediated gene transfer of human phenylalanine hydroxylase into NIH 3T3 and hepatoma cells. *Proc Natl Acad Sci USA* 1986;83:409–413.

68. Rubin EM, Lu RH, Cooper SL, et al: A mouse model for sickle cell anemia. *Am J Hum Genet* 1986;39:A216.
69. DeMayo JL, Sifers RN, Carlson JA, et al: Expression of normal and mutant human α1-antitrypsin genes in transgenic mice. *Am J Hum Genet* 1986;39:A195.
70. Constantini F, Chada K, Magram J: Correction of urine β-thalassemia by gene transfer into the germ line. 1986; *Science* 233:1192.
71. Izant JG, Weintraub H: Constitutive and conditional suppression of exogenous and endogenous genes by anti-sense RNA. *Science* 1985;229:345–352.
72. Holt JT, Gopal TV, Moulton AD et al: Inducible production of c-fos antisense RNA inhibits 3T3 cell proliferation. *Proc Natl Acad Sci USA* 1986;83:4794–4798.
73. Thomas KR, Capecchi MR: Introduction of homologous DNA sequences into mammalian cells induces mutations in the cognate gene. *Nature* 1986;324:34–38.
74. Adcock MW, O'Brien WE: Molecular cloning of cDNA for rat and human carbamyl phosphate synthetase I. *J Biol Chem* 1984;259:13471–13476.
75. Robson KJH, Ross TC, MacGillivray RTA, et al: Purification of phenylalanine hydroxylase mRNA from rat liver and cloning of its cDNA. *Proc Natl Acad Sci USA* 1982;79:4701–4705.
76. Kraus JP, Rosenberg LE: Purification of low-abundance messenger RNAs from rat liver by polysome immunoadsorption. *Proc Natl Acad Sci USA* 1982;79:4015–4019.
77. Chandra T, Kurachi K, Davie EW, et al: Induction of α1-antitrypsin mRNA and cloning of its cDNA. *Biochem Biophys Res Comm* 1981;103:751–758.
78. Royer-Pokora B, Kunkel LM, Monaco AP, et al: Cloning the gene for an inherited human disorder—chronic granulomatous disease—on the basis of its chromosomal location. *Nature* 1986;322:32–38.
79. Himeno M, Mueckler MM, Gonzalez FJ, et al: Cloning of DNA complementary to ornithine aminotransferase mRNA. *J Biol Chem* 1982;257:4669–4672.
80. Woo SLC, Lidsky AS, Guttler F, et al: Cloned human phenylalanine hydroxylase gene allows prenatal diagnosis and carrier detection of classical phenylketonuria. *Nature* 1983;306:151–155.
81. Nathans J, Thomas D, Hogness DS: Molecular genetics of human color vision: The genes encoding blue, green, and red pigments. *Science* 1986;232:193–202.
82. Monaco AP, Neve RL, Colletti-Feener C, et al: Isolation of candidate cDNAs for portions of the Duchenne muscular dystrophy gene. *Nature* 1986;323:646–650.
83. Friend SH, Bernards R, Rogelj S, et al: A human DNA segment with properties of the gene that predisposes to retinoblastoma and osteosarcoma. *Nature* 1986;323:643–646.
84. Horwich AL, Fenton WA, Williams KR, et al: Structure and expression of a complementary DNA for the nuclear coded precursor of human mitochondrial ornithine transcarbamylase. *Science* 1984;224:1068–1074.
85. Fenton WA, Levy E, Furtak K, et al: Isolation and characterization of the human gene encoding ornithine transcarbamylase. *Am J Hum Genet* 1986;39:A198.
86. Valerio D, Duyvesteyn MGC, Dekker BMM, et al: Adenosine deaminase: Characterization and expression of a gene with a remarkable promoter. *EMBO* 1985;4:437–443.
87. Chu ML, deWet W, Bernard M, et al: Human proαl(I) collagen gene structure reveals evolutionary conservation of a pattern of introns and exons. *Nature* 1984;310:337–340.
88. Chu ML, deWet W, Bernard M, et al: Fine structural analysis of the human pro-αl(I) collagen gene. Promoter structure. AluI repeats and polymorphic transcripts. *J Biol Chem* 1985;260:2315–2320.
89. Gitschier J, Wood WI, Goralka TM, et al: Characterization of the human Factor VIII gene. *Nature* 1984;312:326–330.
90. Myers RM, Larin Z, Maniatis T: Detection of single base substitutions by ribonuclease cleavage at mismatches in RNA:DNA duplexes. *Science* 1985;230:1242–1246.

91. Gibbs RA, Caskey CT: Detection of new mutations at the HPRT gene locus by RNase A cleavage analysis. *Am J Hum Genet* 1986;39:A93.
92. Fischer SG, Lerman LS: DNA fragments differing by single base pair substitutions are separated in denaturing gradient gels: Correspondence with melting theory. *Proc Natl Acad Sci USA* 1983;80:1579-1583.
93. Myers RM, Fischer SG, Lerman LS, et al: Nearly all single base substitutions in DNA fragments joined to a GC-clamp can be detected by denaturing gradient gel electrophoresis. *Nucl Acid Res* 1985;13:3131-3145.
94. Wilson JM, Stout JT, Palella TD, et al: A molecular survey of hypoxanthine-guanine phosphoribosyltransferase deficiency in man. *J Clin Invest* 1986;77:188-195.
95. Wiginton DA, Adrian GS, Friedman RL, et al: Cloning of cDNA sequences of human adenosine deaminase. *Proc Natl Acad Sci USA* 1983;80:7481-7485.
96. Daddona PE, Shewach DS, Kelley WN, et al: Human adenosine deaminase. *J Biol Chem* 1984;259:12101-12106.
97. Daddona PE, Davidson BL, Perignon JL, et al: Genetic expression in partial adenosine deaminase deficiency: mRNA levels and protein turnover for the enzyme variants in human B-lymphoblast cell lines. *J Biol Chem* 1985;260:3875-3880.
98. O'Dowd BF, Klavins MH, Willard HF, et al: Molecular heterogeneity in the infantile and juvenile forms of Sandhoff disease (O-Variant G_{M2} Gangliosidosis). *J Biol Chem* 1986;261:12680-12685.
99. DiLella AG, Ledley FD, Rey F, et al: Detection of phenylalanine hydroxylase messenger RNA in liver biopsy samples from patients with phenylketonuria. *Lancet* 1985;1:160-161.
100. Lamhonwah A-M, Gravel R: personal communication.
101. Gautron S, Daegelen D, Mennecier F, et al: Molecular mechanisms of McArdle's disease (muscle glycogen phosphorylase deficiency): RNA and DNA analysis. *J Clin Invest* 1987;79:275-281.
102. deVerneuil H, Grandchamp B, Romeo PH, et al: Molecular analysis of uroporphyrinogen decarboxylase deficiency in a family with two cases of hepatoerythropoietic porphyria. *J Clin Invest* 1986;77:431-435.

CHAPTER 6

Gene Therapy of Somatic Cells: Status and Prospects

Stuart H. Orkin, MD, and
David A. Williams, MD

The molecular basis of human genetic disorders is being defined with increasing precision using recombinant DNA methods that have been developed over the past decade. This new knowledge has had a profound influence on our understanding of genetic heterogeneity and mutation in man and on prenatal diagnosis. For the most part, however, few insights have been gained that can be translated readily into new approaches to the management of affected patients. But given the availability of many cloned genes whose products are absent or altered in clinically significant genetic disorders and the methodology to introduce them into mammalian cells in a functional state, attention has been focused recently on the potential of "gene therapy" as a new mode of treatment. Prior to the substantial research into gene structure and function that has occurred in the last several years, scenarios for gene therapy were highly speculative. More recently, however, advances in gene transfer technology have encouraged the formation of more specific and realistic goals. In this chapter we will describe the framework in which current studies that have been developed illustrate the potential strengths and problems with ongoing approaches to genetic management of inherited disease.

POTENTIAL STRATEGIES FOR GENE THERAPY

In principle, genes might be introduced either during embryonic (or fetal) life *(germline therapy)* or only into specific somatic cells of an individual *(somatic gene therapy)*. The intent in either instance would be to provide a normal, functional gene to an individual affected with a serious inherited disorder. In germline therapy, the introduced gene would be passed on to subsequent generations if it were integrated into germ cells (as opposed to only somatic cells of the embryo or fetus). In somatic gene therapy, genetically modified DNA would be present only during the lifetime of the individual.

Whichever approach was chosen, investigators would ultimately prefer to correct a defective gene in situ, that is, remove the mutant gene or a specific segment and replace it with the normal version. Of course, this necessitates precise knowledge of the gene involved in the disorder and, most likely, its particular mutation. In situ correction of a mutant gene would ensure normal regulation of the corrected gene, as all the genetic elements required for its expression (promoter, enhancers intervening sequences) would be present. Although experimentally quite feasible in yeast,[1] directed insertion (or recombination) in mammalian cells appears to occur very infrequently as opposed to nonspecific, random integration of exogenous genetic material.[2,3] For example, Smithies and co-workers have demonstrated targeted integration into the human β-globin gene region at a level approximately three orders of magnitude below random integration. Capecchi and associates have shown specific recombination at a rate about tenfold higher than Smithies using microinjection of DNA into the nucleus. In either instance, random integration of foreign DNA occurs more frequently than targeted insertion under current protocols. Given the current inability to target genes more efficiently to specific chromosomal sites introduction of genes into human embryos or fetuses is precluded for the foreseeable future. Ethical considerations also argue strongly against this approach at present. These include disruption of some genes by insertion of the foreign gene, possible oncogenes due to interaction next to an oncogene, and the necessity to interfere with the fetus in vitro.

An alternative is the introduction of appropriately regulated, intact genes into the germline (or somatic cells) without replacement of the abnormal gene(s) that resides in the genome. In *Drosophila* the use of P-element plasmids is particularly effective.[4] Although several genes have been successfully introduced into the germline of mice and been shown to be appropriately regulated in resulting progeny (transgenic mice),[5] insertional mutagenesis due to random integration of foreign DNA into critical regions of the genome again precludes this approach to the treatment of human disorders.

As currently envisioned, therefore, potential gene therapy in man must be restricted to random introduction of normal gene copies into somatic cells that already harbor mutant alleles of the gene. This would be imperfect therapy by design in that the introduced genes would not be subject to the controls influencing the expression of a normal gene in situ. These general limitations are particularly relevant to consideration of genetic disorders, which might most realistically benefit from somatic therapy. Disorders that are most common worldwide and are associated with significant medical burden, such as the thalassemias, may be among the least suitable candidates.

In principle, virtually all somatic cells of the body might be suitable recipients for foreign genes. Major cellular compartments include the bone marrow, skin, liver, and brain. Bone marrow stem cells represent a particularly attractive target, since bone marrow is readily accessible for sampling, in vitro manipulation, and reinfusion. Moreover, stem cells have the potential to differentiate and, thereby, repopulate hematopoietic tissue completely in a suitable host environment. Also, many genetic disorders specifically affect bone-marrow-derived cells. The successful application of allogeneic bone marrow transplantation to a variety of genetic diseases is a testament to the proliferative and differentiative capacities of hematopoietic stem cells.

Over the past decade many techniques have been developed for the introduction of DNA into mammalian cells. In theory, any of the existing methods could be applied to bone marrow stem cells. These include microinjection, coprecipitation of DNA and calcium phosphate[7] or DEAE-dextran,[8] electric shock,[9] modified DNA (SV40 and adeno-)[10] and RNA (retro-) viruses. In practice, however, the low concentration of stem cells in bone marrow (10–30 cells per 10^5 nucleated marrow cells) severely limits the application of many of these methods for potential somatic therapy in that they are inherently either inefficient or cumbersome. Attention most recently, therefore, has focused on the potential use of retroviruses to provide highly efficient transfer and integration of foreign genetic material into such cells. Although most current work has centered on this general approach, it should be noted that one report has recently described the introduction of foreign DNA into human hematopoietic progenitor cells using electric shock (electroporation).[11] If these data are confirmed and extended to hematopoietic stem cells, electroporation may represent an alternative to the strategies described below.

GENE TRANSFER BY RETROVIRUSES

Evolution has specifically tailored retroviruses for efficient delivery of their genomes to cells, subsequent integration within the host cell genome, and high-level expression of their internal sequences. In an effort to take advantage of many of these features, various laboratories have constructed defective retroviral vectors in which sequences essential for virus production have been removed to allow for insertion of foreign DNA sequences.[12–14]

Aspects of the life cycle of retroviruses that are relevant to the development of this gene transfer system have been reviewed recently[15] and are summarized in Figures 6.1 and 6.2. It should suffice to note the following:

1. Integration of the DNA copy of the RNA viral genome in an infected cell is very efficient; it is directed by sequences within the retroviral long-terminal repeats (LTR), and the overall structure of the transferred genome is preserved.

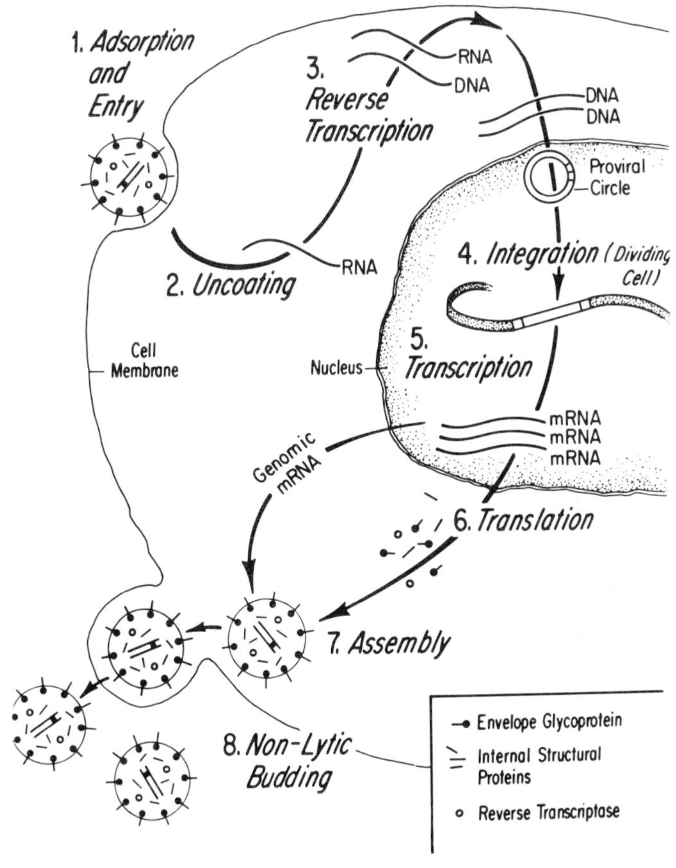

FIGURE 6.1 Life cycle of wild retrovirus. Steps in the life cycle include (1) adsorption and entry; (2) the uncoating of the virion particle; (3) production of a DNA copy of the viral genome by viral-encoded reverse transcriptase; (4) integration of provirus after entry of provirus into the nucleus; (5) transcription of new genome with the subsequent production of messenger RNA; (6) translation of messenger RNA into new glycoproteins, internal structural proteins, and reverse transcriptase; and (7) nonlytic budding of new particles after assembly.

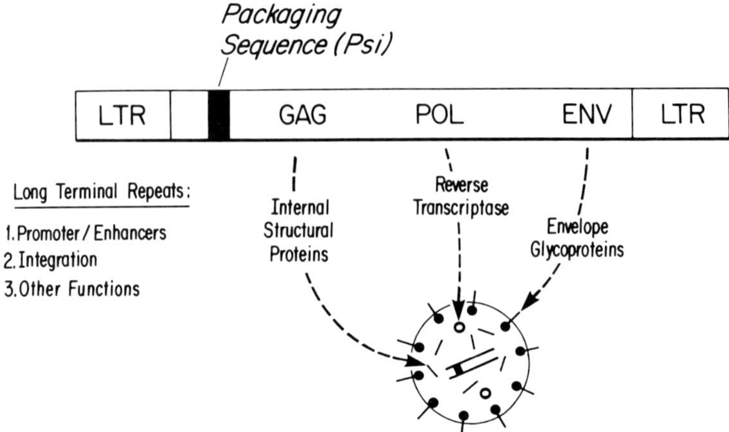

FIGURE 6.2 Genome of wild retrovirus. Long terminal repeats (LTR) including the viral promoter, enhancers, and sequences important for integration; Psi, packaging sequence required in *cis* for packaging of genomic RNA into virion particles; GAG, gene encoding internal structural proteins of virion core; POL, gene encoding reverse transcriptase; ENV, gene encoding envelope glycoproteins present on virion membrane.

2. Virion proteins that are essential for viral production (eg gag, pol, and env) can be supplied in *trans* (ie, by an infected cell).
3. The integrated proviral genome behaves as a cellular gene and is transferred to all progeny of an originally infected cell.
4. Budding of virus is nonlytic, which permits establishment of permanent cell lines that produce recombinant retroviruses in culture.

Recombinant retrovirus vectors maintain sequences that are needed in *cis* (ie, on the recombinant molecule itself) for infection, integration, and transcriptional control of the proviral genome (contained in the LTR) and a sequence termed psi that is required for packaging of genomic RNA into virions.[16] Viral sequences whose functions can be supplied in *trans* (gag-pol and env) are deleted from these vectors. In their place dominant, selectable markers, such as G418-resistance (neo),[14] hypoxanthine phosphoribosyl-transferase (HPRT),[17] or dihydrofolate reductase (methotrexate-resistance),[18] have been introduced to permit selection of recombinant viruses.

Recombinant defective retrovirus can be generated using specific "packaging" cell lines.[16,18,19] These murine cell lines harbor defective, integrated retroviral genomes that supply gag-pol and env functions in *trans* and package "defective" recombinant molecules that cannot make the proteins needed for viral assembly. The retroviral DNA is introduced in plasmid form by standard transfection into these cells. Drug selection is imposed to isolate clones of cells that may produce the desired recombinant virus. Retrovirus can be obtained with surface coats for infection of either murine or human cells. The recombinant virus can be titered from the producer cells by transfer of medium to mouse or human fibroblasts and subsequent drug selection. By use of such packaging cells helper-free recombinant retrovirus can be routinely produced. Such recombinant virus can infect and integrate into the DNA of tissue culture or primary cells but cannot give rise to additional infectious virus, since it does not produce gag-pol and env in the infected cell. Continued spread of recombinant virus in culture or in an animal is thereby avoided by this general approach.

GENE TRANSFER INTO HEMATOPOIETIC CELLS

Excluding the skin, bone marrow cells are the most accessible somatic cells for possible genetic manipulation. Moreover, hematopoietic cells can be easily removed, manipulated in vitro, and then returned to an intact animal or human. Both in vivo and in vitro assays have been developed that permit assessment of the developmental pathway of hematopoiesis. Several severe genetic disorders are manifested primarily in bone marrow-derived cells, a fact of particular relevance to potential genetic therapy. Therefore, transfer of genes into hematopoietic stem cells represents an attractive system for somatic therapy and for experimental cellular biology.

Gene transfer into primary hematopoietic cells has been demonstrated in several studies. Although Cline and co-workers first reported introduction of foreign genes into murine bone marrow by calcium phosphate coprecipitation,[20] the low and variable efficiency of gene transfer by this approach (¼ 1/1000 cells) greatly limits its applicability. Recently, in an effort to achieve more efficient and reproducible transfer into pluripotent hematopoietic cells, most research groups have turned to the use of recombinant retroviruses.

The basic experimental approach involves co-cultivation of murine bone marrow cells with retrovirus producer cells and subsequent reinjection of the marrow cells into lethally irradiated syngeneic recipient mice (or into the mutant strain W/W^V without irradiation). Within 10 to 14 days marrow reinfusion colonies (CFU-S) form in the spleen.[21] These colonies contain hematopoietic cells of all lineages, although lymphoid cells may be distributed throughout the stroma and not concentrated within the colonies themselves. Southern blot analysis of the DNA isolated from spleen cells or individual CFU-S permits assessment of the success of gene transfer into marrow cells.

The first demonstration of reconstitution of mice with transduced marrow cells using recombinant retrovirus was reported by Williams et al.[22] Using a high-titer retrovirus, approximately 15% of CFU-S contained the foreign proviral sequences. Reinjection of CFU-S into secondary mice established that gene transfer into a self-renewing, pluripotent stem cell had occurred. More recent work by Dick et al,[23] Keller et al,[24] and Lemishka et al[25] showed that the stem cell containing the inserted gene may be long-lived, that is, present up to 4 months after reinfusion, and totipotent, that is, gives rise to both lymphoid and myeloid progeny. Efficient transfer of retroviral sequences into murine marrow has also been described by Eglitis et al.[26] Drug selection during or just after co-cultivation with the virus-producing cells in vitro has been noted to increase the proportion of CFU-S that contains a foreign sequence.

Genes that have been transferred into intact mice by retroviruses include G418 (neomycin-resistance gene), HPRT, DHFR (methotrexate-resistance), and human adenosine deaminase (ADA). At present, with current technology it appears that gene transfer into a significant fraction of hematopoietic stem cells is feasible using retroviral vectors.

Retrovirus-mediated gene transfer into human hematopoietic cells using helper-virus containing viral stocks was described by Gruber et al.[27] More recently, Hock and Miller[28] reported production of drug-resistant CFU-GM with a helper-free retrovirus.

GENE EXPRESSION FOLLOWING TRANSFER INTO HEMATOPOIETIC CELLS

Naturally, the goal of current efforts is to attain high-level expression of foreign genes within marrow-derived cells following transplantation. The success of somatic genetic therapy, as well as biologic experiments aimed at examining hematopoiesis, clearly depends on both the regularity and the level of this expression. Quantitative data on gene expression following transfer are less abundant at present than data on transfer per se. Although experience so far is somewhat limited and additional results sure to be obtained soon, it appears that potential difficulties reside in the area of gene expression. These difficulties, moreover, may be specifically related to the target cells, that is, primary hematopoietic stem and progenitor cells.

Miller et al[17] first reported data on the expression of human HPRT in mice that received marrow infected with helper virus and a retrovirus carrying human HPRT. Although the spleens of most mice appeared to contain human HPRT DNA sequences by Southern blot analysis, HPRT enzyme expression was observed in only a few mice and at a very low level.

Recently, Dick et al,[23] reported the recovery of G418-resistant bone marrow progenitor cells (CFU-GM) from animals transplanted with cells infected with a G418 resistance gene. Even though all stem cells contained the G418 resistance gene, only a fraction (about 3%) expressed sufficient neotransferase activity to survive in vitro selection in a progenitor assay. Similarly, Keller et al[24] demonstrated G418 resistance of progenitors recovered from transplanted mice. Yet, upon reinjection of positive CFU-S cells into a second mouse, the level of functional resistance to selection diminished with time. The general impression is that expression attained in these studies so far has been relatively low and, furthermore, that it is extinguished with time, even though the proviral sequences are still present in the host cell DNA.

Our own experiments illustrate the biologic differences between primary hematopoietic cells and cultured cells that are generally used to assess the ability of specific retroviral constructs to express a product. We have constructed a series of retroviruses that harbor the human adenosine deaminase (ADA) gene. A construction that affords expression in cell culture is termed zip-DHFR-SV40ADA.[29] Dihydrofolate reductase is transcribed from the retroviral LTR and permits selection of infected cells with methotrexate. Translatable human ADA RNA is transcribed from an internal SV40 viral promoter. Expression of human ADA enzyme is equal to or greater than mouse endogenous enzyme in all cultured cells that can be infected with the virus. Of note, murine lymphoid cells of both T- and B-cell origin express human ADA enzyme following infection. Therefore, the SV40 promoter is functional in these hematopoietic cells. Using the same virus, we have failed to observe human ADA enzyme expression in murine CFU-S that contains integrated proviral sequences. Furthermore, RNA analysis reveals that only about 50% of retrovirus-DNA-positive spleens or spleen foci of transplant recipients contained retrovirus-directed RNA transcripts. Where present, the level of these transcripts is variable and on average very much lower than that seen in tissue culture cells infected in vitro.

Several possible explanations might account for the apparent difficulties encountered in obtaining adequate expression from retroviral constructions in vivo. For one, these problems very likely reflect intrinsic biologic differences between tissue culture cell lines and hematopoietic stem cells and progenitors. Cells might differ in their choice of suitable transcriptional and enhancer elements or, possibly, in factors that might facilitate RNA processing or stabilize specific RNA sequences. At present, data are insufficient to permit definite conclusions to be drawn. The failure of several strong promoter and enhancer elements to function in teratocarcinoma cells provides a precedent for stem cells in which specific transcriptional units (eg, SV40 promoter or LTR) do not function.[30] Whether observations in such cells, particularly with respect to repression of transcription by retrovirus LTR sequences, are relevant to findings in hematopoietic cells is under study.

At present, experiments in this area are largely empiric as investigators search for recombinant vectors that yield more satisfactory results. As one approach to this problem, in our laboratory we have simplified retroviral constructs carrying human ADA cDNA to a unit in which a constitutively expressed promoter (for the human phosphoglycerate kinase [PGK] gene) drives ADA cDNA expression within a retrovirus disabled by a deletion within its LTR sequences. Initial experiments have documented human ADA expression in murine hematopoietic progenitors and CFU-S infected with such a construction. These results lead us to conclude that appropriate design and empiric testing of a variety of constructions will ultimately yield useful retroviruses for human ADA and other gene sequences. More problematic, perhaps, is whether general rules for the design of vectors capable of adequate expression in vivo will emerge. Recently, Belmont and colleagues[31] have described expression of human ADA in murine progenitors infected with a recombinant retrovirus.

ADDITIONAL EXPERIMENTAL CONSIDERATIONS

By necessity most investigation in this general area has been undertaken in murine hematopoietic cells, largely because techniques for handling these cells and for marrow reconstitution are readily available. The extent to which apparent difficulties in expression of retroviral constructs in vivo may relate specifically to murine cells and not to primate cells is uncertain. Perhaps study of dogs and monkeys reconstituted with infected marrow cells will assist in answering this question. At a minimum, such investigations will provide useful experience in extending gene transfer in hematopoietic cells to larger animals. Careful experimental work remains to be performed on the nature of the hematopoietic stem cells into which foreign genes are inserted by retroviruses. Although a self-renewing, multipotential stem cell, the CFU-S of the mouse may bear little relevance to the cells required for long-term reconstitution of an animal after marrow transplantation.[32] This may explain why the number of progeny cells containing a foreign gene some months after transplant is uniformly low (either by functional assay or by DNA analysis of stem cells remaining within bone marrow) irrespective of how efficient the gene transfer into CFU-S is initially. The extent to which marrow stem cell kinetics may affect the potential for a subpopulation of marrow containing a transferred gene to compete with other marrow populations during the stress of reconstitution is unknown. In mice specific hematopoietic stem cell clones may variably contribute to overall hematopoiesis, and particular lineages, over time.[25] Therefore, the expression of a transferred gene within the host might not be stable and might rather unpredictably either increase or decrease, depending on the number of cycling stem cells containing (and expressing) the foreign sequence.

DISORDERS SUITABLE FOR INITIAL GENE THERAPY ATTEMPTS

Our incomplete understanding of gene regulation and limitations in somatic cells that are accessible for gene introduction severely restrict disorders that might be considered suitable for genetic intervention. At first approximation, only conditions for which allogeneic bone marrow transplantation is beneficial stand to profit from gene transfer into hematopoietic cells.[15,33] A logical first step in evaluating the potential of a disorder for gene therapy is treatment of the condition with bone marrow transplantation. If clinical improvement ensues, then gene therapy might accomplish the same result. If not, it is unrealistic to expect that gene transfer into marrow cells could yield a positive clinical result. Whether gene introduction into other somatic cells, for example, hepatic or skin cells, will be useful in selected diseases or deficiency states remains to be explored. Gene transfer into skin cells might be particularly useful in hormonal deficiencies or clotting-factor deficiencies.

By nearly general consensus the severe immunodeficiency states due to either ADA or purine nucleoside phosphorylase (PNP) deficiency[15,34] would appear to be among the best candidates for genetic therapy. Both diseases are the result of enzyme deficiency within bone marrow-derived cells.[35] Both enzymes are single-chain polypeptides that undergo essentially no intracellular processing and for which the respective human genes have been cloned. Tissue-specific regulation of gene expression is likely not to be critical in these instances and subnormal amounts of enzyme (roughly 10% of normal) may be sufficient to correct the disorders clinically.

Among other disorders due to the deficiency of a product in hematopoietic cells and manifest strictly as a hematologic disorder, chronic granulomatous disease (CGD) is a condition worthy of consideration from this standpoint.[33,36] In CGD, a defect within the NADPH-oxidase of phagocytic cells (granulocytes, monocytes, eosinophils) prevents intracellular killing of ingested microorganisms.[36] Bone marrow transplantation, although infrequently performed in this situation, is curative.[33] The gene that is abnormal in the classical, X-linked variety of CGD has recently been isolated.[37] Introduction of this gene into bone marrow cells offers a new approach to correction of this disease. Although not considered as severe as the immunodeficiency states noted above, CGD often causes significant morbidity due to the inability to eradicate indolent infections. Our laboratory is currently examining the potential for genetic therapy for this disorder.

Many other inherited disorders are being evaluated as potential candidates as well. These include storage disorders, aminoacidurias,[38,39] and the Lesch-Nyhan syndrome.[17] Patients in whom central nervous system abnormalities occur are not likely to respond to gene transfer into bone marrow, although this remains to be more fully evaluated principally by analysis of bone marrow transplantation results. It is unrealistic to suppose that gene transfer into marrow for these disorders could surpass standard bone marrow transplantation from a metabolic perspective.

Most inherited disorders noted above are relatively uncommon. Genetic therapy of these inborn errors would be a first step and represents an important proving ground for the technology. The extension of gene therapy to hemoglobin disorders—thalassemia or sickle cell anemia—would stand in marked contrast. Until our understanding of gene regulation permits high-level and regulated expression of eukaryotic genes upon transfer into hematopoietic cells, the treatment of these common conditions may not be feasible. Nevertheless, given the pace of progress over the past several years, we should not be too pessimistic about even these possibilities.

CONCLUSION

The ethics of gene therapy and specific details of human experimentation have not been addressed in this review of current research. A consensus exists that initial trials should proceed only after careful local and national review of experiments and protocols.[34,40] Exposition of these points has been presented, and has been restated by NIH advisory panels.

Recently it has been frequently said that gene therapy in man is imminent.[41] That such proclamations have not been borne out by current work should not be taken as a failure of current technology, but merely as a reflection of the natural enthusiasm of both investigators and those who report on their affairs. The prevailing wisdom would suggest that such human experimentation will come, but at what pace is uncertain. What is learned at a basic level about expression in vivo from retroviruses will direct ongoing efforts. The development of alternative methods for gene transfer or radically improved approaches to site-directed gene repair could immediately alter the mode by which genetic therapy might occur.

REFERENCES

1. Hinnen A, Hicks JB, Fink GR: Transformation of yeast. *Proc Natl Acad Sci USA* 1978;75:1929–1933.
2. Smithies O, Gregg RG, Boggs SS, et al: Insertion of DNA sequences into the human chromosomal beta-globin locus by homologous recombination. *Nature* 1985; 317:230–234.
3. Thomas KR, Folger KR, Capecchi MR: High frequency targeting of genes to specific sites in the mammalian genome. *Cell* 1986;44:419–428.
4. Rubin GM, Spradling AC: Genetic transformation of Drosophila with transposable element vectors. *Science* 1982;218:348–353.
5. Palmiter RD, Brinster RL, Hammer RE, et al: Dramatic growth of mice that develop from eggs microinjected with metallothionein-growth hormone fusion gene. *Nature* 1982;300:611–615.
6. Brinster RL, Chen HY, Traumbauer M: Differential regulation of metallothionein-thymidine kinase fusion genes in transgenic mice and their offspring. *Cell* 1982;29:701–710.
7. Wigler M, Silverstein S, Lee LS, et al: Transfer of purified herpes virus thymidine kinase gene to cultured cells. *Cell* 1982;11:223–232.
8. Sompayrac LM, Danna KT: Efficient infection of monkey cells with DNA of simian virus 40. *Proc Natl Acad Sci USA* 1981;78:7575–7578.
9. Potter H, Weis L, Leder P: Enhancer-dependent expression of human kappa-immunoglobulin genes introduced into mouse pre-B lymphocytes by electroporation. *Proc Natl Acad Sci USA* 1984;81:7161–7165.
10. Mulligan RC, Howard BH, Berg P: Synthesis of rabbit beta-globin in cultured monkey kidney cells following infection with SV40 beta-globin recombinant genome. *Nature* 1979;227:108–114.
11. Toneguzzo F, Keating A: Stable expression of selectable genes introduced into human hematopoietic stem cells by electric field-mediated DNA transfer. *Proc Natl Acad Sci USA* 1986;83:3496–3499.
12. Shimotohno K, Temin H: Formation of infectious progeny virus after insertion of herpes simplex thymidine kinase gene into DNA of an avian retrovirus. *Cell* 1981;26:67–77.
13. Stuhlmann H, Cone R, Mulligan RC, et al: Introduction of a selectable gene into different animal tissues by a retrovirus recombinant vector. *Proc Natl Acad Sci USA* 1984; 81:7151–7155.
14. Cepko C, Roberts BE, Mulligan RC: Construction and application of a highly transmissible murine retrovirus shuttle vector. *Cell* 1984;31:1053–1062.
15. Williams DA, Orkin SH: Somatic gene therapy: Current status and future prospects. *J Clin Invest* 1986;77:1053–1056.
16. Mann R, Mulligan RC, Baltimore D: Construction of a retrovirus packaging mutant and its use to produce helper-free defective retrovirus. *Cell* 1983;33:153–159.
17. Miller AD, Eckner RJ, Jolly DJ, et al: Expression of a retrovirus encoding human HPRT in mice. *Science* 1984;225:630–632.
18. Miller AD, Law MF, Verma IM: Generation of a helper free amphotropic retrovirus that transduces a dominant-acting methotrexate-resistant dihydrofolate reductase gene. *Mol Cell Biol* 1985;5:431–437.
19. Cone R, Mulligan RC: High efficiency gene transfer into mammalian cells: Generation of helper-free recombinant retrovirus with broad mammalian host range. *Proc Natl Acad Sci USA* 1984;81:6349–6353.
20. Cline MJ, Stang H, Morse L, et al: Gene transfer in intact animal. *Nature* 1980; 284:422–425.

21. Till JE, McCulloch EA: A direct measurement of the radiation sensitivity of normal mouse bone marrow cells. *Radiat Res* 1961;14:213–218.
22. Williams DA, Lemischka IR, Nathan DG, et al: Introduction of new genetic material into pluripotent hematopoietic stem cells of mice. *Nature* 1984;310:476–480.
23. Dick JE, Magli ML, Huszar D, et al: Introduction of a selectable gene into primitive stem cells capable of long-term reconstitution of the hemopoietic system of W/W^v mice. *Cell* 1985;42:71–79.
24. Keller G, Paige C, Gilboa E, et al: Expression of a foreign gene in myeloid and lymphoid cells derived from multipotent haematopoietic precursors. *Nature* 1985;318:149–154.
25. Lemischka I, Raulet DH, Mulligan RC: Developmental potential and dynamic behavior of hematopoietic stem cells. *Cell* 1986;45:917–927.
26. Eglitis MA, Kantoff P, Gilboa E, et al: Gene expression in mice following high efficiency retroviral-mediated gene transfer. *Science* 1985;230:1395–1398.
27. Gruber HE, Finley KD, Hershberg RM, et al: Retroviral vector-mediated gene transfer into human hematopoietic progenitor cells. *Science* 1985;230:1057–1061.
28. Hock RA, Miller AD: Retrovirus-mediated transfer and expression of drug resistance genes in human haematopoietic progenitor cells. *Nature* 1986;320:275–277.
29. Williams DA, Orkin SH, Mulligan RC: Retrovirus-mediated transfer of human adenosine deaminase sequences into cells in culture and into murine hematopoietic cells in vivo. *Proc Natl Acad Sci USA* 1986;83:2566–2570.
30. Gorman CM, Rigby PWJ, Lane DP: Negative regulation of viral enhancers in undifferentiated embryonic stem cells. *Cell* 1985;42:519–526.
31. Belmont JW, Henkel-Tiggers J, Chang SMW, et al: Expression of human adenosine deaminase in murine hematopoietic progenitor cells following retroviral transfer. *Nature* 1986;322:385–387.
32. Magli MC, Iscove NN, Odartehenko N: Transient nature of early haematopoietic spleen colonies. *Nature* 1982;295:527–529.
33. Parkman R: The application of bone marrow transplantation to the treatment of genetic diseases. *Science* 1986;232:1373–1378.
34. Anderson WF: Prospects for human gene therapy. *Science* 1984;226:401–409.
35. Kredich NM, Hershfield MS: Immunodeficiency diseases caused by adenosine deaminase deficiency and purine nucleside phosphorylase deficiency. Stanbury JB, Wyngaarden JB, Fredrickson DS, (eds): *The Metabolic Basis of Inherited Disease.* New York, McGraw-Hill, 1983, 1157 pp.
36. Tauber AI, Borregaard M, Simons E, et al: Chronic granulomatous disease: a syndrome of phagocyte oxidase deficiencies. *Medicine* 1983;62:286–309.
37. Royer-Pokora B, Kunkel LM, Monaco AP, et al: Cloning the gene for an inherited human disorder (chronic granulomatous disease) on the basis of its chromosomal location. *Nature* 1986;322:32–38.
38. Woods PA, O'Brien WE, Beaudet AL: Development of citrullinemia as a model for gene therapy. *Am J Human Genet* 37(abstr):542.
39. Ledley FD, Grenett HE, McGinnis-Shelnutt M, et al: Retroviral-mediated gene transfer of human phenylalanine hydroxylase into NIH 3T3 and hepatoma cells. *Proc Natl Acad Sci USA* 1986;83:409–413.
40. *Federal Register.* 1986, pp 23210–23211.
41. Budiansky S: US clinical trails imminent. *Nature* 1984;312:393.

CHAPTER 7

Prenatal Diagnosis and Carrier Detection by DNA Analysis

Corinne D. Boehm, BS, MS

Since 1976 over 500 prenatal diagnoses have been accomplished by analysis of fetal DNA samples.[1-5] In the majority of these cases the fetus was at risk of having sickle cell anemia, thalassemia, or another hemoglobinopathy. However, the number of single gene disorders to which DNA technology can be applied for prenatal diagnosis for selected couples continues to grow. Currently, this list includes α_1-antitrypsin deficiency,[6,7] phenylketonuria (PKU)[8,9] hemophilia A (Factor VIII deficiency or classical hemophilia),[10-15] hemophilia B (Factor IX deficiency),[16] ornithine transcarbamylase (OTC) deficiency,[17] Duchenne's muscular dystrophy (DMD),[18-20] and cystic fibrosis.[21-23]

Antenatal diagnosis for some of these disorders has been accomplished by means other than DNA analysis as well. Mid-trimester fetal blood sampling by fetoscopy or placental aspiration has been used with 99% accuracy for diagnosis of the hemoglobinopathies (over 5,000 cases as of May 1984), α_1-antitrypsin deficiency (10 cases), hemophilia A (300 cases), and hemophilia B (30 cases).[5] However, fetoscopy is a specialized procedure and is performed at only 20 or so medical centers worldwide. Even in experienced hands the procedure carries a 3 to 4% risk of fetal mortality.[24]

Fetuses at risk for OTC deficiency have been diagnosed in utero by determination of OTC activity in fetal liver biopsy samples obtained through fetoscopy,[25,26] and PKU could be diagnosed similarly by determination of phenylalanine hydroxylase activity in fetal liver. Quantification of fetal serum creatine phosphokinase (CPK) levels was used to predict DMD status in 61 at risk male fetuses, but because of four false-negative results (7% of the 61 cases), the fetal serum CPK level was deemed unreliable as a prenatal diagnostic test for DMD and is no longer in use.[5]

The introduction of DNA methods to the field of prenatal diagnosis has been well received for three main reasons. First, the fetal sampling techniques for obtaining DNA samples represent vast improvements over those used for obtaining fetal blood or liver biopsy samples. Fetal DNA can be isolated from amniocytes obtained by amniocentesis at 16 weeks of gestation (fetal loss rate of less than 0.5%).[27] Recently, the development of chorion villus sampling as a technique for obtaining fetal tissue at 9 to 11 weeks of gestation has given many couples an attractive alternative to both amniocentesis at 16 weeks and fetoscopy at 18 weeks of gestation.[28-30] Second, because gene expression is not necessary for diagnosis, DNA analysis is not limited by problems relating to gene activity, with respect to either tissue specificity or fetal developmental stage. Third, DNA methods hold great potential for diagnosis of conditions that could not be diagnosed in utero previously because the primary defect is unknown. Many research groups have isolated DNA probes that detect random polymorphisms, and linkage maps for many of these probes have been determined. Pedigree analysis of large families in which certain single gene disorders are segregating have proven useful in identifying pieces of DNA linked to the loci for Huntington disease.[31] Duchenne's muscular dystrophy,[18] and cystic fibrosis,[21-23] among others. Even though the primary cause of these disorders is not known, the pieces of linked DNA may be used for diagnosis.

Diagnosis by DNA analysis can be achieved through several different methods, including those by which the disease—producing mutation itself is detected in the fetus (direct detection) and a method by which fetal inheritance of a mutation is deduced by following the inheritance pattern of a closely linked DNA polymorphism (indirect detection). Although direct detection methods are usually considered preferable to indirect methods, their exclusive use is not practical at this time for disorders caused by any of a number of different mutations, such as β-thalassemia in North America and detrimental X-linked disorders like DMD and hemophilia. In addition, direct detection methods cannot be applied to diagnosis for disorders in which the gene responsible has not been discovered, such as Huntington's disease and cystic fibrosis. For such disorders the use of linked DNA polymorphisms is the most useful approach to diagnosis in the majority of cases. Polymorphisms, however, are diagnostic in less than 100% of cases. Specifically, they are not diagnostic in instances in which a parent is not informative at a linked polymorphic site. Currently, the use of polymorphisms is diagnostic in about 93% of pregnancies in which the fetus is at risk for β-thalassemia,[32] slightly more than 90% for DMD,[19,20] and close to 100% for hemophilia A.[10,11,33] Family studies initiated prior to fetal sampling are necessary to identify couples for whom polymorphisms will be useful for prenatal diagnosis and to determine which polymorphism(s) should be used in analysis of each fetal sample. Sometimes direct detection methods can be used for families in which polymorphisms are not diagnostic.

Sickle cell anemia, α_1-antitrypsin deficiency (homozygosity for the Pi Z allele), and most cases of α^o-thalassemia are disorders for which direct detection methods can be routinely applied because of the homogeneous molecular nature of each disorder. Thus, diagnosis can be achieved in essentially 100% of pregnancies at risk for any of these three disorders.

The most commonly used DNA methods will be described in this chapter, as will their applicability to prenatal testing for certain single gene disorders. The accuracy of the testing is in general quite high, but depends on several factors that need to be clearly defined for each couple being studied.

DNA TECHNIQUES USEFUL FOR DIAGNOSIS

Since a full complement of DNA is present in each cell nucleus, virtually any nucleated cell should be suitable for DNA analysis regardless of whether the gene in question is being transcribed. Thus, white blood cells, amniocytes, and chorion villi are all candidate cells for DNA analysis. Currently, DNA diagnosis relies almost exclusively on two methods. These are the Southern blot technique[34] and oligonucleotide probe analysis.[35] However, other methods are being developed and several have potential for use in diagnosis. These include a system designed to detect single nucleotide differences by electrophoresis of double-stranded DNA fragments in a denaturing gradient gel,[36] and detection of a point mutation by amplification of a specific stretch of DNA followed by hybridization with an end-labeled oligonucleotide.[37]

Southern Blot Analysis

In the widely used Southern blot analysis technique, double-stranded, high-molecular-weight DNA is digested by a restriction endonuclease chosen because of its ability to detect either a DNA polymorphism or a pathologic, disease-producing mutation. Restriction endonucleases are isolated from bacteria, each of which cleaves DNA nonrandomly after encountering a specific sequence of several nucleotides that constitutes that enzyme's recognition sequence. After endonuclease digestion the resulting DNA fragments are separated by size using electrophoresis in an agarose gel. The DNA in the gel is then denatured to create single-stranded DNA molecules available for hybridization with a probe. After the DNA fragments are transferred out of the gel onto a filter, specific filter-bound DNA fragments can then be detected by hybridization with a radiolabeled DNA or RNA probe that has sequence homology to the DNA fragment of interest. Subsequent autoradiography produces an x-ray film with banding patterns that indicate the locations on the filter, and therefore the fragment sizes, of the DNA sequences homologous to the probe.

Use of DNA Polymorphisms for Diagnosis (Indirect Detection of Mutation)

DNA alterations that affect a restriction endonuclease site by either creating a new site or obliterating a previously existing one can be detected on a Southern blot as changes in the size of the relevant DNA fragment. Many of these recognition site changes are biologically neutral and represent normal inherited variations. These are referred to as restriction site polymorphisms. DNA fragment sizes can also be altered by small insertions or deletions, again many of which are neutral and have been referred to as hypervariable regions (HVRs). Both restriction site polymorphisms and HVRs are referred to by the general name of restriction fragment length polymorphisms (RFLPs) since they affect DNA fragment lengths.

In 1978 the first human RFLP useful for diagnosis was discovered by Kan and Dozy.[38] They found that at a point about 5,000 bp 3′ to the β-globin gene one of two normal sequences appears. One sequence contains a recognition site for the endonuclease Hpa I and the β-globin gene in chromosomes of this type resides in a 7.6-kb fragment after Hpa I digestion. On chromosomes lacking this Hpa I site, the β-globin gene resides in a 13-kb fragment. There is also an infrequent variant in which the β-globin gene lies within a 7.0-kb Hpa I fragment. Thus, each individual either is homozygous for one of the polymorphism types or is heterozygous with one chromosome containing the polymorphic Hpa I site and the other lacking it. Although the polymorphism is unrelated to the β-globin gene in any functional sense, its proximity to the gene means that it will almost always be inherited together with the gene as a single unit. When parents at risk for a child with a β-chain hemoglobinopathy are heterozygous at the Hpa I site (or any other closely linked β-globin polymorphism), family studies are usually successful in determining which form of the polymorphism is segregating with their normal β-globin gene and which with their variant β-globin gene. Then, once the polymorphism type of a fetus is known, the fetal β-globin genotype can be deduced. An example of the use of a polymorphism for prenatal diagnosis of β-thalassemia is shown in Figure 7.1.

Meiotic recombination, the interchromosomal exchange of homologous DNA sequences during meiosis, has the potential to destroy the established association between a gene and the linked polymorphism type by replacing the polymorphism type on one chromosome with that from the other chromosome. Such an event could cause an error in diagnosis. The

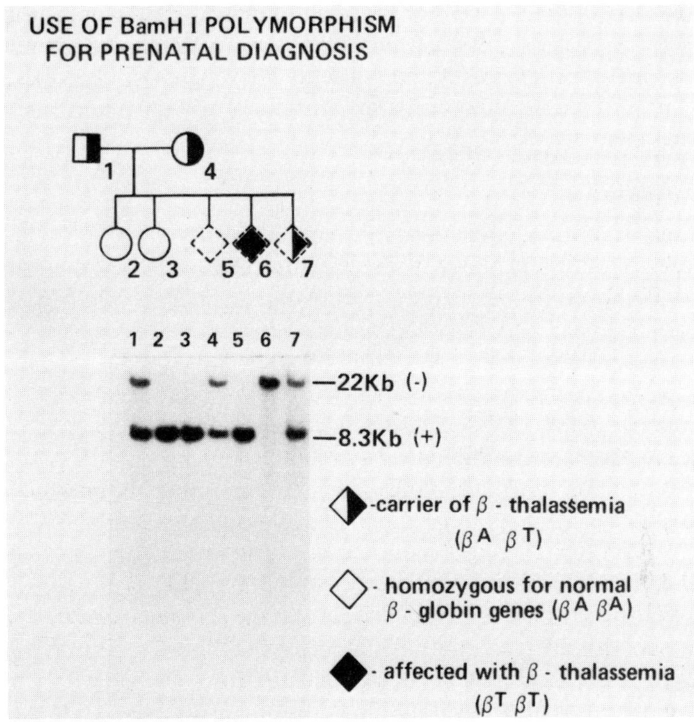

FIGURE 7.1 Example of the use of a DNA polymorphism for prenatal diagnosis of β-thalassemia. The two forms of the polymorphism 3′ to the β-globin gene are detected as the presence (+) and absence (−) of a BamH I restriction site. BamH I restriction patterns show heterozygosity at this polymorphic site (+/−) in both the father (1) and mother (4) who are carriers of β-thalassemia and homozygosity (+/+) in their normal daughters (2,3). BamH I restriction patterns of any potential fetus (5,6,7) with indicated genotype is also shown.

chance of this occurring is a function of how tightly linked the gene and polymorphic loci are; the degree of linkage has a direct effect on the accuracy of a diagnosis. For instance, the chance that a recombination will occur between the β-globin gene and the polymorphic Hpa I site in any particular meiosis is estimated to be 1 in 2,000.[39] Thus, the Hpa I polymorphism is a highly accurate predictor of inheritance at the β-globin locus.

Prenatal diagnosis of β-thalassemia by DNA analysis relies heavily on the use of linked polymorphisms as does diagnosis of DMD and hemophilia A and B. This reliance exists because in world populations these disorders result from many different mutations. Thirty-six point mutations producing β-thalassemia have been described,[40–43] and the relatively high mutation rate for DMD especially, but also for hemophilia A and B, means that the molecular causes of these disorders are numerous. The generalized nature of DNA polymorphisms makes them useful for diagnosis regardless of the specific mutation, as long as the mutation is tightly linked to the polymorphism.

Family Studies

Correct use of family data in determining the linkage phases between alleles at the disease locus and alleles at the polymorphic locus is also essential for accurate diagnosis. Some examples of the use of pedigree analysis for both autosomal recessive and X-linked recessive disorders follow.

Autosomal Recessive Disorders. Figure 7.1 provides an example of prenatal diagnosis by linkage analysis in a simple pedigree. However, pedigree analysis may be more complicated. For example, both parents may be heterozygous at a polymorphic site, but their polymorphic alleles and β-globin alleles may be in opposite coupling phases as at site 1 in Pedigree 7.1, below. Here, one parent's β^A gene is coupled with the + allele at site 1 and that parent's β^{thal} gene with the − allele; the coupling phases in the other parent are the opposite (β^A gene with the − allele and the β^{thal} gene with the + allele). In this case, both affected and normal fetuses will have the same polymorphism type at site 1. Use of an additional site (site 2, Pedigree 7.1) at which one of the parents is heterozygous allows the diagnosis to be made in cases in which the other site alone is inconclusive, as for fetuses C and D.

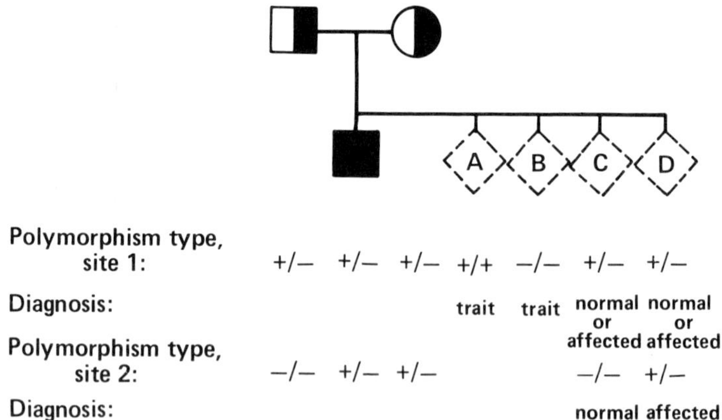

PEDIGREE 7.1 Autosomal recessive disorder. Both parents are heterozygous at site 1 but their polymorphic alleles and β-globin alleles are in opposite coupling phases. Thus, diagnosis is not possible by use of site 1 alone in fetuses C and D. Inclusion of site 2 at which one parent is also heterozygous allows diagnosis to be made for fetuses C and D.

Heterozygotes for β-thalassemia can be discovered by population screening, but for those autosomal recessive disorders for which there is no test by which carriers can be identified, such as PKU and cystic fibrosis (CF), it is only through the birth of an affected child that a couple is known to be at risk. If an affected child is dead, prenatal diagnosis by DNA analysis might still be possible if the parents are heterozygous at polymorphic site(s), and parental polymorphism haplotypes can be determined through study of unaffected offspring (Pedigree 7.2). A polymorphism haplotype describes the particular combination of polymorphic alleles that exist on a given chromosome. Two or more polymorphic sites are necessary to construct a haplotype. The haplotype is constructed by examining inheritance patterns within the family. For instance, in Pedigree 7.2 the first unaffected daughter inherited the mother's − allele at site 1 and her + allele at site 2. Thus, in the mother the polymorphism haplotype on one chromosome is −+ (site 1, site 2) and, by deduction, +− on the other chromosome. The father's two haplotypes can be readily determined without any other family considerations, since he is heterozygous at only one site. If four distinct parental haplotypes can be identified, any fetus with the same two parental haplotypes as an unaffected child will be unaffected. In Pedigree 7.2, three of the four combinations of parental haplotypes are represented among the three unaffected children. The fetus has the fourth combination and thus is affected.

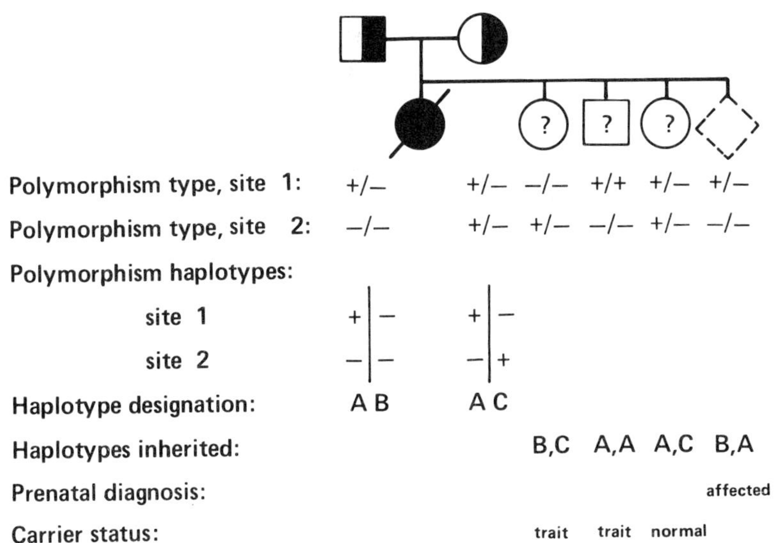

PEDIGREE 7.2 Autosomal recessive disorder for which no carrier test is available for general population screening. Although the affected child is deceased, carrier testing and prenatal testing can be performed for this family since the 3 unaffected children have 3 of the 4 possible haplotype combinations.

Carrier testing by DNA analysis of siblings of an affected individual is often possible, as shown in Pedigree 7.3, but might not be helpful if screening methods did not exist for determining carrier status in a potential mate. For siblings in which a diagnosis of non-carrier is made, concern about occurrence of the autosomal recessive disorder in their children will be alleviated. However, for siblings shown to be carriers (statistically, two-thirds of the siblings would be carriers), concern may be increased. Without the possibility of a potential mate being tested for carrier status, the risk of their having an affected child is raised to one-fourth of the carrier frequency. However, prenatal testing by DNA analysis would be able to determine only whether the mutant gene had been inherited from the carrier parent. If so, the chance that the fetus is affected would increase to one-half of the carrier frequency. These couples would have to consider several points in their family planning as it relates to the possibility of having children with this inherited disorder. The risk of the disorder, their perception of the burden of the disorder, and their feelings about terminating a pregnancy in which the fetus is probably unaffected would all have to be weighed.

X-Linked Recessive Disorders. Pedigree analysis for X-linked disorders differs in several ways from that for autosomal recessive disorders. For instance, the occurrence of a new mutation is more often observed in genetically lethal X-linked disorders than in autosomal recessive disorders. In 1935 Haldane suggested that for genetically lethal X-linked diseases such as DMD, perhaps one-third of the isolated cases represent new mutations.[44] In contrast, new mutations in autosomal recessive disorders are rarely observed. Also, carrier testing for X-linked disorders is sometimes less conclusive than for autosomal recessive disorders. For instance, Emery observed obligate DMD carrier females with normal creative phosphokinase (CPK) levels and estimated that only two-thirds of carrier women have elevated

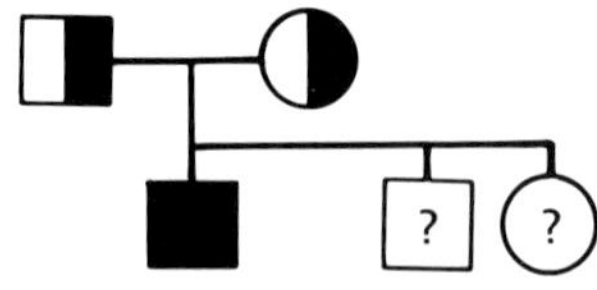

Polymorphism type: +/– –/– +/– +/– +/+

Diagnosis: carrier non-carrier(normal)

PEDIGREE 7.3 Autosomal recessive disorder for which no carrier test is available for general population screening. For family with an affected member, determination of carrier status in unaffected siblings is achieved through DNA analysis.

serum CPK levels.[45] This phenomenon may be the result of X chromosome inactivation; perhaps carrier females who have a majority of their cells with the X chromosome carrying the DMD mutation inactivated will have more normal serum CPK levels than will other carriers. Gale and Murphy similarly concluded that grossly elevated serum CPK levels can be diagnostic of the carrier state in at-risk females, but normal or borderline levels cannot distinguish carriers from non-carriers.[46] Sometimes carrier testing by DNA analysis is of more diagnostic value. Such is the case when a female has not inherited the same polymorphism haplotype as an affected male relative (or, in some cases, the same as an unaffected male). However, results showing inheritance of the same polymorphism haplotype as an affected male in a family with no previous history of DMD by itself will be inconclusive with respect to carrier status. In this situation, Bayesian analysis should be relied upon for the most accurate prediction of carrier status.[47] In such an analysis, CPK values, the family pedigree, and the polymorphism typing are all taken into account. In Pedigree 7.4, a sister's heterozygosity at the polymorphic site is consistent with her being either a carrier or a non-carrier. When she is

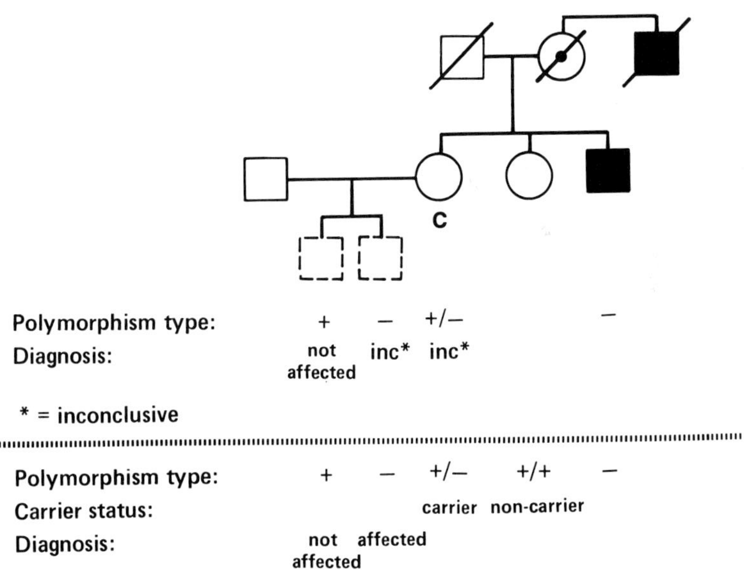

PEDIGREE 7.4 X-linked disorder. **Top Panel:** Although determination of carrier status can not be made for at risk female (consultand), prenatal testing is conclusive for her male fetus who has a different allele type than her affected brother. **Bottom panel:** By inclusion of another sister in the study, carrier testing is now possible for consultand and prenatal testing conclusive for both male fetuses.

carrying a male fetus that has inherited the allele different from her brother's, a diagnosis of an unaffected fetus (with accuracy depending on the recombination rate) can be made even if her carrier status is not known. However, if the male fetus inherits the same polymorphic allele as the affected brother, the results from DNA analysis would be inconclusive, and Bayesian analysis would provide her with the statistically calculated chance that the fetus is affected based on the best available information. When her sister is included in the study, we gain the information that the two sisters' X-chromosome derived from their father carries a + polymorphic allele. Once that + allele is accounted for in the sisters, it is clear that their mother was heterozygous at the polymorphic site and the sister who is pregnant has inherited the same allele as her affected brother and is therefore a carrier. A diagnosis of DMD, not possible previously, can now be made in the fetus.

Polymorphism haplotypes can sometimes provide more information than can be gathered by examination of each polymorphic site independently, as shown in Pedigree 7.5. The consultand was concerned both about her carrier status and about whether her 14-month-old son had DMD. Independent analyses of sites 1 and 2 provide inconclusive results with respect to her carrier status. It is only with haplotype information, obtained by studying the consultand's son, that the conclusion that she is not a carrier can be reached. Also, since her son has a − allele at site 1, he is known not to have inherited the DMD gene present in his uncle. This can be confirmed by the finding of normal CPK values in the son.

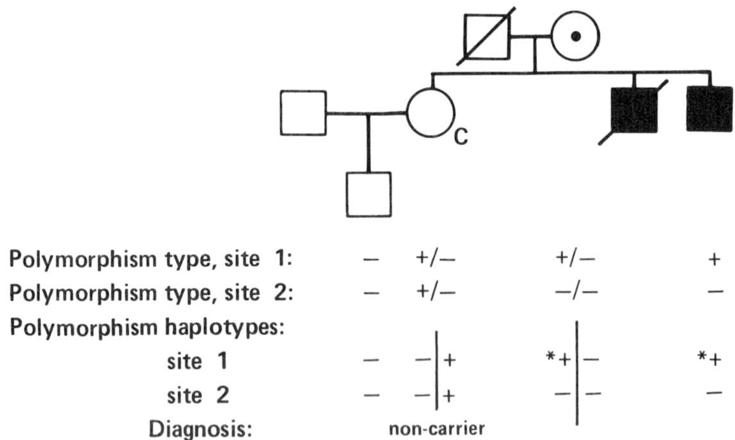

PEDIGREE 7.5 X-linked disorder. By use of sites 1 and 2 separately, carrier testing for consultand (C) is not possible. However, use of the 2 sites together through creation of polymorphism haplotypes identifies her as a noncarrier.

For both autosomal recessive and X-linked recessive pedigrees, haplotypes should always be constructed for the purpose of optimizing the diagnostic potential. Use of haplotypes also optimizes the chance of detecting meiotic recombination or false paternity, events that, if undetected, could result in an error in diagnosis.

Use of Direct Detection Methods for Diagnosis

When a disease-producing mutation can be directly detected and distinguished from the normal state, an accurate prenatal diagnosis can be made in all instances. At the present time, this is possible in situations in which (1) a restriction site is changed by the disease-producing mutation (see for example, Fig. 7.2), (2) the mutation is a result of a deletion (see, for example, Fig. 7.3), or (3) the mutation is one for which an oligonucleotide probe exists (see the next section and Fig. 7.4). In the first and second instances, DNA fragment sizes would be changed as a direct result of the mutation, and results from Southern blot analysis would be diagnostic. Extended-family studies and pedigree analysis are not necessary for diagnosis, although analysis of parental samples in parallel with the fetal sample is advised.

For deletions to be detected in the heterozygous state, at least one endpoint of the deletion must be within a stretch of DNA for which a probe is available. This allows for detection of the deletion as an abnormally sized fragment rather than simple absence of a band on the autoradiogram. In many cases, absence of a band cannot be accurately detected in individuals whose other allele is not deleted. In Pedigree 7.6 (p. 155), the father is a carrier of a $\gamma\delta\beta$-thalassemia allele in which the entire β-globin region is deleted, and the endpoint of the deletion cannot be detected with any available probe. Although the genotypes of the son and daughter are different, their restriction patterns are identical. The difference is that the son is hemizygous and the daughter homozygous for the $-$allele. This quantitative difference may not always be detectable in a Southern blot. Similarly, the diagnosis in fetus 2 may not be possible since it is not known whether it has inherited its father's deletion or normal β-globin allele. In fetus 1, inheritance of the deletion from the father can be deduced since the polymorphic $-$allele was not inherited.

Sometimes a fetus is at risk for a compound heterozygous state, such as Hb S/β-thalassemia, in which the prenatal diagnosis may be achieved by direct methods for the detection of one parent's variant allele and by polymorphism analysis for detection of the other parent's variant allele. Family studies may still be necessary for the prospective parent with the directly detectable allele when that parent is heterozygous at the polymorphic site being used for determination of inheritance from the other parent. An example is shown in Pedigree 7.7 (p. 155).

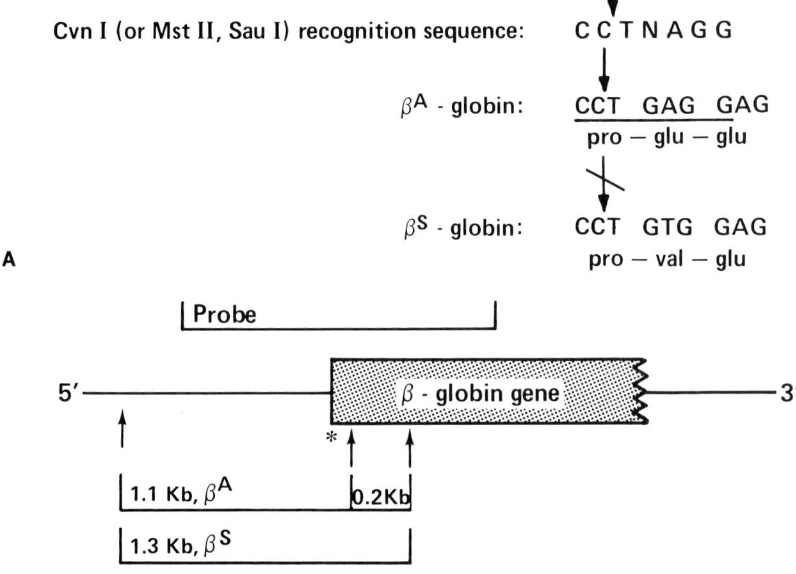

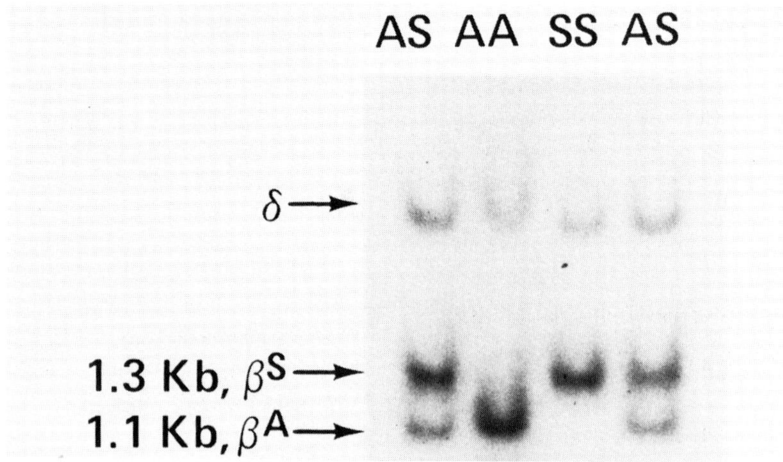

FIGURE 7.2 A: This figure shows that the sickle cell mutation destroys a Cvn I endonuclease recognition site. In the top line is the 7-nucleotide recognition sequence for Cvn I in which N represents any nucleotide. The arrow demonstrates the location at which Cvn I will cleave the DNA. The normal β-globin sequence for codons 5,6, and 7 (pro-glu-glu) contains a Cvn I recognition site (underlined). The β^S mutation, a single nucleotide A to T substitution in the middle of codon 6, substitutes val for glu and destroys the Cvn I recognition sequence. Cvn I will not cleave this sequence, as demonstrated by the arrow with the slash through it. **B:** In this map arrows indicate the locations of Cvn I restriction sites flanking and within the 5′ portion of normal (β^A) and sickle cell (β^S) globin genes. The resulting fragments are detectable with a probe of the indicated sequences. Endonuclease digestion of these DNAs with Cvn I produces the indicated DNA fragments which differ in length (kb). **C:** Autoradiogram shows Cvn I restriction patterns from individuals with sickle cell trait (AS), normal β-globin genes (AA), and sickle cell anemia (SS). β^S-globin genes reside in a 1.3-kb fragment and β^A-globin genes in a 1.1 or, rarely, 1.05-kb fragment (**not shown**). The probe cross-hybridizes with a δ-globin gene fragment.

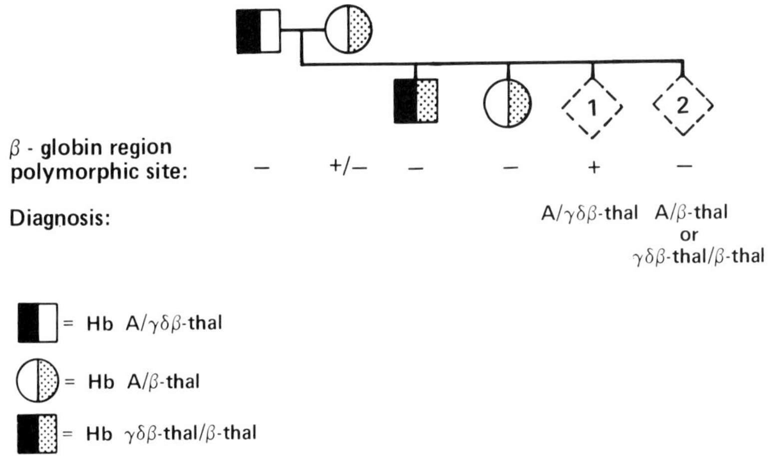

PEDIGREE 7.6 Father carries a large deletion of sequences from the β-globin gene region and the endpoints of this deletion are not detectable with any available probes. In fetus 1, inheritance of the deletion is deduced since no polymorphism type has been inherited from the father. The pattern in fetus 2 is consistent with its being either homozygous for the – polymorphic allele (and thus not having inherited the deletion) or hemizygous for the polymorphic allele (and thus having inherited the deletion).

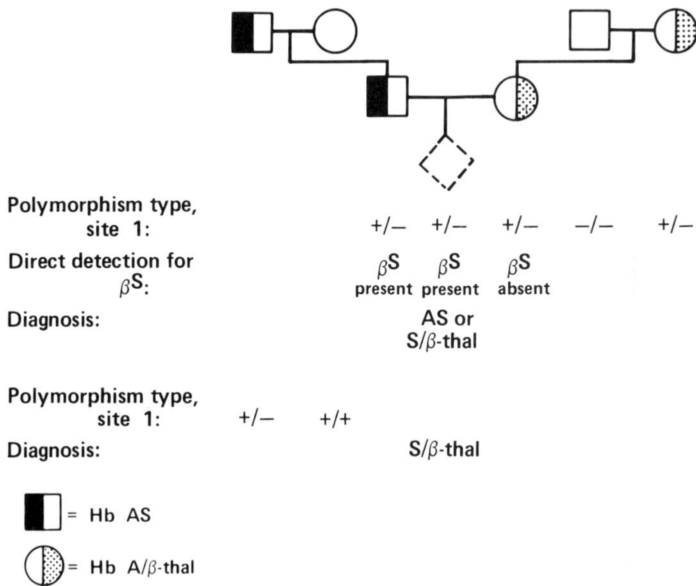

PEDIGREE 7.7 Fetus at risk for Hb S/β-thalassemia. Although the presence or absence of the Hb S allele can be determined in the fetus by direct detection (nonlinkage) methods, it is still necessary to perform family studies on the paternal side of the family since the father and the fetus are heterozygous at the polymorphic site being used for determining allele type inheritance from the mother.

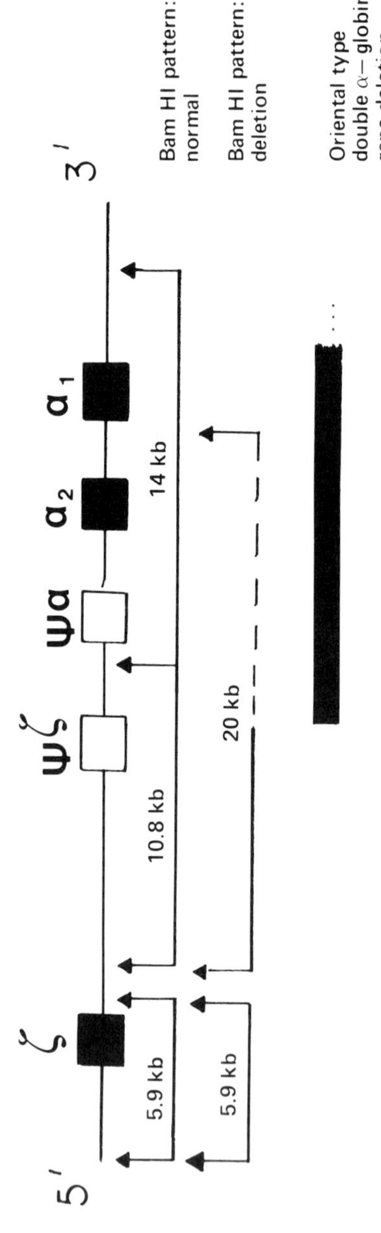

5'
3'
ζ
ψζ
ψα
$α_2$
$α_1$
5.9 kb
5.9 kb
10.8 kb
14 kb
20 kb
Bam HI pattern: normal
Bam HI pattern: deletion
Oriental type double α– globin gene deletion
A

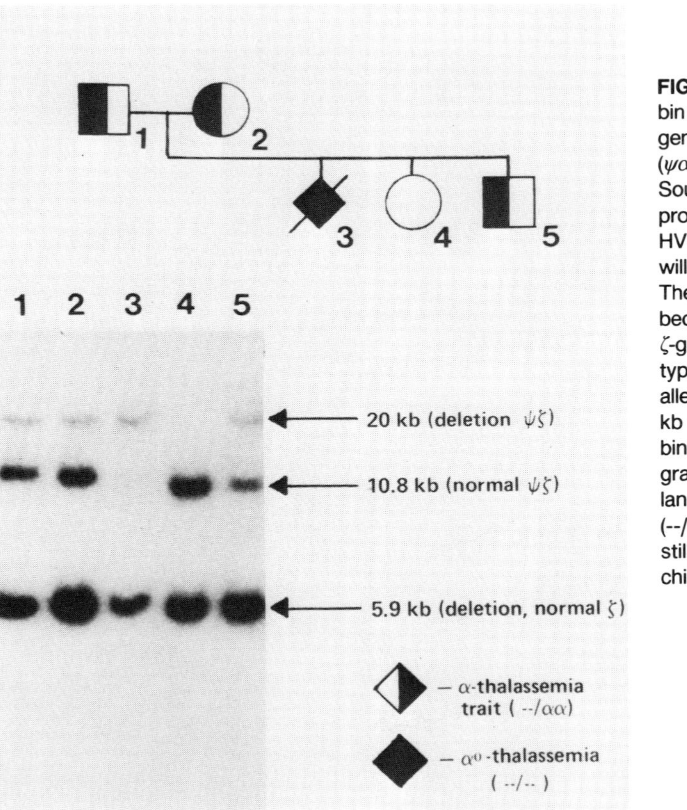

FIGURE 7.3 A: The 30-kb α-globin gene cluster includes one functional ζ-globin gene, two functional α-globin genes (α_2 and α_1) and two inactive pseudogenes, one related to the ζ-globin gene ($\psi\zeta$), and one to the α-globin gene ($\psi\alpha$). Also shown is the BamH I restriction pattern in this gene cluster. A Southern blot of BamH-I-digested DNA when hybridized against a ζ gene probe normally demonstrates 5.9-kb and 10.8-kb fragments. Because of an HVR (hypervariable region) within the 10.8-kb fragment, one of three alleles will exist on any given chromosome (approximately 10.8, 11.5, or 10.0 kb). The 14-kb α-globin-containing fragment is not observed with a ζ-globin probe because of the lack of homology between sequences in this fragment and the ζ-globin probe. The darkened block represents sequences deleted in the typical form of the double α-globin gene deletion in Orientals. In this deletion allele, the 5.9-kb hybridizing fragment is retained and the approximately 10.8-kb fragment is enlarged to 20 kb. The dashed line (----) represents non α-globin-region sequences that are brought in by the deletion. **B:** The autoradiogram shows BamH-I-digested DNA probed with ζ-globin sequences. The lanes represent DNA from parents both of whom are carriers of α-thalassemia (--/$\alpha\alpha$) (lanes 1 and 2), their affected hydropic infant, which was delivered stillborn (lane 3), and their carrier (lane 5) and homozygous normal (lane 4) children.

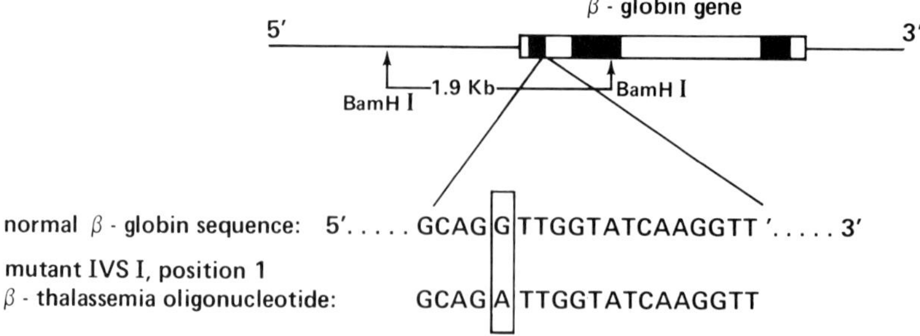

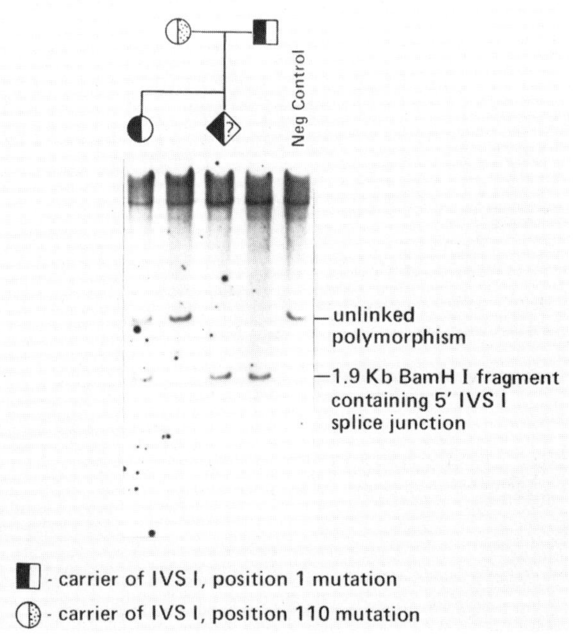

FIGURE 7.4 A: Coding sequences within the β-globin gene are shown as solid boxes (■) and intervening sequences and untranslated 5′ and 3′ parts of the gene are shown as open boxes (□). Below the gene is shown its normal sequence for a 19-nucleotide stretch including the first nucleotide of intervening sequence I (IVS-I) which is boxed. A single nucleotide change of G to A at nucleotide 1 within IVS-1 produces a β^{o}-thalassemia allele. DNA from genes harboring this mutation will hybridize to the oligonucleotide probe shown in the bottom line, but DNA from genes (normal or thalassemia) that do not contain this mutation will not hybridize. The BamH-I restriction sites shown by the arrows delineate the 1.9-kb BamH I fragment within which this sequence lies. **B:** An autoradiogram shows BamH-I-digested DNA hybridized with the mutant oligonucleotide probe (**A**). In the family depicted in the pedigree the father is shown to have this IVS-1 nt 1 mutation, whereas the mother does not. The mother was shown to have the IVS-1 nt 110 β-thalassemia allele in a separate oligonucleotide hybridization experiment. The fetus has inherited the IVS-1 nt 1 allele from the father, as has the carrier child. The carrier child, therefore, has inherited the normal β-globin allele from the mother. Further analysis of the fetal sample, either by hybridization with an oligonucleotide probe for the IVS-1 nt 110 mutation or by polymorphism typing, is required to complete the prenatal diagnosis. A polymorphism unrelated to the β-globin gene region and present in a larger BamH I fragment is detected with the IVS-I nt 1 oligonucleotide probe.

Oligonucleotide Probe Analysis

Oligonucleotide probe analysis is much like Southern blot analysis in that DNA is digested and electrophoresis is carried out. It differs in that a drastically shorter probe, termed an oligonucleotide probe, is used for hybridization (see Fig. 7.4).[35] Each single-stranded oligonucleotide probe is chemically synthesized and is about 20 bases in length, shorter than probes used for Southern blotting by a factor of 10 to 100. Because of their short length, they do not hybridize under appropriate conditions to genomic DNA sequences that differ by even a single nucleotide. Thus, a probe can be designed to detect any variant once the specific nucleotide change and the sequence surrounding the change are known. Rather than a difference in fragment sizes being the distinguishing feature as it is in Southern blot analysis, it is the presence or absence of bands on the autoradiogram that is the diagnostic feature and that indicates whether a particular sequence is present or absent in an individual. Because an individual whose DNA shows hybridization with an oligomer may be either heterozygous or homozygous for that sequence, the use of an oligonucleotide probe to the normal sequence will be necessary for prenatal diagnosis when both parents are carrying the same mutation.

DISORDERS TO WHICH DNA ANALYSIS CAN BE APPLIED FOR DIAGNOSIS

Hemoglobinopathies

Sickle Cell Anemia

The single nucleotide change that produces sickle cell anemia when present in homozygous form also obliterates a normally existing Cvn I recognition site (as well as Dde I, Mst II, and Sau I sites).[48-50] This results in enlargement of what is normally a 1.1-kb fragment to 1.3 kb. The difference in fragment size of 0.2 kb can be detected readily on a Southern blot (see Fig. 7.2). Thus, all fetuses at risk for sickle cell anemia can be diagnosed by use of this endonuclease. To help avoid an error due to an unexpected polymorphism, parental samples should be studied concurrently.

α^o-Thalassemia

Hydrops-fetalis-associated α^o-thalassemia in Orientals is due to homozygosity for a null allele in which both α-globin genes are deleted (— —/— —) (see Fig. 7.3).[51,52] Usually the deletion has a 5′ endpoint within the ξ-globin gene region and results in an abnormally sized ξ-globin fragment.[53,54] This variant is easily detected in a Southern blot using any of several endonucleases and a

ξ-globin probe (see Fig. 7.3). In some Filipinos with α-thalassemia trait ($--/\alpha\alpha$), the deletion spans the entire α-globin gene complex, including both α-globin genes, the $\psi\alpha$, $\psi\xi$, and ξ-globin genes. Some non-deletion α-globin variants alter restriction endonuclease sites,[55,56] but others, including Hb Constant Spring, do not,[57] and their inheritance from one generation to the next can be detected indirectly by use of DNA polymorphisms (both HVRs and restriction site polymorphisms) within the α-globin gene cluster[58–61] or, if they are available, oligonucleotide probes.

δβ-Thalassemia

Most $\delta\beta$-thalassemia alleles result from deletions which include part or all of the δ- and β-globin genes but not the γ- or ε-globin genes.[62] These deletions can be detected by altered DNA fragment sizes, some with a γ-globin probe and some with a β-globin probe, depending on the extent of the deletion.

Hb Lepore

This β-thalassemia allele is a hybrid of the δ- and β-globin genes ($5'\delta$-$3'\beta$) and is accompanied by the loss of the structurally intact δ- and β-globin genes on that chromosome. Because endonuclease sites flanking the δ and β loci differ, the Hb Lepore deletion can be detected directly with any of several endonucleases.[63]

HbO^{Arab} and HbD^{Punjab}

These β-globin variants each cause an amino acid substitution for the glutamic acid at position 121. In HbO^{Arab}, it is replaced by glutamine and in HbD^{Punjab} it is replaced by lysine. Both single nucleotide substitutions delete a normally present EcoRI site and change normal 5.3-kb and 3.2-kb β-globin-specific fragments to a single 8.5-kb fragment. Thus, these variants can be detected directly.[64]

β-Thalassemia

More than 35 point mutations, most of which do not affect restriction endonuclease sites, are known to cause β-thalassemia in world populations.[40–43] In the United States, Canada, Great Britain,[65] and Sicily,* the existence of many different β-thalassemia alleles within the gene pool necessitates the use of a general approach to prenatal diagnosis. Accordingly, linked polymorphisms can be used for predicting the inheritance at the β-globin locus.[32] In contrast, in Sardinia, 95% of β-thalassemia major is due to homozygosity for a nonsense mutation at codon 39. In Sardinia oligonucleotide probes for this

*Kazazian H: Personal communication.

mutation and the corresponding normal sequence have been used for prenatal diagnosis in at least 94 cases.[4]

In the United States and Canada, 93% of members of couples at risk for a child with β-thalassemia are heterozygous at at least one of ten polymorphic sites that are detectable with the following endonuclease and probe: Hind III with a γ-globin probe (2 sites),[66,67] Hinc II (2 sites)[68] and Ava II[69] with a $\psi\beta_1$-globin probe; one site each with Hinf I[70] and Rsa I[71] and a 5′ β-globin probe; one Ava II site[68,72] and one BamH I site[73] with a β-globin probe; and one Hind III site with a 3′ β-globin probe.[74] Because of the high degree of polymorphism heterozygosity within this region, in 87% of at-risk couples both members are heterozygous at one or more polymorphic sites and, assuming family studies will provide the information necessary for establishing coupling phases, all fetuses of these couples can be diagnosed with respect to β-thalassemia status (see Fig. 7.1). For the remaining 13% of couples for whom heterozygosity cannot be found in one of the two parents, sufficient information will have been gathered through polymorphism studies to construct an extensive polymorphism haplotype associated with that parent's β-thalassemia allele.[32] It has been shown that, within a specific ethnic group, most β-thalassemia alleles are associated with only one or two polymorphism haplotypes, presumably because of their relatively recent origin.[32,40,75–77] Thus, once a β-thalassemia-associated haplotype is known, an educated guess can be made as to the mutation that individual carries. This guess can be tested with an appropriate direct detection method (oligonucleotide probe or restriction endonuclease, depending on the mutation), and if that mutant is found this method can in turn be used for prenatal diagnosis. Assuming the other parent is not carrying this same variant, the fetus is also tested at the DNA polymorphic site for which that parent is heterozygous to determine which β-globin allele has been inherited from that parent.

Because carriers of β-thalassemia can be accurately identified by their microcytic red blood cells and elevated levels of Hb A_2, linkage studies do not require that an affected child be available for study. Inheritance patterns may be determined through unaffected children, prospective grandparents, or other relatives of the couple. In our last 2 years' experience, approximately 55% of the couples we studied had not had an affected child but were known to be at risk because they had been screened. Thirty-two percent had no children. Linkage studies were conclusive in 87% of childless couples. One of three family situations will usually be sufficient for linkage analysis. In addition to studying the prospective parents, the study should include (1) an affected or homozygous normal child, (2) all four grandparents of the fetus or (3) one set of grandparents of the fetus and a carrier child of the at-risk couple. The only family situation in which it can be guaranteed a priori that linkage relationships can be determined is one that includes study of either an affected or homozygous normal child and a carrier child. Thus, in most instances, there is no way to predict with absolute assurance ahead of time which relatives will be the informative ones. Linkage relationships will sometimes be determined through study of a surprisingly small number of relatives (such as one parent from each member of a couple) whereas in other situations many more relatives will be required.

Several β-thalassemia mutants can be directly detected because an endonuclease site has been affected by the mutation. These include (1) a C-G change at IVS-2, position 745 of the β-globin gene, which creates a Rsa I site;[75] (2) a G-A change at IVS-2, position 1, which destroys an Hph I site;[78,79] (3) a deletion of the same nucleotide that is substituted in the β^S allele, which destroys the same Cvn I site;[80] and (4) a C-T change in codon 39, which creates a Mae I site.[81] Several deletions large enough to affect fragment sizes to an extent detectable by Southern blotting are known to exist,[28] but only one,[83] a 619-bp deletion of the 3′ part of the β-globin gene and flanking 3′ sequences, is present in any great frequency. This allele accounts for about 30% of β-thalassemia alleles in Indians and is found in Pakistanis as well.

Disorders of Coagulation

Hemophilia A (Classic Hemophilia, Factor VIII:C Deficiency)

Approximately one of every 10,000 males is born with this X-linked recessive disorder. Recently, a human cDNA of the Factor VIII:C gene, the gene affected in hemophilia A, was constructed from mRNA isolated from a human liver.[84] The gene itself is quite large, 186 kb long, and contains 26 exons.[85] To date, two DNA polymorphisms have been found that can be detected with a cDNA probe. One is detected by the endonuclease Bcl I[11] and the other by Bgl I.[86] Approximately 60% of obligate carrier females are heterozygous at one or the other of these two intragenic sites. Three additional polymorphisms that lie outside the gene have been described. A Bgl II polymorphism is detectable with the DX13 probe.[87] Family studies have demonstrated a low rate of recombination between this polymorphic site and the Factor VIII:C gene.[11,87] Winter et al report that the 95% confidence limits place the rate of recombination between this polymorphism and the Factor VIII:C gene at less than 4.5% per meiosis.[15] Approximately 50% of females are heterozygous at this site.[87] Two other linked polymorphisms can be detected with Taq I and Msp I and the ST14 probe.[33] Ninety percent of females are heterozygous at the ST14 locus. The 95% confidence limits for the chance of recombination between ST14 and the Factor VIII:C gene are 0 to 6.5%.[11,33] At least two recombinants have been observed between ST14 and hemophilia-producing mutations.* In one of these two cases an affected male fetus was incorrectly predicted to be unaffected.

Close to 100% of females are heterozygous at at least one of the polymorphic sites described above and, therefore, the applicability of DNA analysis to prenatal and carrier testing is quite high, although it may be accompanied by error rates of up to 5% if a polymorphism detected with either DX13 or ST14 is used. Diagnosis achieved by use of polymorphisms within the Factor VIII:C gene should be quite reliable with an error rate not expected to exceed 1%. Several instances of prenatal and carrier testing through use of the Bcl I[11-14] and Bgl II[10,15] polymorphisms have been described. It is hoped that genomic probes that include the intervening sequences will identify additional polymorphisms that can be used for prenatal and carrier testing, since polymorphisms within the gene are probably more accurate indicators of inheritance of hemophilia A mutations than are polymorphisms less tightly linked to the gene.

Several molecular defects responsible for hemophilia A have been identified within the Factor VIII:C genes of persons with this disease. In three instances, in-phase stop codons have been initially detected by the loss of Taq I restriction sites and then subsequently confirmed by nucleotide sequencing (two cases)[88] and oligonucleotide analysis (one case).[86] These nonsense mutations have been found in exon 24, exon 26,[88] and exon 18.[86] Intragenic deletions have also been detected. Two are in the 3′ end of the gene and are 30 kb and 21.9 kb long each.[88] One is in the middle of the gene and is 80 kb in length.[86] In a recent report of the molecular defects in another six hemophilia genes, it is suggested that 20% of the disease-producing mutations can be identified by screening of the DNA with three endonucleases and two probes.[89]

Hemophilia B (Christmas Disease, Factor IX Deficiency)

Hemophilia B is also an X-linked recessive disorder and affects about one of every 50,000 males born. cDNA gene probes for the Factor IX gene were first isolated in 1982 and 1983.[90-92] An intragenic Taq I polymorphism, which is diagnostic in about 40% of cases,[93,94] has been used several times for prenatal diagnosis and carrier detection.[16,94,95] Three other intragenic polymorphisms that can be detected with the full-length cDNA probe have been described.[96,97] One alters a Xmn I recognition site, and another, which is actually the presence or absence of a 50-bp sequence that probably arose through duplication, can be detected by either Hinf I or Dde I.[96] Recently, an Msp I polymorphism has also been described.[97] Three of the polymorphisms (Xmn, Taq, and Hinf I) lie within a 6.5-kb stretch of the gene. The four

*Phillips D, Kazazian H: Personal communication.

polymorphisms together are useful for diagnosis in approximately 66% of cases, despite the existence of linkage disequilibrium among the sites.[96] Because the polymorphisms are all intragenic, their accuracy as predictive indicators of Factor IX deficiency in informative families is approximately 99%.

Factor IX gene deletions were specifically looked for in a small subset of hemophilia B patients who had produced anti-Factor IX antibodies.[98] Five patients were examined and four of the five had gross rearrangements of the gene. Two had deletions greater than 18 kb in length, one of which had a residual section of the gene, the other had no gene sequences detectable with a full-length cDNA probe. The third had a deletion larger than 9 kb long with part of the gene clearly still present, and the fourth had some type of unidentified gross alteration of the gene. Three further cases of at least partial deletion of the Factor IX gene have been described and the deletions used for carrier detection in the three families in which the respective deletions were segregating.[99-101] In addition, one instance of a splice junction mutation has been described.[102]

Duchenne Muscular Dystrophy

In 1982 and 1983, linkage of the DMD locus with two anonymous X-chromosome probes was described.[103-105] The two DNA clones, designated RC8 and L1.28, appeared to flank the DMD locus, one on each side, and each appeared to be about 15 cM from the DMD locus.[105] Taq I polymorphisms were found with each probe, and females were heterozygous 22% of the time for the polymorphism detected with the RC8 probe and 45% of the time for the polymorphism detected with the L1.28 probe. Use of one polymorphism alone for carrier detection or prenatal testing was not recommended because of the approximately 15% chance of an error due to meiotic recombination. However, the polymorphisms could be useful in situations in which the known carrier females were heterozygous at both polymorphisms. This would reduce the chance of a diagnostic error due to recombination to situations in which recombination had occurred twice, once between the DMD locus and the RC8 polymorphic site and again between the DMD locus and the L1.28 polymorphic site. The likelihood of this occurrence per mieosis would be approximately $.15 \times .15$, or 2%.[106,107] Since only a small percentage of females would be heterozygous at both sites, the applicability of these two sites for diagnosis was low.

Subsequently, a number of other DMD-linked clones were identified (including the OTC locus)[107-112] at distances from the DMD locus ranging from 3 to 20 cM. Summaries of the polymorphisms detectable with these clones, their locations relative to one another and the DMD locus, the frequencies of their polymorphic alleles,[18,113,114] and their use in carrier determination and prenatal diagnosis and in documentation of a new mutation have been published.[18]

Recently, two groups independently have reported the cloning of sequences apparently closer yet to the DMD locus. The approach taken by Kunkel and colleagues was to clone sequences homologous to those absent in a male with a cytogenetically visible deletion who had three X-linked recessive disorders of which one was DMD.[115] Of 81 clones isolated, one, designated pERT 87, identified deletions of at least 38 kb in 5 of 57 unrelated males with DMD.[19] Within this clone a number of polymorphisms have been identified that are believed to be approximately 95% accurate in predicting inheritance of alleles at the DMD locus.* Five of these polymorphisms confer heterozygosity on approximately 90% of females, making them quite useful for prenatal diagnosis and carrier detection. These are an Xmn I polymorphism detectable with clone pERT 87-1, Bst XI with 87-8, Xmn I, Taq I, and Bam HI polymorphisms each detectable with 87-15, Bgl II with 87-30, and Bam HI with j-Bir. In another laboratory, Ray and associates have cloned sequences involved in an X/21 chromosome translocation associated with DMD in a female carrying the balanced translocation.[20] The two laboratories have exchanged DNA samples from their patients with DMD and report slightly less than total concurrence for deletions detected with their respective probes. A Taq I polymorphism has been detected with the clone XJ-1.1 which was isolated from the translocation, and this polymorphism, too, for which 41% of females are heterozygous, is useful for prenatal diagnosis and carrier detection. The most accurate use of these polymorphisms in diagnosis will be achieved in instances in which women are heterozygous at several of the polymorphic sites. The risk of an error due to meiotic recombination will be reduced when longer stretches of this complex can be determined to have been inherited apparently free of recombination. Great effort is now focused on identifying the gene affected in DMD.

α_1-Antitrypsin Deficiency

Severe α_1-antitrypsin deficiency is an autosomal recessively inherited condition in which about 80% of homozygotes for the Pi^Z allele develop degenerative lung disease and pulmonary emphysema. In addition, about 14% develop cirrhosis of the liver as infants which is often fatal. The Pi^Z allele results from a single amino acid substitution (lysine for glutamic acid) at position 52 from the carboxyl terminus of the α_1-antitrypsin gene.[116,117] Synthetic oli-

*Kunkel L: Personal communication.

gonucleotide probes can be used to identify individuals homozygous for the normal allele (MM), homozygous for the defective allele (ZZ), and heterozygous (MZ).[118] The use of these oligonucleotides for prenatal diagnosis has been reported.[6] In addition, the Pi^Z allele is strongly associated (54/54 ZZ individuals) with a particular allele at an Ava II polymorphism 3′ to the α_1-antitrypsin gene; this allele has not been observed in 32 unaffected (ie, not ZZ) individuals.[7] Because of this strong linkage disequilibrium, this polymorphism also can have great applicability to prenatal diagnosis of α_1-antitrypsin deficiency.

Classical Phenylketonuria

A human phenylalanine hydroxylase (PAH) cDNA was isolated in 1983,[119] and 10 restriction site polymorphisms have been identified with this cDNA.[8] Southern blots prepared from DNA of individuals with classical phenylketonuria (PKU) almost never detect any major structural rearrangements in affected genes.* This suggests that most PKU mutations are due to single nucleotide substitutions or small insertions or deletions, as is the case with β-thalassemia. The observation that multiple polymorphism haplotypes are coupled with PAH-deficient genes[120] and that studies of PAH mRNA in liver from patients with PKU[121] suggest that multiple mutations may be responsible for the disorder in world populations.

Because the PAH gene is expressed only in liver, there is no biochemical assay suitable for use as a generalized screening test for carrier detection. Thus, the diagnostic potential for this disease is currently restricted to the use of linked polymorphisms in families in which there is an affected child. Because of the high heterozygosity rate at the polymorphic loci, use of the polymorphisms for prenatal diagnosis for fetuses of parents of affected children and/or carrier testing for unaffected siblings is possible for approximately 90% of families.[8] Several prenatal diagnoses have been achieved through use of these polymorphisms,[9] but it is expected that many couples in which both partners are known carriers may decline prenatal testing because dietary control can effectively minimize or eliminate mental retardation in affected persons, the main complication of the disease.

The phenotype of hyperphenylalaninemia may also be expressed through mutations at loci other than the phenylalanine hydroxylase gene, such as in persons with dihydropteridine reductase deficiency or a defect in dihydrobiopterin synthesis.[122] In these conditions, the PAH genes are thought to be normal. Thus, in families in which these disorders are segre-

*Woo SLC: Personal communication.

gating, the PAH-associated polymorphisms cannot be used to indicate inheritance or noninheritance of the hyperphenylalaninemia phenotype.

Ornithine Transcarbamylase Deficiency

A human cDNA to the X-linked ornithine transcarbamylase (OTC) gene was isolated in 1984.[123] Two Msp I polymorphisms have been identified with this probe that together confer heterozygosity on 69% of females, thus making available prenatal diagnosis and/or carrier detection for the majority of families.[124] Of the four polymorphism haplotypes theoretically possible with these two Msp polymorphisms, all four were found among 15 OTC-deficient genes, indicating that multiple mutations are probably responsible for this disease. This is not unexpected, since one-third of the cases for this lethal X-linked disease are probably due to new mutations.[44] In another instance, OTC deficiency was accompanied by a deletion large enough to be visible on chromosome analysis in an affected boy. In a subsequent pregnancy for the mother of this child, OTC deficiency was ruled out by virtue of the presence of OTC-hybridizing sequences in a male fetus.[17]

Of 15 OTC-deficient genes examined by Rozen and co-workers,[124] only one gene deletion was identified, indicating that most mutations are probably due to single nucleotide substitutions or small insertions or deletions. Two cases of the loss of the same Taq I restriction site associated with OTC deficiency in unrelated boys have been reported. It was possible to identify the source of the mutation in both families, demonstrating the independent origins of these two alleles. The exact nucleotide change in each has not been determined, but it is possible that both of these changes represent the creation of a new stop codon within the gene.[125]

Cystic Fibrosis

Recently, several groups have reported linkage of the cystic fibrosis (CF) phenotype with polymorphic loci on chromosome 7.[21,23,126,127] One anonymous locus, DOCRI-917, shows an approximately 15% recombination rate with the CF gene in 39 families.[23,126] Another, the met oncogene, maps between q21 and q31 on chromosome 7[127] and shows 0% recombination in 13 families (21). In June 1986, it was reported by another group that out of 100 informative meioses only one recombinant was seen, indicating extremely tight linkage.[128] Another locus, J3.11, assigned to chromosome 7 cen-q22 also shows tight linkage with the CF gene (22); no recombinants out of 27 meioses were seen. By using a total of six polymorphic sites (Taq I and Ban I with met D oncogene probe, Taq I and Msp I with the met H oncogene probe, and Msp I and Taq I with the J3.11 probe) 75 to 80% of couples with

CF children will be fully informative, and prenatal diagnosis can be carried out in all pregnancies. In the remaining 20 to 25% of couples, one member will usually be heterozygous at one or more sites and an affected fetus can be ruled out in approximately 50% of their pregnancies. Thus, the total diagnostic rate using polymorphisms detected by either the met oncogene or J3.11 is 85 to 90%.

No evidence has been found of nonlinkage of a CF gene with these chromosome 7 polymorphic loci.

SOURCES OF ERROR IN DNA DIAGNOSIS BY SOUTHERN BLOTTING

Contamination of Genomic DNA with Probe DNA

After 6 years of experience with prenatal diagnosis in several labs, it is clear that the most common source of error has been contamination of fetal DNA with probe DNA sequences.[129] This has occurred in several different labs and, as a result, several fetuses with sickle cell anemia have been incorrectly diagnosed as having sickle cell trait. The probes being used were originally constructed from β^A alleles and, therefore, when digested with Cvn I, yielded the normal, β^A-sized fragment. The autoradiograms with the diagnostic errors displayed both a β^S-sized fragment, which originated from fetal DNA, and a β^A-sized fragment, which originated from probe DNA. This source of error can be eliminated through use of a probe that, should it be introduced into a fetal DNA sample, could not be confused with fetal fragments. One way to achieve this is to construct a probe that has one endpoint within sequences present in the genomic DNA fragment that is detected by the probe. In this case, digested plasmid DNA would yield a fragment size clearly distinguishable from any genomic fragments. If contamination were to occur, it would be evident on the autoradiogram, but an incorrect interpretation of the results would not occur because of it. In some instances, cDNA probes can be helpful in avoiding this type of error because there are gaps in homology between the genomic DNA and the probe cDNA at points where the introns have been removed.

Incomplete Endonuclease Digestion of DNA

Occasionally, an endonuclease will not cleave genomic DNA at all possible sites. When this happens, some of the bands on an autoradiogram may be of normal size, but not indicative of the pattern from the individual being studied. Presence of the larger fragment, or absence of the smaller, could lead to misinterpretation of the restriction pattern. Some probes may provide useful internal controls for detection of incomplete digestion. For instance, a β-globin cDNA probe cross-hybridizes with δ-globin-containing fragments. Incomplete digestion at the polymorphic Hpa I site 3′ to the β-globin gene will often be accompanied by incomplete digestion at a nonpolymorphic Hpa I site within the δ-globin gene. The presence of a δ-globin fragment of abnormal size could indicate that digestion at the Hpa I site 3′ to β may be incomplete. Comparison of the relative intensities of the polymorphic bands with other constant bands on the autoradiogram might also be helpful in detecting incomplete digestion.

While grossly incomplete DNA digestion will be obvious on an autoradiogram, the tell-tale signs of partial digestion, which is the form of incomplete digestion most likely to cause misdiagnosis, are more subtle. They consist of unexpected, larger than normal band(s) in the presence of normal sized bands. These subtle changes can be most readily detected on autoradiograms in which the background signal is minimal. This is especially important when working with fetal samples, which often contain less DNA than desired.

Linkage Analysis

There are three sources of error unique to linkage analysis.

Meiotic Recombination

Meiotic recombination between the polymorphic site and the disease locus can cause an error in diagnosis. In general, when the informative polymorphic sites are within the affected gene, the likelihood of meiotic recombination is lower than when sites outside the gene are used. However, some genes are quite large (Factor VIII is 186 kb and phenylalanine hydroxylase is 100 kb), and meiotic recombination may be more likely within these genes than within the smaller genes, such as β-globin, which is 1.5 kb long. It is known that the likelihood of meiotic recombination between two sites is not only a function of the distance between the sites, although this is certainly a major factor. For instance, the chance of recombination between the β-globin gene and a polymorphic Hinc II site 13 kb in the 5′ direction is estimated to be 1/350, whereas that between the gene and a polymorphic Bam HI site 9 kb in the 3′ direction is about 1/2000.[39,68] Thus, empiric data are an important factor in determining recombination rates.

When polymorphic sites are somewhat removed from a disease site, use of polymorphisms on both sides of a disease locus can reduce the possibility of an error drastically since two recombination events (one on either side of the disease locus) would be necessary for an error to go undetected. This approach was used for DMD testing with an anonymous polymorphism 15 cM from the gene on one side and another polymorphism 15 cM on the other side of the gene. By using these polymorphic sites on either side of the DMD locus, the chance of error due to recombination was reduced to the chance of recombination between the disease site and both polymorphisms, which is $.15 \times .15$, or about 2%.[106,107]

False Paternity

When a polymorphism is used to track the inheritance of a mutation, correct identification of the biologic father is essential for test accuracy. False assumptions of biologic paternity can result in identification of the wrong polymorphism type as being associated with the mutant gene and, therefore, in a mistake in the prenatal diagnosis (Fig. 7.5). As the number of family members necessary for establishing a linkage phase increases, the greater the chance is that false paternity will have occurred at some point in the pedigree. This, in turn, increases the chances of an error in the prenatal diagnosis due to false paternity. For autosomal recessive disorders for which carrier testing exists, a family study for DNA analysis might include grandparents or aunts and uncles or even cousins of a fetus because the presence or absence of the mutant gene can be detected in these individuals, and the inheritance of the mutant gene with the key polymorphism can be determined. However, when carrier testing is not possible for an autosomal recessive disorders, only DNA from members within the immediate family will be helpful in establishing which polymorphism has been coinherited with the mutant gene. Thus, the chance that false paternity might result in an error in a diagnosis increases as

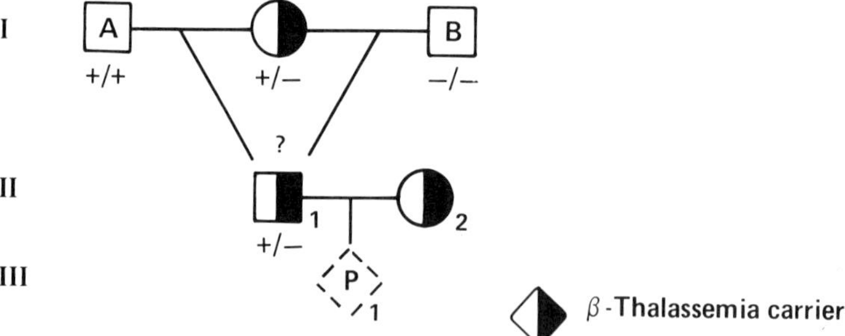

FIGURE 7.5 An example of how false paternity can produce an error in a prenatal diagnosis. Restriction patterns at a single polymorphic site linked to the β-globin gene are shown for individuals in this pedigree. If the prospective father's father is individual A, it is deduced that II-1's β-thalassemia allele is coupled with his polymorphic − allele. However, if it is individual B, it is deduced that II-1's β-thalassemia allele is coupled with his polymorphic + allele. If this polymorphism is used for linkage studies in the fetus (III-1) an error will be made in the prenatal diagnosis if the non-biologic father of II-1 has been used in the study.

the number of family members included in the study increases, and it is for autosomal recessive disorders with carrier tests that analysis of large pedigrees for linkage studies is sometimes undertaken. For X-linked recessive disorders, false paternity in a fetus or male offspring is not a source of error in diagnosis, but false paternity can cause an error in determination of carrier status and establishment of linkage phases in females. Although the issue of paternity can be an uncomfortable topic to discuss with families undergoing linkage analysis, it is a potential source of error about which they should be informed. At the same time, they can be made aware of any alternative methods of prenatal diagnosis in which the accuracy of the test is not dependent on paternity issues, such as fetoscopy for β-thalassemia and the coagulation disorders. Perhaps this crucial information can be most easily given by the counselor and accepted by the consultand during a preliminary intake phone call when other family members are not yet involved.*

Interlocus Heterogeneity

For DNA polymorphisms to be used in making accurate diagnoses, one requirement absolutely must be met: the polymorphism being used must be closely linked to the disease locus. Some single gene disorders are genetically more complicated than others in the sense that mutations within different, unlinked genes are responsible for disease states that appear identical clinically. Osteogenesis imperfecta (OI) type II is such a disorder.[130] In one family this disease state has been shown to result from mutation in the pro-α1 collagen gene (located on chromosome 17),[131] and in another family from mutation in the pro-α2 collagen gene (located on chromosome 7).[132] Use of polymorphisms linked to the pro-α1 gene would have no relevance at all to inheritance of the OI type II phenotype in the second family. In addition, the original pro collagen transcript undergoes several posttranslational modification steps that are directed by different enzymes, any of which might also produce the same disease state if altered.[133] Thus, the application of DNA polymorphisms to the prenatal diagnosis of OI type II will be restricted to families for whom an investigator has undertaken the task of characterizing the specific defect responsible for OI type II in their family. Alternatively, OI type II may often be diagnosable in utero by sonography in the midtrimester of pregnancy.

After the initial recognition of a disease state as being linked to a polymorphic site, subsequent testing will often be necessary to determine whether mutations in more than one gene can produce the phenotypically identical single gene disorder. By establishing that the disease-producing locus is linked to the same site in numerous unrelated families, the chance

*Hutton E: Personal communication.

that a diagnostic error will be made because of nonlinkage will decrease. Such studies are currently being undertaken in efforts to establish that the gene responsible for Huntington's disease is always linked to the G8 locus on chromosome 4 and the gene responsible for cystic fibrosis is always linked to the 311-met oncogene complex of loci on chromosome 7q. This type of correlation is especially important for disorders in which the primary defect has not yet been determined, for example, Huntington's disease and CF.

THE JOHNS HOPKINS EXPERIENCE

Between 1978 and April 1986 our laboratory has studied 632 pregnancies for diagnosis of a hemoglobinopathy (sickle cell anemia, 363; β-thalassemia, 150; α^{o}-thalassemia, 37; SC disease, 22; S/β-thalassemia, 15; E/β-thalassemia 2; S/O^{Arab}, 1; β-thalassemia/$\delta\beta$-thalassemia, 1). Thirty-eight pregnancies have been studied for hemophilia A, and three for Duchenne muscular dystrophy. Diagnosis was possible for 93% of the cases.

Two errors have been made. One was in a prenatal diagnosis for sickle cell anemia. An affected fetus was incorrectly diagnosed as having sickle cell trait. This error was due to contamination of the fetal DNA with probe DNA sequences prior to Mst II digestion. Since the discovery of this mistake the probe we use has been shortened and an Mst II site has thus been removed. The other mistake was in a fetus at risk for β-thalassemia. This fetus, which was a carrier for β-thalassemia, was incorrectly diagnosed as being affected. The result was due to a faulty linkage assumption based on results from a diagnosis made in a previous pregnancy.

Forty-eight couples have requested more than one prenatal diagnosis. Of these, 43 have had two pregnancies studied, four have had three pregnancies studied, and one has had four. Of this total, 15 were studied for sickle cell anemia, 27 for β-thalassemia, 5 for α^{o}-thalassemia, and 1 for S/β-thalassemia.

Of the last 50 families studied because of β-thalassemia risk, only 19 (38%) had a previously affected child. Many couples were identified as being at risk through screening programs. In almost all of these couples, family members were informative for the establishment of polymorphism coupling phases.

Follow-up information has been difficult to obtain, and many families have been lost to follow-up. This is unfortunate because the validity of new tests such as these is dependent on obtaining follow-up studies. Of 208 pregnancies studied in which subsequent posttermination or postnatal study has been possible, the prenatal diagnosis was found to be correct in 206 (99%).

ACKNOWLEDGMENTS

I would like to thank Dr. Haig Kazazian, Jr., for his help and guidance in the writing of this manuscript. Also, I would like to thank Mrs. Emily Pasterfield for her patience and efforts in its preparation.

REFERENCES

1. Kan YW, Golbus MS, Dozy AM: Prenatal diagnosis of α-thalassemia: Clinical application of molecular hybridization. *N Engl J Med* 1976;295:1165–1167.
2. Kan YW, Dozy AM: Antenatal diagnosis of sickle cell anemia by DNA analysis of amniotic fluid cells. *Lancet* 1978;2:910–912.
3. Boehm CD, Antonarakis SE, Phillips JA, III, et al: Prenatal diagnosis using DNA polymorphisms: Report on 95 pregnancies at risk for sickle cell disease or β-thalassemia. *N Engl J Med* 1983;308:1054–1058.
4. Rosatelli C, Tuveri T, DiTucci A, et al: Prenatal diagnosis of β-thalassemia with the synthetic-oligomer technique. *Lancet* 1985;1:241–243.
5. Alter BP: Antenatal diagnosis of thalassemia: A review. *Annals of the New York Academy of Sciences* 1985;445:393–407.
6. Kidd JV, Golbus MS, Wallace BR, et al: Prenatal diagnosis of α_1-antitrypsin deficiency by direct analysis of the mutation site in the gene. *N Engl J Med* 1984;310:639–642.
7. Cox DW, Mansfield T: Prenatal diagnosis for alpha$_1$-antitrypsin deficiency. *Lancet* 1985;1:230.
8. Lidsky AS, Ledley FD, DiLella AG, et al: Extensive restriction site polymorphism at the human phenylalanine hydroxylase locus and application in prenatal diagnosis of phenylketonuria. *Am J Hum Genet* 1985;37:619–634.
9. Lidsky AS, Guttler F, Woo SLC: Prenatal diagnosis of classical phenylketonuria by DNA analysis. *Lancet* 1985;1:549–551.
10. Tonnessen T, Sondergaard F, Mikkelsen M, et al: X-chromosome-specific probe DX13 for carrier detection and first trimester prenatal diagnosis in haemophilia A. *Lancet* 1984;2:1269–1270.
11. Gitschier J, Drayna D, Tuddenham EGD, et al: Genetic mapping and diagnosis of hemophilia A achieved through a Bcl I polymorphism in the Factor VIII gene. *Nature* 1985;314:738–740.
12. Gitschier J, Lawn RM, Rotblat F, et al: Antenatal diagnosis and carrier detection of haemophilia A using Factor VIII gene probe. *Lancet* 1985;1:1093–1094.
13. Antonarakis SE, Carpenter RJ, Jr., Hoyer LW, et al: Prenatal diagnosis of haemophilia A by Factor VIII gene analysis. *Lancet* 1985;1:1407–1409.
14. Din N, Schwartz M, Kruse T, et al: Factor VIII gene specific probe for prenatal diagnosis of haemophilia A. *Lancet* 1985;1:1446–1447.
15. Winter RM, Harper K, Goldman E, et al: First trimester prenatal diagnosis and detection of carriers of haemophilia A using the linked DNA probe DX13. *Br Med J* 1985;291:765–769.
16. Tonnessen T, Sondergaard F, Guttler F, et al: Exclusion of haemophilia B in a male fetus by chorionic villus biopsy. *Lancet* 1984;2:932.
17. Old JM, Purvis-Smith S, Wilcken B, et al: Prenatal exclusion of ornithine transcarbamylase deficiency by direct gene analysis. *Lancet* 1985;1:73–75.
18. Bakker E, Goor N, Wrogemann K, et al: Prenatal diagnosis and carrier detection of Duchenne muscular dystrophy with closely linked RFLPs. *Lancet* 1985;1:655–658.

19. Monaco AP, Bertelson CJ, Middleworth W, et al: Detection of deletions spanning the Duchenne muscular dystrophy locus using a tightly linked DNA segment. *Nature* 1985;316:842–845.
20. Ray PN, Belfall B, Duff C, et al: Cloning of the breakpoint of an X;21 translocation associated with Duchenne muscular dystrophy. *Nature* 1985;318:672–675.
21. White R, Woodward S, Leppert M, et al: A closely linked marker for cystic fibrosis. *Nature* 1985;318:382–384.
22. Wainwright BJ, Scambler PJ, Schmidtke J, et al: Localization of cystic fibrosis to human chromosome 7 cen-q22. *Nature* 1985;318:384–385.
23. Buchwald M, Barker D, Braman JC, et al: Cystic fibrosis locus defined by a genetically linked polymorphic DNA marker. *Science* 1985;230:1054–1057.
24. Alter BP: Prenatal diagnosis of hemoglobinopathies: A status report. *Lancet* 1981; 2:1152–1155.
25. Rodeck CH, Patrick AD, Pembrey ME, et al: Fetal liver biopsy for prenatal diagnosis of ornithine carbamyl transferase deficiency. *Lancet* 1982;2:297–300.
26. Holzgreve W, Golbus MS: Prenatal diagnosis of ornithine transcarbamylase deficiency. *Am J Hum Genet* 1984;36:320–328.
27. NICHD National Registry for Amniocentesis Study Group. Midtrimester amniocentesis for prenatal diagnosis: Safety and accuracy. *JAMA* 1975;236:1471–1476.
28. Simoni G, Brambati B, Danesino C, et al: Diagnostic application of first trimester trophoblast sampling in 100 pregnancies. *Hum Genet* 1984;66:252–259.
29. Jahoda MGJ, Vosters RPL, Sachs ES, et al: Safety of chorionic villus sampling. *Lancet* 1985;2:941–942.
30. Jackson JG: First-trimester diagnosis of fetal genetic disorders. *Hosp Pract* 1985; 20:39–48.
31. Gusella JF, Wexler NS, Conneally PM, et al: A polymorphic DNA marker genetically linked to Huntington's disease. *Nature* 1983;307:234–238.
32. Boehm CD, Kazazian HH, Jr: Use of restriction site polymorphism for prenatal diagnosis of hemoglobinopathies. In Loukopoulos D (ed): *Prenatal Diagnosis of Thalassemia*. Boca Raton, FL, CRC Press, to be published.
33. Oberle I, Camerino G, Heilig R, et al: Genetic screening for hemophilia A (classic hemophilia) with a polymorphic DNA probe. *N Engl J Med* 1985;312:682–686.
34. Southern EM: Gel electrophoresis of restriction fragments. *Meth Enzymol* 1979; 68:152–176.
35. Wallace RB, Schold M, Johnson MJ, et al: Oligonucleotide directed mutagenesis of the human β-globin gene. A general method for producing specific point mutations in cloned DNA. *Nucl Acids Res* 1981;9:3647–3656.
36. Meyers RM, Lumelsky N, Lerman LS: Detection of single base substitutions in total genomic DNA. *Nature* 1985;313:495–498.
37. Saiki RK, Bugawan TL, Horn ET, et al: Analysis of enzymatically amplified β-globin and HLA-DQα-DNA with allele-specific oligonucleotide probes. *Nature* 1986;324:163–166.
38. Kan YW, Dozy AM: Polymorphism of DNA sequences adjacent to human β-globin structural gene: Relationship to sickle mutation. *Proc Natl Acad Sci USA* 1978;75:5631–5635.
39. Chakravarti A, Buetow KH, Antonarakis SE, et al: Non-uniform recombination within the human β-globin gene cluster. *Am J Hum Genet* 1984;36:1239–1258.
40. Orkin SH, Kazazian HH, Jr: The mutation and polymorphisms of the human β-globin gene and its surrounding DNA. *Ann Rev Genet* 1984;18:131–171.
41. Kazazian HH, Jr: The Nature of Mutation. *Hosp Pract* 1985;20:55–69.
42. Kazazian HH, Jr, Orkin SH, Boehm CD, et al: Characterization of a spontaneous mutation to a β-thalassemia allele. *Am J Hum Genet*, to be published.

43. Boehm CD, Dowling CE, Waber PG, et al: Use of oligonucleotide hybridization in the characterization of a β^{0}-thalassemia gene ($\beta^{37\ TGG\text{-}TGA}$) in a Saudi Arabian. *Blood* 67, to be published.
44. Haldane JBS: *J Genet* 1935;31:317-326.
45. Emery AEH: Genetic counselling. *Scot Med J* 1969;14:335-347.
46. Gale AN, Murphy EA: The use of serum creatine phosphokinase in genetic counseling for Duchenne muscular dystrophy. *J Chron Dis* 1978;31:101-109.
47. Murphy EA, Chase GA: *Principles of Genetic Counseling,* Chicago, Year Book Medical Publishers, 1975.
48. Geever RF, Wilson LB, Nallaseth FS, et al: Direct identification of sickle cell anemia by blot hybridization. *Proc Natl Acad Sci USA* 1981;78:5081-5085.
49. Orkin SH, Little PFR, Kazazian HH, Jr, et al: Improved detection of the sickle mutation by DNA analysis. *N Engl J Med* 1982;307:32-36.
50. Chang JC, Kan YW: A sensitive new prenatal test for sickle cell anemia. *N Engl J Med* 1982;307:30-32.
51. Ottolenghi S, Lanyon WG, Paul J, et al: The severe form of α-thalassemia is caused by a haemoglobin gene deletion. *Nature* 1974;251:389-391.
52. Taylor JM, Dozy A, Kan YW, et al: Genetic lesion in homozygous alpha thalassemia (hydrops fetalis). *Nature* 1974;251:392-393.
53. Lauer J, Shen C-KJ, Maniatis T: The chromosomal arrangement of human α-like globin genes: Sequence homology and α-globin gene deletion. *Cell* 1980;20:119-130.
54. Pressley L, Higgs DR, Clegg JB, et al: Gene deletions in α-thalassemia prove that the 5′ zeta locus is functional. *Proc Natl Acad Sci USA* 1980;77:3586-3589.
55. Orkin SH, Goff SC, Hechtman RL: Mutation in an intervening sequence splice junction in man. *Proc Natl Acad Sci USA* 1981;78:5041-5045.
56. Pirastu M, Saglio G, Chang JC, et al: Initiation codon mutation as a cause of α-thalassemia. *J Biol Chem* 1984;259:12315-12317.
57. Higgs DR, Pressley L, Aldridge B, et al: Genetic and molecular diversity in nondeletion HbH disease. *Proc Natl Acad Sci USA* 1981;78:5833-5837.
58. Higgs DR, Goodbourn SEY, Wainscoat JS, et al: Highly variable regions of DNA flank the human α-globin genes. *Nucl Acids Res* 1981;9:4213-4224.
59. Beutler E, Kuhl W, Johnson C: A common mutant EcoRI restriction endonuclease site in the 5′ flanking portion of the human α-globin gene. *Proc Natl Acad Sci USA* 1981; 78:7056-7058.
60. Goodbourn SEY, Higgs DR, Clegg JB, et al: Molecular basis of length polymorphism in the human ζ-globin gene complex. *Proc Natl Acad Sci USA* 1983;80:5022-5026.
61. Wainscoat JS, Higgs DR, Kanavakis E, et al: Association of two DNA polymorphisms in the α-globin gene cluster: Implications for genetic analysis. *Am J Hum Genet* 1983; 35:1086-1089.
62. Weatherall DJ, Clegg JB: Thalassemia revisited. *Cell* 1982;29:7-9.
63. Flavell RA, Kooter JM, DeBoer E, et al: Analysis of the β-δ-globin gene loci in normal and Hb Lepore DNA: Direct determination of gene linkage and intergene distance. *Cell* 1978;15:25-41.
64. Phillips JA, III, Kazazian HH, Jr: Globin gene analysis by restriction endonuclease mapping, in Fairbanks VR (ed): *Current Hematology.* New York, Wiley Medical, 1981, p. 24.
65. Thein SL, Old JM, Fiorelli G, et al: Feasibility of prenatal diagnosis of β-thalassemia with synthetic DNA probes in two Mediterranean populations. *Lancet* 1985;2:345-347.
66. Jeffreys AJ: DNA sequence variants in the ${}^{G}\gamma$-, ${}^{A}\gamma$-, δ-, and β-globin genes of man. *Cell* 1979;18:1-10.
67. Tuan D, Biro PA, DeRiel JK, et al: Restriction endonuclease mapping of the human γ-globin gene loci. *Nucl Acids Res* 1979;6:2519-2544.

68. Antonarakis SE, Boehm CD, Giardina PJV, et al: Nonrandom association of polymorphic restriction sites in the β-globin gene cluster. *Proc Natl Acad Sci USA* 1982; 79:137–141.
69. Wainscoat DH, Thein SL, Old JM: A new DNA polymorphism for prenatal diagnosis of β-thalassemia in Mediterranean populations. *Lancet* 1984;2:1299–1301.
70. Moschonas N, deBoer E, Flavell R: The DNA sequence of the 5′ flanking region of the human β-globin gene: Evolutionary conservation and polymorphic differences. *Nucl Acids Res* 1982;10:2109–2120.
71. Semenza GL, Malladi P, Poncz M, et al: Detection of a novel DNA polymorphism in the β-globin cluster and evidence for site-specific recombination. *Ped Res* 1984;18:225a.
72. Driscoll MC, Baird M, Bank A, et al: A new polymorphism in the human β-globin gene useful in antenatal diagnosis. *J Clin Invest* 1981;68:915–919.
73. Kan YW, Lee KY, Furbetta M, et al: Polymorphism of DNA sequence in the β-globin gene region: Application to prenatal diagnosis of β^o-thalassemia in Sardinia. *N Engl J Med* 1980;302:185–188.
74. Tuan D, Feingold E, Newman M, et al: Different 3′ endpoints of deletions causing δβ-thalassemia and HPFH. *Proc Natl Acad Sci USA* 1983;80:6937–6941.
75. Orkin SH, Kazazian HH, Jr, Antonarakis SE, et al: Linkage of β-thalassemia mutations and β-globin gene polymorphisms with DNA polymorphisms in the human β-globin gene cluster. *Nature* 1982;296:627–631.
76. Kazazian HH, Jr, Orkin SH, Antonarakis SE, et al: Molecular characterization of seven β-thalassemia mutations in Asian Indians. *EMBO J* 1984;3:593–596.
77. Kazazian HH, Jr, Orkin SH, Markham AF, et al: Quantification of the close association between DNA haplotypes and specific β-thalassemia mutations in Mediterraneans. *Nature* 1984;310:152–154.
78. Treisman RA, Proudfoot JB, Shander M, et al; A single base change at a splice site in a β^o-thalassemic gene causes abnormal RNA splicing. *Cell* 1982;29:903–911.
79. Baird M, Driscoll C, Schreiner H, et al: A nucleotide change at a splice junction in the human β-globin gene is associated with β^o-thalassemia. *Proc Natl Acad Sci USA* 1981;78:4218-4221.
80. Kazazian HH, Jr, Orkin SH, Boehm, CD, et al: β-thalassemia due to deletion of the nucleotide which is substituted in sickle cell anemia. *Am J Hum Genet* 1983; 35:1028–1033.
81. Thein SL, Wainscoat JS, Lynch JR, et al: Direct detection of β^o 39 thalassemia mutation with Mae I. *Lancet* 1985;2:1095.
82. Padanilam BJ, Felice AE, Huisman THJ: Partial deletion of the 5′ β-globin gene region causes β^o-thalassemia in members of an American black family. *Blood* 1984;64:942–944.
83. Orkin SH, Old JM, Weatherall DJ, et al: Partial deletion of β-globin gene DNA in certain patients with β^o-thalassemia. *Proc Natl Acad Sci USA* 1979;76:2400–2404.
84. Toole JJ, Knopf JL, Wozney JM, et al: Molecular cloning of a cDNA encoding human antihaemophilic factor. *Nature* 1984;312:342–347.
85. Gitschier J, Wood WI, Goralka TM, et al: Characterization of the human Factor VIII gene. *Nature* 1984;312:326–330.
86. Antonarakis SE, Waber PG, Kittur SD, et al: Hemophilia A: Detection of molecular defects and of carriers by DNA analysis. *N Engl J Med* 1985;313:842–848.
87. Harper K, Pembrey ME, Davies KE, et al: A clinically useful DNA probe closely linked to haemophilia A. *Lancet* 1984;2:6–8.
88. Gitschier J, Wood WI, Tuddenham EGD, et al: Detection and sequence of mutations in the Factor VIII gene of hemophiliacs. *Nature* 1985;315:427–430.

89. Youssoufian H, Antonarakis SE, Phillips DG, et al: Detection of six new mutations in hemophilia A. *Clin Res* 1986;34:654A.
90. Choo KH, Gould KG, Rees DJG, et al: Molecular cloning of the gene for human anti-haemophilic Factor IX. *Nature* 1982;299:178–180.
91. Kurachi I, Davie EW: Isolation and characterization of a cDNA coding for human Factor IX. *Proc Natl Acad Sci USA* 1982;79:6461–6464.
92. Jaye M, De la Salle H, Schamber F, et al: Isolation of a human anti-haemophilic Factor IX cDNA using a unique 52-base synthetic oligonucleotide probe deduced from the amino acid sequence of bovine Factor IX. *Nucl Acids Res* 1983;11:2325–2335.
93. Camerino GK, Grzeschik KH, Jaye M, et al: Regional localization on the human X chromosome and polymorphism of coagulation Factor IX gene (hemophilia B locus). *Proc Natl Acad Sci USA* 1984;81:498–502.
94. Giannelli G, Choo KH, Winship PR, et al: Characterization and use of an intragenic polymorphic marker for detection of carriers of haemophilia B (Factor IX deficiency). *Lancet* 1984;1:239–241.
95. Grunebaum L, Cazenave JP, Camerino G, et al: Carrier detection of hemophilia B by using a restriction site polymorphism associated with the coagulation Factor IX gene. *J Clin Invest* 1984;73:1491–1494.
96. Winship PR, Anson DS, Rizza CR, et al: Carrier detection in hemophilia B using two further intragenic restriction fragment length polymorphisms. *Nucl Acids Res* 1984; 12:8861–8872.
97. Camerino G, Oberle I, Drayna D, et al: A new Msp I restriction fragment length polymorphism in the hemophilia B locus. *Hum Genet* 1985;71:79–81.
98. Gianneli F, Choo KH, Rees DJG, et al: Gene deletions in patients with haemophilia B and anti-factor IX antibodies. *Nature* 1983;303:181–182.
99. Peake IR, Furlong BL, Bloom AL: Carrier detection by direct gene analysis in a family with hemophilia B (Factor IX deficiency). *Lancet* 1984;1:242–243.
100. Chen SH, Chance P, Yoshitake S, et al: Factor IX deficiency: Partial internal gene deletion in a family and the value of cDNA probe for genetic analysis. *Clin Res* 1985;33: 117A.
101. Hassan JH, Leonardi A, Guerriero R, et al: Hemophilia B with inhibitor: Molecular analysis of the subtotal deletion of the Factor IX gene. *Blood* 1985;66:728–730.
102. Rees DJ, Rizza CR, Brownlee GG: Hemophilia B caused by a point mutation in a donor splice junction of the human Factor IX gene. *Nature* 1985;316:643–645.
103. Davies KE, Young B, Elles R, et al: Cloning of a representative genomic library of the human X chromosome after sorting by flow cytometry. *Nature* 1981;293:374–386.
104. Murray JM, Davies KE, Harper PS, et al: Linkage relationships of a cloned DNA sequence on the short arm of the X chromosome to Duchenne muscular dystrophy. *Nature* 1982;300:69–71.
105. Davies KE, Pearson PL, Harper PS, et al: Genetic analysis of the short arm of the X chromosome defined by two random cloned DNA sequences flanking Duchenne muscular dystrophy. *Nucl Acids Res* 1983;11:2303–2311.
106. Harper PS, O'Brien T, Murray JM, et al: The use of linked DNA polymorphism for genotype prediction in families with Duchenne muscular dystrophy. *J Med Genet* 1983;20:252–254.
107. Wieacker P, Davies KE, Pearson PL, et al: Carrier detection in Duchenne muscular dystrophy by use of cloned DNA sequences. *Lancet* 1983;1:1325–1336.
108. Kunkel LM, Tantravali U, Eisenhard M, et al: Regional localization on the human X of DNA sequences cloned from flow-sorted chromosomes. *Nucl Acids Res* 1982; 10:1557–1561.

109. Alridge J, Kunkel L, Bruns G: A strategy to reveal high-frequency RFLPs along the human X chromosome. *Am J Hum Genet* 1984;36:546–564.
110. Hofker MH, Wapenaar MC, Goor N, et al: Isolation of probes detecting RFLPs from X chromosome-specific libraries: Potential use for diagnosis of DMD. *Hum Genet* 1985;70:148–156.
111. Rozen R, Fox J, Fenton WA, et al: Gene deletion and RFLPs at the human ornithine transcarbamylase locus. *Nature* 1985;313:815–817.
112. Davies KE, Briand P, Ionasescu V, et al: Gene for OTC: Characterization and linkage to DMD. *Nucl Acids Res* 1984;13:155–165.
113. Wilcox DE, Affara NA, Yates JRW, et al: Multipoint linkage analysis of the short arm of the human X chromosome in families with X-linked muscular dystrophy. *Hum Genet* 1985;70:365–375.
114. Brown CS, Thomas NST, Sarfarazi M, et al: Genetic linkage relationships of seven DNA probes with Duchenne and Becker muscular dystrophy. *Hum Genet* 1985;71:62–74.
115. Kunkel LM, Monaco AP, Middlesworth W, et al: Specific cloning of DNA fragments absent from the DNA of a male patient with an X chromosome deletion. *Proc Natl Acad Sci USA* 1985;82:4778–4782.
116. Jeppsson JO: *FEBS Lett* 1976;65:195–197.
117. Yoshida A, Lieberman J, Gaidulis L, et al: Molecular abnormality of human alpha$_1$-antitrypsin variant (Pi-ZZ) associated with plasma activity deficiency. *Proc Natl Acad Sci USA* 1976;73:1324–1328.
118. Kidd VJ, Wallace RB, Itakura K, et al: α_1-Antitrypsin deficiency detection by direct analysis of the mutation in the gene. *Nature* 1983;304:230–234.
119. Woo SLC, Lidsky AS, Guttler F, et al: Cloned human phenylalanine hydroxylase gene allows prenatal diagnosis and carrier detection of classical phenylketonuria. *Nature* 1983;306:151–155.
120. DiLella AG, Ledley FD, Woo SLC: Prenatal diagnosis and carrier detection of phenylketonuria by gene mapping, In Koprowski H, Ferrone S. Albertini A (eds): *Biotechnology in Diagnostics.* New York, Elsevier 1985, pp 295–307.
121. DiLella AG, Ledley FD, Rey F, et al: Detection of phenylalanine hydroxylase messenger RNA in liver biopsy samples from patients with phenylketonuria. *Lancet* 1985; 1:160–161.
122. Tourian A, Sidbury JB: Phenylketonuria and Hyperphenylalaninemia in Stanbury JB, Wyngaarden JB, Fredrickson DS, et al (eds): *The Metabolic Basis of Inherited Diseases.* New York, McGraw-Hill, 1983, 5th ed.
123. Horwich AL, Fenton WA, Williams KR, et al: Structure and expression of a complementary DNA for the nuclear coded precursor of human mitochondrial ornithine transcarbamylase. *Science* 1984;224:1068–1974.
124. Rosen R, Fox J, Fenton WA, et al: Gene deletion and restriction fragment length polymorphisms at the human ornithine transcarbamylase locus. *Nature* 1985;313:815–817.
125. Nussbaum RL, Boggs BA, Beaudet AL, et al: New mutation and prenatal diagnosis in ornithine transcarbamylase deficiency. *Am J Hum Genet* 1986;38:149–158.
126. Knowlton RG, Cohen-Haguenauer O, Cong NV, et al: A polymorphic DNA marker linked to cystic fibrosis is located on chromosome 7. *Nature* 1985;318:380–382.
127. Dean M, Park M, LeBreau M, et al: The human met oncogene is related to the tyrosine kinase oncogenes. *Nature* 1985;318:385–388.
128. Beaudet AL, Rosenbloom C, Spence JE, et al: Linkage of cystic fibrosis (CF) and the met oncogene. *Pediatr Res* 1986;20:470A(#1859).
129. Boehm CD, Kazazian HH, Jr: Error in prenatal diagnosis by DNA analysis. *N Engl J Med* 1984;311:58.

130. Byers PH, Bonadio JF, Steinmann B, et al: Molecular heterogeneity in perinatal lethal osteogenesis imperfecta (OI type II). *Am J Hum Genet* 1983;35:39a.
131. Steinmann B, Rao VH, Vogel A, et al: Cystein in the triple-helical domain of one allelic product of the $\alpha1$(I) gene of type I collagen produces a lethal form of osteogenesis imperfecta. *J Biol Chem* 1984;259:11129–11138.
132. DeWet NJ, Pihlajaniemi T, Myers J, et al: Synthesis of a shortened pro $\alpha2$(I) chain and decreased synthesis of pro $\alpha2$(I) chains in a proban with ostengenesis imperfecta. *J Biol Chem* 1983;258:7721–7728.
133. Prockop DJ: Genetic defects of Collagen. *Hosp Pract* 1986;21:125–140.

CHAPTER 8

Recombinant DNA Analysis of Multifactorial Disease

Barton Childs, MD, and
Arno G. Motulsky, MD

The medical applications of recombinant DNA techniques so far reviewed have been limited to disorders engendered by the actions of genes at single loci. This work has been so successful that optimism has been expressed about rewards to be expected in the application of these methods to multifactorial diseases.[1] Such optimism is generated by the prospect of finding precisely defined genetic risk factors for the diseases of adult life. It is also based on the assumption that the origins of such diseases are in many ways similar to those caused by genes at one locus. These expectations are appropriate, but differences in complexity between monogenic and multifactorial inheritance are such as to beget the prediction that progress in unravelling the latter will be less rapid at the very least.

Some insight into what lies ahead may be gained by a contrast between the properties of monogenic and multifactorial conditions. Probably the principal difference is the extent of our ignorance of the identity and nature of either genetic or environmental contribution to most multifactorial diseases. The term *multifactorial* refers to multiple factors in the causation of disease. It is inferred that some of these are environmental while others are genetic, and that genes at more than one locus are involved. In many cases, neither the environmental nor the genetic factors are known. The term *multifactorial inheritance* is often used when straightforward mendelian transmission cannot be demonstrated, even though little or nothing is known about the mechanism of inheritance.

Such a definition might seem to be offering an alternative to the mendelian mode, but in fact there is no true discontinuity between monogenic and multifactorial inheritance. The latter is merely a special case of the former, and while it is easy to point to polar examples of each, there are many others in which ambiguity is expressed in phenotypes that show degrees of familial aggregation varying all the way from something resembling mendelian modes to the sporadic distribution that cannot be differentiated from non-genetic variation. And this irregularity of transmission appears within diseases no less than between them. For example, although we expect some phenotypic and genetic heterogeneity in such monogenic disorders as Tay-Sachs disease and phenylketonuria, it is possible to study patients with these diseases knowing that what differentiates them from unaffected people are genes at a single locus. We cannot be so confident apropos, say, of gout, where in a population of cases there is a continuous decline in familial aggregation with age at onset.[2] Such within-disease variability is inevitable even when alleles at only one or two loci furnish the genetic source and one or two experiences or conditions supply the non-genetic ingredients. Indeed, differences in cause of the same disorder may exist even within families; one person's susceptibility may be enhanced by a concentration of all the relevant genes available in the family, while a sib who has fewer of them may get the disease because of a more intense and prolonged exposure to some precipitating factor.

Other differences are shown in Table 8.1. As popularly defined, monogenic diseases are many and rare, multifactorial diseases fewer but common. Furthermore, most monogenic disorders have their onset in infancy and childhood.[3] More than 90% declare themselves before puberty, and although there are multifactorial disorders that appear in childhood, most such diseases occur later in life. Presumably, the more disruptive of development and homeostasis the genetic effect is, the earlier it is likely to be observed. In contrast, the genetic influence in the multifactorial disorders of adult life is less salient, and more likely to produce cumulative changes that are expressed only after reproduction or when the early effects of aging supervene. Or these genes may merely set the stage for the adverse influences of experi-

TABLE 8-1 Some Factors That Tend to Differentiate Monogenic from Multifactorial Diseases

	Monogenic	Multifactorial
Age at onset	Prepubertal	Postpubertal
Frequency	Rare	Common
Latency	Short	Long
Sex difference	Occasional	Frequent
Influence of migration	No	Yes
Secular change	No	Yes
Effects of SES	No	Yes

ences and conditions of living. For example, the incidence and prevalence of diseases of later life are much more likely to be affected by socioeconomic status, geographic location, and secular change, all evidences of the participation in cause of non-genetic elements. Furthermore, such variations in prevalence must be reflected in uncertainty as to the *actual* risk for each individual carrying genes conferring susceptibility.

THE ANALYSIS OF MULTIFACTORIAL DISEASES

In trying to comprehend the multiple factors that contribute to complex phenotypes, the natural way to proceed is by way of the reductionist approach that has proved so successful with monogenic diseases.[4–6] We might begin with an epidemiologic study aiming at the identification of subgroups, each distinguished by clinical, physiological or biochemical properties that appear to characterize families and that could give leads to the identity of relevant genes, which, together with specific experiences, might account for most of the variation within the subgroup. Such a strategy was exploited with notable effect by Goldstein and Brown who, starting with an ill-defined phenotype—heart attacks in men under 60 years of age—proceeded by logical steps first to isolate a subgroup characterized by familial hypercholesterolemia, and then to show that the abnormality in the metabolism of cholesterol in such patients was associated with failure of their cells to take it up owing to lack of a lipoprotein receptor.[7] The receptor was then characterized, its gene was located, and the mutations associated with disease were defined by sequence analysis. This reductionist strategy proceeds by a series of approximations; in the genetic case, from some distal, or peripheral, phenotypic level to the next, more proximal one, aiming at explanations in terms of each, and ending with a description of the qualities of the gene itself.

Each such distal level has properties not necessarily predicted by the characteristics of that proximal to it; that is, new qualities of physiology and behavior emerge as a result of the enlarged empirical content of the more distal phenotype. This emergent complexity may make it difficult to decide in what direction to pursue the reductionist strategy. Perhaps it is at just this point that recombinant DNA methods will be most helpful, especially as the map density increases, but even this most incisive approach may be handicapped by several aspects of phenotypic complexity: (1) the names of diseases often disguise the diversity of their cause; (2) the causes of a disease with variable age at onset are likely to differ with age; (3) individuality is likely to modify gene effects variably.

The Lack of Diagnostic Specificity

We sometimes forget that diseases have no intrinsic being; that their names represent only convenient rubrics, classes that have logistical uses but no precise conceptual content, particularly as to cause. So diagnostic labels range in power of definition from such straightforward phenotypes as phenylketonuria to the clinically overlapping and imprecisely defined forms of mental illness, such as schizophrenia, in which efforts to erect a system of subtypes have proved frustrating, and for research purposes a "best-estimate" diagnosis may require the deliberations of a committee. There is a continuum of diagnostic specificity within diseases too, and such is the range of variation of both genes and experiences that it may be said with accuracy that every case of every disease is unique. But our job, even while acknowledging this degree of variability, is to discover the salient genes and specific experiences that account for *most* of the variation for both the diagnostic class and the individual patients it embraces.[5,6] For each patient it will be the *particular combination* of these most prominent factors that must be described; even if one had a comprehensive list of all risk factors for a particular disease, it would be of little use except in relation to how they are distributed in particular individuals.

Age at Onset

It is a part of the lore of human genetics that early onset of a disease with a broad span of onsets is associated with greater severity of expression and increased familial aggregation of affected persons.[8] These variations are likely to be due to differences in cause; early onset may be promoted by one or two genes of especially adverse effect, whereas cases of later onset are more likely to be a product of more intense or prolonged exposure to precipitating experiences or conditions. Thus, genetic risk factors can be expected to be most obvious in the cases of earliest onset.

Modifying Influences

And then there is the individual in whom the gene-environment transaction takes place; an individual with a particular developmental and social history, a person in whom biologic and cultural factors have mingled to produce an individuality that is a testing ground for any given gene-environment interaction.[8] So the true individual risk for many gene-environment interactions cannot be determined in the absence of some knowledge of the factors that constitute this individuality. For example, it has been suggested that the pathogenesis of multiple sclerosis is initiated by a viral infection in children at 5 to 10 years of age.[9] The emergence of the disease 30 or more years later must be influenced not only by how the original infection was handled, a process involving genetically variable elements, but also by aspects of development, themselves subject to genetic variation, as well as by some of the innumerable experiences that intervene between the original infection and the time when the disease becomes overt.

THE GENES OF MULTIFACTORIAL DISEASE

What are the genes? They cannot be a special kind, unrelated to those that produce single-gene diseases. But they do differ in being under less intense negative selection, and they are, therefore, more common in the population, often reaching polymorphic levels and likely to be harmful only under modern conditions of abundance or surfeit.

But what of the genes of undoubted bad effect; those which in homozygotes produce inborn errors, and some of which in heterozygotes reach polymorphic frequencies: can they be exonerated? Not altogether; for example, it has been reported that some heterozyogotes for homocystinuria are prone to arterial occlusive diseases,[10] and some carriers of a gene promoting osteogenesis imperfecta may be liable to early osteoporosis.[11] These examples suggest that under conditions of stress, some heterozygotes may develop symptoms, either akin to those observed in the homozygotes or perhaps others representing delayed or cumulative effects of a relatively unresponsive homeostasis. But not much is known of such expressions. Vogel has made an exhaustive search for reports of heterozygous effects of genes causing recessive disorders, and although some effects are frequently observed in tolerance tests or in measures of enzyme activity, such genes are not much implicated in common multifactorial diseases.[12] Kacser and Burns have suggested why genes specifying enzymes that work in pathways are unlikely, in heterozygotes, to be associated with common disease.[13,14] The reason is that the other enzymes in the pathway can accommodate to reduction in activity of any one. In genetic terms the "wild" allele acts as a dominant so that the heterozygote effect is more or less equal to that of the normal homozygote. The mechanism for this "evolution of dominance" remains unclear despite its having been the object of the attention of population geneticists for 50 years.[15] Somehow the genes endow homeostatic mechanisms with broad flexibility to resist threats from within as well as without.

So, if not recessive, the genes associated with the diseases of later life would be expected to act as dominants (that is, to produce their effects more or less equally in both heterozygotes and homozygotes) or at least not to act as recessives. These conditions are presaged in studies in drosophila in which the most deleterious gene effects are recessive, whereas those that are expressed merely in reduced viability are dominants.[16]

Some support for these ideas appears in observations on human diseases. Most of the monogenic disorders with onset during infancy and childhood are recessive, whereas many of those that occur in adult life are dominants.[3] This accords with observed burdens; it is the recessives that are characterized by early death, as well as infertility and handicap for survivors, while the dominants may become clinically manifest only after puberty or even after reproduction is complete. As for the genes of multifactorial disease, these are in the main dominants, some more completely so than others. Examples are: (1) LDL receptor defects lead to heart attacks between the ages of 35 to 60 in heterozygotes, whereas homozygotes suffer heart attacks as young adults, or even in childhood.[7] (2) There is little clinical difference between patients with insulin-dependent diabetes who are homozygous for the HLA alleles DR3 or DR4 and those who are heterozygous for these and any other of the HLA alleles.[17–18] (3) Many other autoimmune disorders are associated with alleles of the HLA loci, usually but not always in the heterozygous state.[19] (4) Several of the frequent diseases of lipid metabolism, some of which promote premature heart attacks, appear to segregate as autosomal dominants.[20,21] (5) Many disorders are associated with alleles of the blood groups, especially ABO.[22]

However these blood group genes function in, say, duodenal ulcer or in infections, they seem to do it independently of gene dosage. It should be added that if the literature is ambiguous on this issue of dominance, it is because it is given so little attention. Gene dosage is often not mentioned at all, and the relationship of clinical expression to the heterozygous and homozygous states is usually unreported.

RECOMBINANT DNA ANALYSIS OF MULTIFACTORIAL PHENOTYPES

This brief review recounts the gaps in our knowledge of causes of multifactorial diseases and suggests a need for the following: (1) the resolution of complex phenotypes into rather more homogenous entities for which lists of risk factors, including both genes and experiences, can be composed; (2) precise definition of the residual heterogeneity of cause within each subgroup; (3) definition of distributions of risk factors in affected individuals in each subgroup and in their relatives, both affected and unaffected.

With such information in hand it may be possible to define susceptibility individually, giving probabilities for each person in the light of his or her private list of risk factors. We may expect that the application of recombinant DNA methods to the study of questions such as these will be rewarding in three ways: in the discovery of new genes and markers, in the resolution of heterogeneity, and in the elucidation of pathogenesis.

New Genes

New genes may be expected to be specific genes and gene fragments either associated with disease or directly involved in pathogenesis. Those merely associated with disease may be alleles at linked loci capable of acting as markers in family studies. Genes actually involved in pathogenesis should be more illuminating, especially in revealing the relationships of the different kinds of mutation to clinical expression. Strategies employed in finding them depend upon whether or not the phenotype includes a specific protein.

With Candidate Proteins

We are in the best position when the details of the homeostatic system involved in pathogenesis are known so that the component proteins suggest candidate genes. One such homeostatic system is that of lipid transport and disposition. It is well known that heart attacks in individuals below 50 to 55 years of age are likely to be a consequence of defects, or at least variations, of one or more components of this system. Table 8.2 lists the apolipoproteins that constitute important elements of the system.[23,24] All have been mapped to chromosomes, monogenic deficiencies expressed in various forms of hyperlipidemia and atherosclerotic heart disease are known, and the proteins themselves are the focus of a good deal of investigation just now. In addition, restriction fragment length polymorphisms (RFLPs) have been found for all, and we are going to be confronted by the necessity to fit such new informa-

TABLE 8-2 Some Characteristics of the Apolipoproteins

Apolipoprotein	Predominant Lipoprotein Type	Chromosome	Protein Polymorphism	RFLP
AI	HDL	11	−	+
AII	HDL	1	−	+
AIV	HDL	11	+	+
B	LDL	2	+	
CI	HDL, VLDL	19	−	−
CII	VLDL	19	−	+
CIII	VLDL	11	+	+
E	VLDL	19	+	−

tion into an already complex composition of both clinical variety and risk factors.

Since the dyslipoproteinemias are well defined risk factors in coronary heart disease, much attention is being given to a more detailed analysis of the molecular biology of the apolipoproteins. In the procedure for investigation, various DNA variants (RFLPs and minisatellites) of the apolipoproteins are used and estimates are made of their frequency in populations with coronary heart disease, with various dyslipoproteinemias or in individuals with both traits. It is presumed that DNA variants that are tightly linked to an adjacent apolipoprotein gene would show different frequencies among individuals who carry a mutant apolipoprotein gene that is involved in a dyslipoproteinemia or in coronary heart disease; the DNA variants in this design are used as markers to tag a closely linked genetic abnormality of an apolipoprotein gene. Elicitation of the underlying defect would require cloning of the involved gene and a study of its structure and function to determine the pathogenetic abnormality. It is essential when comparing normals with a given patient population that there is careful ethnic matching since DNA markers (no less than other genetic markers) may have different frequencies in various populations.

Some suggestive results have been obtained. At the Apo I-CIII locus, an Sst I polymorphism has been shown to be associated with severe hypertriglyceridemia.[25] Other investigators, however, were not able to demonstrate this association.[26–29] A higher frequency of this Sst variant was also seen in British patients with myocardial infarction[30] and in a Seattle population.[31] A strong association between myocardial infarction and a Pst I polymorphism at the AI-CIII locus was reported from Boston.[32] It is noteworthy that this apparently unselected population of patients with coronary heart disease had much lower HDL levels (58% of the Boston patients had HDL levels below the 10th percentile) than Seattle patients with angiocardiographically proven coronary heart disease where no association between the Pst I variant and coronary heart disease could be demonstrated.[31] Since the AI-CIII locus is involved in the control of HDL level, the discrepancy could possibly be explained by this finding.

Conflicting results have also been obtained with DNA markers at the Apo B locus. Since high apolipoprotein B levels are often seen in coronary heart disease, some underlying lesions at the apo B locus might be expected. Breslow and his group found abnormal frequencies of RFLPs at the Xba I and Eco RI sites, and at a minisatellite gene at the downstream (3′) end of the apo B gene in patients with coronary heart disease.[33] In Seattle, a correlation of coronary heart disease with the minisatellite marker was detected but not with the Xba I and Eco RI variants or with two additional variants at the apo B locus (Taq I, Pvu II).[31] It is also interesting that the various apo B associations were with coronary heart disease only and not with quantitative lipid levels. Given the current state of knowledge, one might expect that susceptibility to coronary heart disease would be mediated by the intervening variable of a quantitative lipid abnormality such as that found with the Pst association and HDL levels at the AI-CIII locus. However, if a predisposition to coronary heart disease mediated by an apolipoprotein marker can be confirmed in the presence of normal lipid levels, one would need to postulate intrinsic properties of mutant apolipoprotein molecules that render such particles atherogenic. Such a result would be a most important finding, since it could account for certain cases of atherosclerosis because of qualitative rather than quantitative lipid abnormalities.

Without Candidate Proteins

These apolipoproteins were bound to be subjected immediately to restriction enzyme analysis not only because of the frequency and gravity of the diseases with which they are associated, but also because the proteins and their roles in homeostasis were well known. But there are other multifactorial diseases associated with heavy impacts for which no candidate genes can be suggested; the major psychoses are often mentioned. Is there a strategy likely to be useful in such instances? At the moment there is none beyond expensive and time-consuming "fishing expeditions." One possible expedient is that of looking for chromosomal polymorphisms or other variations that might be associated with the disease and that could suggest, therefore, what part of which chromosome to examine. But in general, the search is unlikely to prosper until the map density is such as to provide highly polymorphic markers every 20 cm or so.[34] Even then, large numbers of families might be needed to establish linkage. Lander and Botstein have shown how such numbers can be reduced by new strategies: interval mapping, in which the presumed locus lies in an interval of known size between two markers, and simultaneous search, in which several loci are examined simultaneously.[35] If there is heterogeneity between families, the simultaneous search is likely to detect at least one marker segregating with each different kind of family. Most investigators agree that large multiplex families represent the most favorable hunting ground. It is to be expected, however, that families with several affected cases will be uncharacteristic of all, differing genetically from each other and from the more common families with only one, or occasionally a second, case.

But there is much to be done before the map can be used for exploration. So the interval between now and the time a workable map is available may be filled with profit by epidemiologic studies seeking subtypes, with further characterization of each by the discovery of reliable biochemical or other markers. Many marker candidates have been turned up in studies of schizophrenia and affective disorder,[30] but their usefulness, if any, has been bedeviled by the assumption that the marker ought to characterize all cases of schizophrenia, say, when the specificity of such a diagnosis remains very much in doubt. Subtyping on clinical and demographic grounds is a necessary preliminary to any detailed search for heterogeneity.

Genetic Heterogeneity

Diagnostic precision is a cardinal aim in medicine, and incisive definition is a principal virtue of a genetic analysis. Evidence of the participation of genes, however vague, gives an etiologic clue, but difficulties in the pursuit of this desirable end are encountered when the point of entry of the analysis is very far distal to the gene product. That is, the degree of heterogeneity of cause is directly related to the distance of the phenotype from the gene. Clinical expressions give the least useful information, whereas variations in amino acid sequence or activity of some gene product, or in its immunologic characteristics, are more informative. But direct examination of the DNA is likely to provide the ultimate precision in sorting out genetic and phenotypic subtypes. Some examples follow.

The Apolipoproteins

What the relationships between the apolipoprotein variants and their clinical expression will turn out to be is unclear. It may become apparent that clinical differences will depend upon the kind of mutation, or it may be that different mutations will be associated with very similar phenotypes, or most likely both. So we shall be learning whether or not, and to what degree, such phenotypes as heart attack and dyslipoproteinemia can be differentiated by allelic variation, and if such distinctions are possible we will wish to know to what degree allelic variation is reflected in the need for specificity in treatment and prevention. It seems likely that even if treatment does not vary according to mutation, prevention will. Some mutations will produce their effects almost independently of the environment, while others will only make a person somewhat more susceptible to adverse experiences. The potentially bad effects of the latter will be more readily prevented.

Insulin-Dependent Diabetes

A similar resolution of genetic heterogeneity is occurring in insulin-dependent diabetes. At least two subtypes can be distinguished on clinical grounds: one form associated with the serologically distinguished HLA allele DR3 is presumed to be of autoimmune origin, whereas a second is thought to be caused by infection by a virus that damages the B cells of the pancreas.[37] The latter is frequently associated with the HLA allele DR4. Some patients have both DR3 and DR4, and these come down with the disease earlier, are more severely affected, and have more affected relatives and a higher monozygotic twin concordance than the homozygotes for either allele alone.[38] Presumably, the HLA DR alleles are in linkage disequilibrium with other genes that impart susceptibility to, or actually promote, the disease, and the two together in a double heterozygote are more diabetogenic than either one alone. Restriction enzyme analysis may be expected to help both in the detection and characterization of the genes presumed to be linked to the HLA alleles, and in sorting out additional heterogeneity.[38] Studies of alleles for both and genes at the DR loci show what can be done. For example, a Bgl II 4.2-kb fragment distinguishes a DR chain allele that types serologically as DR3 and that predominates in type I diabetics from other, serologically identical alleles that are less often found in patients with the disease.[39] Similar allelic heterogeneity has been demonstrated for DR chain alleles also typed as DR3.[40] It must be presumed that the susceptibility genes are linked to these special DR3 alleles rather than to others, so these studies represent a start at isolating them. But there is another virtue of these investigations. Risk figures and odds ratios based solely on serologic comparisons of the frequencies of DR3 and DR4 alleles in patients with those of unrelated controls must be biased; that is, while most of the DR3 and DR4 alleles in the diabetics are linked to the susceptibility genes, most of those of the controls are unlikely to be. In fact, the DR3 allele characterized by the Bgl II 4.2-kb fragment carries a relative risk that is double that of DR3 alleles lacking it.[39]

Other Disorders

There is little doubt that the extreme polymorphism of the MHC loci has to do with the necessity for a versatile and flexible defense against marauding microorganisms.[41] It is, therefore, no surprise that variation at these loci should figure in autoimmune diseases. Serologic evidence for "susceptibility" HLA alleles exists for diabetes, rheumatoid arthritis, systemic lupus erythematosus, celiac disease, some thyroid disorders, and other diseases. Heterogeneity within serologic types is known to exist, and recombinant DNA methods are being used to give the serologic associations with disease more specificity. Probes are available and progress is being made; for example, newly described alleles within the DR4 rubric, characterized by restriction enzyme analysis, have been shown to have affinity for rheumatoid arthritis, but the observations are too scanty to have any epidemiologic meaning.[42–44] But some HLA-disease affinities might be easier to dissect. The class I allele B27 is found in about 90% of patients with ankylosing spondylitis, while the class II DR2 has been observed in 98% of patients with narcolepsy.[45,46] The frequency of ankylosing spondylitis is about 1/500 and of narcolepsy 1/2500, whereas B27 is found in 5 to 8%, and DR2 in 25 to 30%, of US whites. Does the strength of these associations mean that there are relatively infrequent versions of the B27 or DR2 serologic phenotypes that mark genes involved in pathogenesis? Are they effectively monogenic disorders? Or is it that these alleles represent a favorable background over which some unrelated gene or genes work; that is, any B27 or DR2 will do?

Four serologic subtypes of B27 are known.[44] Only 2% of unrelated people with B27 develop the disease, while 10 to 20% of the first degree, B27, relatives of patients with the disorder also get it.[45] This sounds as if not all of the subtypes confer equal susceptibility. Further dissection by restriction enzyme techniques, now in progress, should tell the story.[47]

Narcolepsy is characterized by a decreased latency between wakefulness and REM sleep, and in one report, healthy, randomly assembled individuals with the DR2 serologic phenotype attained REM sleep on average nearly twice as quickly as controls who had other DR alleles.[48] Other investigators have reported the results of recombinant DNA studies: a subtype of DR2—DQR2,6—predominates in people with narcolepsy, suggesting that the patients are drawn from a special subpopulation of individuals with the DR2 serologic phenotype.[49] If so, the DQR2,6 allele may be involved in pathogenesis or may be linked to such a gene, and either way may constitute a risk factor with some authority. But in the study of REM sleep latency all but one of the heathy DR2 individuals also had the DQR2,6 gene.[49] Thus, much remains to be done before the meaning of these strong associations will be clear, either in regard to pathogenesis or risk.

Pathogenesis

Knowing the genes involved in a disease phenotype should enhance our comprehension of the abnormal physiology consequent upon their actions. And the key to treatment and prevention lies in the nature of pathogenesis. But we may be denied that insight even though we have the most detailed knowledge of gene structure because the gene-protein affinity may not be apparent, or it may not be evident where the putative protein fits in homeostasis and what it does there.

For this, reverse genetics is needed, a measure just beginning to be developed.[50] Partial success was achieved in the isolation of transcripts of the gene for chronic granulomatous disease and the prediction of a protein they specify.[51] Unfortunately, what the protein is and does is not immediately apparent. In theory, the application of this method to multifactorial phenotypes is limited only by the necessity to find and elucidate the actions of more than one gene.

CONCLUSION

The promise of recombinant DNA methods in the resolution of the genetic heterogeneity of multifactorial disorders and in the characterization of risk factors and their application to individuals is very great. One can see dimly an immense repository of information bearing upon the medical careers of almost everyone. The benefits are incalculable. We may anticipate otherwise unattainable insights into pathogenesis, homeostasis, development, aging, even human nature and evolution, to say nothing of invaluable hints pointing to novel treatments and prevention. But there is much to be done before this medical millenium is upon us; and it is just as well, because we are far from ready to deal with the impact of such information on either individuals or the whole population. A great deal of epidemiologic work is necessary before it will be apparent what genetic risk factors, singly and in combination, mean to *individuals.* Odds ratios based on case control studies, even when well done, can never stand as precise risks for individuals; they are a relative risk for the population studied, not for each of the individuals of which it is composed. And then it is not apparent what an individual is to do with them — particularly when the provocation that can make a risk a reality is unknown. More generally, we lack a tradition for prevention. It is accorded neither priority nor prestige in the medical school curriculum where emphasis is given to diagnosis and treatment of patients who are already sick. So what we can expect of DNA analysis is a very powerful impetus in the process of developing such a tradition, a context in which both physicians and patients can feel comfortable with risk factors and in which a supporting system is in place to make prevention a reality.

REFERENCES

1. Harris R: Molecular euphoria. *J Med Genet* 1986;23:97–98.
2. Yu TF: Diversity of clinical features in gouty arthritis. *Sem Arth Rheum* 1984;13:360–368.
3. Costa T, Scriver CR, Childs B: The effect of mendelian disease on human health: A measurement. *Am J Med Genet* 1985;21:231–242.
4. Motulsky AG: The 1985 Nobel Prize in physiology or medicine. *Science* 1986;231: 126–128.
5. Motulsky AG: Genetic approaches to common diseases, in Bonne-Tamir B, Cohen T, Goodman RM (eds): *Human Genetics, Part B: Medical Aspects.* New York, AR Liss, 1982, pp 89–95.
6. Motulsky AG: Approaches to the genetics of common diseases. In Rotter JI, Samloff IM, Rimoin DL, (eds): *The Genetics and Heterogeneity of Common Gastrointestinal Disorders.* New York, Academic Press, 1980, pp 3–10.
7. Brown MS, Goldstein JL: A receptor-mediated pathway for cholesterol homeostasis. *Science* 1986;232:34–47.

8. Childs B, Scriver CR: Age at onset and causes of diseases. *Perspec Biol Med* 1986; 29:437–460.
9. Poser CM: Pathogenesis of multiple sclerosis. *Acta Neuropathol* 1986;71:1–10.
10. Boers GHJ, Smals GH, Trijbels FJM, et al: Heterozygosity for homocystinuria in premature peripheral and cerebral occlusive arterial disease. *N Engl J Med* 1985;313:709–715.
11. Prokop DJ: Mutations in collagen genes. *J Clin Invest* 1985;75:783–787.
12. Vogel F: Clinical consequences of heterozygosity for autosomal-recessive diseases. *Clin Genet* 1984;25:381–415.
13. Kacser H, Burns JA: The molecular basis of dominance. *Genetics* 1981;97:639–666.
14. Middleton RJ, Kacser H: Enzyme variation, metabolic flux and fitness: Alcohol dehydrogenase in Drosophila melanogaster. *Genetics* 1983;105:633–650.
15. Charlesworth B: Evidence against Fisher's theory of dominance. *Nature* 1979;278: 848–849.
16. Simmons MJ, Crow JF: Mutations affecting fitness in drosophila populations. *Ann Rev Genet* 1977;11:49–78.
17. Foster DW: Diabetes mellitus. In Stanbury JB, Wyngaarden JB, Fredrickson DS, et al (eds): *Metabolic Basis of Inherited Disease*, ed 5. New York, McGraw Hill, 1983, pp 99–117.
18. MacDonald MJ, Gottschall J, Hunter JB, et al: HLA-DR4 in insulin-dependent diabetic parents and their diabetic offspring: A clue to dominant inheritance. *Proc Natl Acad Sci* 1986;83:7049–7053.
19. Srejgaard A, Platz P, Ryder LP: HLA and disease 1982—a survey. *Immunol Rev* 1983;70:193–218.
20. Schaefer EJ, Levy RI: Pathogenesis and management of lipoprotein disorders. *N Engl J Med* 1985;312:1300–1310.
21. Goldbourt U, Neufeld HN: Genetic aspects of arteriosclerosis. *Arteriosclerosis* 1986;6: 357–377.
22. Mourant AE, Kopec AC, Domaniewska-Sobczak K: *Blood Groups and Diseases*. Oxford, Oxford University Press, 1978.
23. Williams DL: Molecular biology in arteriosclerosis research. *Arteriosclerosis* 1985;5: 213–227.
24. Breslow JL: Apolipoprotein defects. *Hosp Pract* Dec. 15, 1985, pp 43–49.
25. Rees A, Stocks J, Shoulders CC, et al: DNA polymorphism adjacent to human apoprotein AI gene: Relation to hypertriglyceridemia. *Lancet* 1983;1:444.
26. Kessling AM, Borsthemke B, Humphries SE: A study of DNA polymorphisms around the human apolipoprotein AI gene in hypertriglyceridemic and normal individuals. *Clin Genet* 1985;28:296–306.
27. Kessling AM, Berg K, Mockleby E, et al: DNA polymorphisms around the apo AI gene in normal and hyperlipidaemic individuals selected for a twin study. *Clin Genet* 1986;29: 485–490.
28. Morris SW, Price WH: DNA sequence polymorphisms with apolipoprotein A-I/C-III gene cluster. *Lancet* 1985;2:1127–1128.
29. Rees A, Stocks J, Paul H, et al: Haplotypes identified by DNA polymorphisms at the apolipoprotein A-I and C-III loci and hypertriglyceridemia. A study in a Japanese population. *Hum Genet* 1986;72:168–171.
30. Ferns GAA, Ritchie C, Stocks J, et al: Genetic polymorphisms of apolipoprotein C-III and insulin in survivors of myocardial infarction. *Lancet* 1985;2:300–303.
31. Deeb S, Failor A, Brown BG, et al: Molecular genetics of apolipoproteins and coronary heart disease, in *Cold Spring Harbor Symposia on Quantitative Biology*, Vol 51: Molecular Biology of Homo Sapiens. Cold Spring Harbor, New York, Cold Spring Harbor Laboratory, to be published.

32. Ordovas JM, Schaefer EJ, Salem D, et al: Apolipoprotein A-I gene polymorphism associated with premature coronary artery disease and familial hypoalphalipoproteinemias. *N Engl J Med* 1986;314:671–681.
33. Hegele RA, Huang L-S, Herbert PN, et al: Apolipoprotein B-gene DNA polymorphisms associated with myocardial infarct. *N Engl J Med* 1986;315:1509–1515.
34. Lander E, Botstein D: Mapping complex genetic traits in humans: New methods using a complete RFLP map. In press.
35. Lander ES, Botstein D: New strategies for studying heterogeneous genetic traits in humans using an RFLP linkage map. *Proc Natl Acad Sci* 1986;83:7353–7357.
36. Sturt E, McGuffins P: Can linkage and marker association resolve the genetic aetiology of psychiatric disorders? Review and argument. *Psychol Med* 1985;15:455–462.
37. Rotter JI, Vadheim CM, Raffel LJ, et al: Genetic etiologies of diabetes. *Paediat Adolesc Endocrinol* 1986;15:1–11.
38. Niven MJ, Hitman GA: The molecular genetics of diabetes mellitus. *Biosci Rep* 1986;6:501–512.
39. Stetler D, Grumet FC, Erlich HA: Polymorphic restriction endonuclease sites linked to the HLA-DR gene: Localization and use as genetic markers of insulin-dependent diabetes. *Proc Natl Acad Sci* 1985;82:8100–8104.
40. Owerbach D, Lernmark A, Platz P, et al: HLA-D region β-chain DNA endonuclease fragments differ between HLA-DR identical healthy and insulin dependent diabetic individuals. *Nature* 1983;303:815–817.
41. Strominger JL: Biology of the human histocompatibility leucocyte antigen (HLA) system and a hypothesis regarding the generation of autoimmune diseases. *J Clin Invest* 1986; 77:1411–1415.
42. Cutbush SD, Ollier W, Awad J, et al: New HLA DNA polymorphisms associated with rheumatoid arthritis. *Dis Mark* 1986;4:173–183.
43. So A, Bodmer J: DNA polymorphisms of the Class II genes in DR4 cells. *Dis Mark* 1986;4:165–172.
44. Nepom GT, Seyfried CE, Holbeck SL, et al: Identification of HLA-DW14 genes in DR^+ rheumatoid arthritis. *Lancet* 1986;2:1002–1004.
45. Van der Linden SM, Khan MA: The risk of ankylosing spondylitis in HLA-B27 positive individuals: A reappraisal. *J Rheumatol* 1984;11:727–728.
46. Parkes JD, Langdon N, Lock C: Narcolepsy and immunity. *Br Med J* 1986;292:359–360.
47. Szots H, Riethmuller G, Weiss E, et al: Complete sequence of HLA-B27 cDNA identified through the characterization of structural markers unique to the HLA-A, B, and C series. *Proc Natl Acad Sci* 1986;83:1428–1432.
48. Schulz H, Geisler P, Pollmaecher T, et al: HLA-DR2 correlates with rapid-eye-movement sleep latency in normal human subjects. *Lancet* 1986;2:803.
49. Marcadet A, Gebuhrer L, Betuel H, et al: DNA polymorphism related to HLA-DRZ DW2 in patients with narcolepsy. *Immunogenetics* 1985;22:679–683.
50. Orkin SH: Reverse genetics and human disease. *Cell* 1986;47:845–850.
51. Royer-Pokora B, Kunkel LM, Monaco AP, et al: Cloning the gene for an inherited human disorder—chronic granulomatous disease—on the basis of its chromosomal location. *Nature* 1986;322:32–38.

CHAPTER 9

Commercial Uses of Recombinant DNA Technology in Human Genetic Disease

Norman Arnheim, PhD, and
Henry A. Erlich, PhD

This chapter will focus on the potential commercial use of recombinant DNA technology in the area of human diseases, especially those with a major genetic component. The nature and size of commercial markets for recombinant DNA products are defined by each biotechnology company as a result of their marketing analyses, and these estimates determine, in part, research and development strategies. In addition, the demonstration of the potential use of a new technology, even in the absence of a clear commercial goal, can be advantageous and affect the public's willingness to make long-term investments in a company. Clearly, however, a biotechnology company must devote most of its resources to areas it believes will provide for its economic growth. Cetus Corporation, for example, has made its major commitment to using this technology for cancer therapeutics, but it is also supporting a significant effort in the area of diagnostics of cancer and infectious and genetic disease. Other biotechnology companies (eg, Genentech) have made a commitment to the area of protein replacement therapy for genetic diseases resulting from the deficiency of a specific polypeptide. Our review will focus on these areas in which recombinant DNA technology may provide advantages for therapy and diagnostics and will discuss projects that have well-defined commercial application as well as those that may eventually lead to clinically useful new products.

HUMAN GENETIC DISEASE

Therapy

Specific deficiencies of proteins or enzymes have been identified for a number of genetic diseases. Some biotechnology companies have selected disorders for which it is either known or considered likely that the administration of the missing protein can ameliorate the disease process. The first project of this type involved human insulin, which is used in therapy for insulin-dependent diabetes, an autoimmune disease with a strong genetic component.[1] The human gene was cloned, expressed in *Escherichia coli*,[2] examined in clinical trials, and its product is currently on the market. A significant motivation for this project was to eliminate the clinical problems associated with the administration of insulins of nonhuman origin. The large-scale production of human insulin, like many other human proteins of therapeutic value, is prohibitively difficult without recombinant DNA technology.

Another example of replacement therapy was the cloning of the gene encoding the blood coagulation protein Factor VIII:C which is nonfunctional in Hemophilia A.[3] The Factor VIII:C gene has recently been cloned and expressed in mammalian cells.[4–6] It is expected that once abundant supplies of recombinant factor VIII:C are available, clinical trials will be initiated. Finally, the commercial development of recombinant human growth hormone (HGH) purified from bacterial cells[7] has received FDA approval following clinical trials and is commercially available. Again, a significant advantage of the recombinant material is, in addition to overcoming the problem of supply, the elimination of the risk of viral infection (Jacob-Crutzfeld disease[8]) associated with HGH derived from human tissue sources.

The three examples of replacement therapy discussed above all involve proteins already known to be clinically efficacious. Clearly, there is a much greater commercial risk to projects involving proteins whose utility in replacement therapy has not yet been demonstrated clinically. Recent studies on $\alpha 1$ antitrypsin illuminate this aspect of the commercial application of protein products for the treatment of disease. The gene was isolated[9] and successfully used as a hybridization probe for the prenatal diagnosis a $\alpha 1$ antitrypsin deficiency.[10] More recently, a cDNA clone encoding the protein has been isolated and expressed in *E. coli* and yeast.[11,12] Clinically, this deficiency is characterized by a high incidence of early-onset emphysema,[13] and it is thought that the gene product itself may have a potential preventative or therapeutic use. Intraveneous administration of the protein might help protect the lung from damage by the proteolytic enzyme elastase, which is liberated from neutrophils.

Even though the clinical utility of this protein has yet to be demonstrated, an improved therapeutic product is already envisaged.[11,12] Structural and functional properties of proteins can be improved using recombinant DNA technology, as demonstrated by the protein engineering of recombinant β interferon to improve its stability when produced in *E. coli*,[14] and of interleukin-2.[15] In the case of $\alpha 1$ antitrypsin, the protein may be partially inactivated in vivo because of the oxidation of a methionine at position 385. Using in vitro mutagenesis, a valine was substituted for the methionine at this position. The altered $\alpha 1$ antitrypsin not only retained its ability to inhibit elastase but was also more resistant to oxidation.[11,12] As with all replacement therapy protocols, there remains some risk that the exogenously administered normal gene product might be immunogenic and elicit an immune response upon long-term use.

Finally, therapeutic approaches in which the normal gene itself is introduced into cells containing a genetic defect have also been envisioned for certain enzyme deficiencies and hemoglobinopathies (see Chapter 6). At this stage, gene therapy remains an exciting and exploratory research area involving complex technical and ethical issues.

Diagnosis

The use of cloned gene probes in the diagnosis of genetic disease was first achieved in the hemoglobinopathies[16] by direct analysis of the altered gene. A new dimension, however, was added by Kan and Dozy in their use of restriction fragment length polymorphisms (RFLPs) for the prenatal diagnosis of sickle cell anemia.[17] Using Southern transfer and hybridization experiments, these workers found a *HpaI* RFLP, one allele of which was in linkage disequilibrium with the β-globin allele (β^S) responsible for the disease. By studying the inheritance of the RFLP in the parents, affected relatives, and the fetus, it was possible to determine whether the latter was homozygous for the sickle cell mutation. This initial approach has been greatly expanded in recent years to many other diseases.[18] Using both disease-specific and random gene probes, RFLPs that are linked (but not necessarily in linkage disequilibrium) with the loci known to cause a particular disease have been discovered. If a polymorphic marker is found to be genetically linked to a particular disease locus, then by analyzing an affected individual and the parents as well as the fetus in question, the genetic makeup of the latter can very often be deduced. This approach has been explored in depth in Chapter 2.

In some genetic diseases, the specific mutation responsible for the disease is known and the same mutant allele is present in most individuals with the disease. In addition to sickle cell anemia, $\alpha 1$ antitrypsin deficiency and some forms of β-thalassemia in certain human populations are characterized by molecular homogeneity.[19–21] In the case of sickle cell anemia, which results from homozygosity of the sickle cell allele (β^S) at the β-globin locus, the T to A mutation in the sixth codon of the β chain results in the loss of a specific restriction enzyme site (*Dde*I, *Mst*II, etc.).[22–25] This mutation can thus be detected directly by Southern blot analysis as a characteristic increase in the length of a specific β-globin restriction fragment, so that the analysis of fetal DNA alone is sufficient for the diagnosis. For most genetic diseases due to single base changes, however, it is expected that the specific mutation responsible for the disease will not alter a restriction enzyme site and therefore cannot be directly diagnosed by Southern blot analysis.

Recently, however, a method utilizing synthetic oligonucleotide probes has been developed to detect the presence of the specific mutation.[19,21,26] For example, this approach is capable of distinguishing between the normal (β^A) and sickle cell (β^S) alleles and is independent of restriction site variation.[26] The method requires the synthesis of a 19-base oligomer complementary to the wild type sequence around the sixth codon of normal β-globin. This oligonucleotide exactly matches the β^A allele but has a one-base mismatch with the β^S allele. Because the nucleotide, which differs between the two alleles, is placed in the middle of the 19-mer, the DNA hybrid formed between the β^A oligomer probe and sickle cell anemia genomic DNA will be unstable under conditions (such as temperature, and salt), where the duplex formed between the probe and wild DNA will be stable. Similarly, a 19-mer probe exactly complementary to the β^S sequence will form, at an appropriate temperature, a stable duplex with sickle cell but not wild-type DNA. In practice, total genomic DNA is cut with a restriction enzyme that produces a unique fragment carrying the β-globin gene. This fragment is the same size for both the β^A and β^S alleles. Two aliquots of the DNA sample are run on an agarose gel, one portion of the dried-down gel is hybridized to the radiolabeled β^A-specific oligomer while the other is hybridized to the radiolabeled β^S-specific probe. This electrophoresis step is necessary because oligonucleotide probes of this length also hybridize to other genomic sequences, and therefore the β-globin DNA fragment must be separated from the rest of the genomic DNA to reduce the level of background signal. If the β-globin fragment hybridizes with both probes, the individual must be AS. If only the β^A-specific probe yields a signal then the DNA must be AA, whereas a positive signal with only the β^S probe identifies an SS individual. This approach, utilizing allele-specific oligonucleotide probes, has also been applied to the analysis of β-thalassemia[19,21] and to α1 antitrypsin deficiency.[10] Although this method is a general one, it requires several μg of genomic DNA, very high specific activity probes, and stringent wash procedures to achieve the requisite sensitivity and specificity; it may, therefore, require some modification for widespread commercial application.

New Technologies

Since the development of Southern transfer and hybridization techniques using radioactively labeled cloned cDNA, genomic, or oligonucleotide probes, a number of new technologies have been developed that have potential commercial application in that they either simplify the diagnostic format or substantially increase the sensitivity, or both.

Nonradioactive Probes. Thus far, genetic analysis using both RFLP and allele-specific oligonucleotide approaches has required ^{32}P-labeled probes to achieve single-copy gene detection. Although highly sensitive, such ^{32}P-labeled probes are unstable and require special procedures for their use and disposal, making them undesirable for widespread clinical diagnosis. The use of DNA probes, labeled with nonisotopic reporter molecules, was pioneered by Ward and his colleagues, who used DNA polymerase I in the nick-translation reaction to incorporate biotinylated nucleotides into specific hybridization probes.[27] The biotin moiety, which was covalently attached by means of a linker to the 5′ carbon of dUTP, has a very high affinity for avidin or streptavidin, allowing detection of the biotin-labeled probe with avidin conjugated to an enzyme. The enzyme, alkaline phosphatase, is capable of converting a colorless soluble substrate to a colored precipitate, forming a discrete band or dot, over the course of several hours. Modifications of this procedure have proved capable of detecting single-copy human genes in Southern blot experiments,[28,29] as have procedures for labeling DNA probes with photobiotin.[30]

A recently developed DNA probe system, based on the single-stranded bacteriophage M13 and a novel labeling reagent, biotinylated psoralen, was reported by Sheldon and co-workers[31] and is illustrated schematically in Figure 9.1. This system, which uses a streptavidin horseradish peroxidase (HRP) conjugate and the substrate tetramethylbenzidine (TMB) has been applied to the RFLP analysis of HLA class II polymorphisms.[31] It is capable of detecting single-copy genes in less than 0.5 μg genomic DNA and of converting substrate for the visualization of colored bands in less than 1 hour (Fig. 9.2). These biotin-labeled HLA class II probes are now commercially available as research reagents and have been used for tissue-typing for bone marrow transplantation, paternity determination, and the study of insulin-dependent diabetes susceptibility, revealing in each case relevant polymorphisms not detected by conventional HLA serologic typing.[31] Specific β-globin probes, labeled and detected similarly, have also been shown to distinguish normal ($\beta^A\beta^A$), sickle cell ($\beta^S\beta^S$) and sickle trait ($\beta^A\beta^S$) individuals by standard RFLP analysis.[32] The sensitivity of this system is thought to result from the large number of reporter molecules (~700 biotins per M13 probe), the high specific activity of HRP, and the ability of the substrate

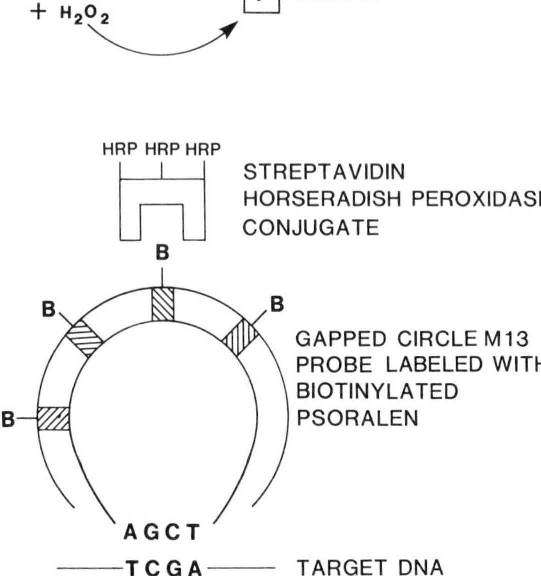

FIGURE 9.1 Nonisotopic probe detection system. The biotinylated M13 probe first hybridizes to the membrane-bound target DNA fragment. After excess probe is washed away, the streptavidin-HRP conjugate is added, which binds the biotin groups on the probe. Next, after excess conjugate is washed away, H_2O_2 and a colorless substrate (TMB) are added and converted to a blue precipitate by the streptavidin-HRP conjugate. Detection of the probe hybridized to a target restriction fragment is seen as a blue band on the Southern blot.

TMB to prevent the inactivation of HRP seen with the conventional substrate, DAB.

In addition to their use in Southern blot analysis, nonradioactive probes labeled with a fluorescent molecule or with biotin have been successfully applied to the in situ hybridization of individual chromosomes[33] and could make a significant contribution to cytogenetic analysis. DNA sequences specific for individual chromosomes can serve as specific probes to help karotyping and identify chromosomes without resorting to banding patterns.

Solution Hybridization Techniques

One approach aimed at simplifying the diagnostic protocol using DNA probes has been reported recently[34] and, unlike standard RFLP analyses, uses a liquid phase hybridization step. This method can detect nucleotide substitutions that occur at a restriction enzyme site. Known as oligomer restriction (OR), it involves hybridization of a labeled oligonucleotide probe with genomic DNA followed by restriction enzyme digestion and is carried out by the serial addition of various reagents to a single tube.

A similar protocol has recently been developed that does not depend upon the mutation affecting a restriction enzyme site. This technology makes use of RNAse A which can cut a DNA/RNA duplex *only* if a base pair mismatch exists.[35] Thus, the digestion of hybrids formed between a mutant DNA sequence and a labeled wild type RNA probe will generate a smaller product that depends upon the position of the mismatch in the DNA/RNA duplex. This method has been demonstrated to work with genomic DNA samples and is also effective in analyzing cloned mutations in plasmids or phage. Sequence alterations in RNA populations using a labeled RNA probe have also been detected by this procedure.[36]

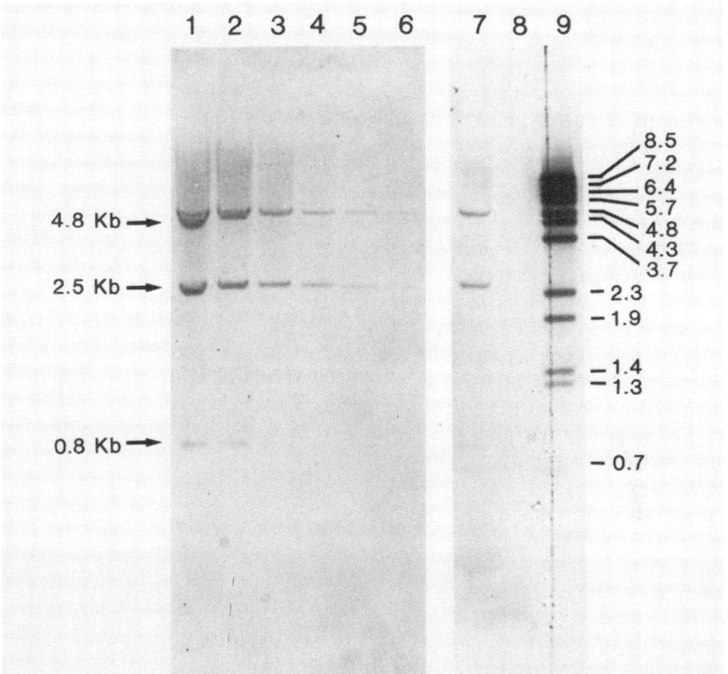

FIGURE 9.2 Detection threshold and specificity of an HLA DQα probe. After digestion with *Hin*dIII, 4, 2, 1, 0.5, 0.25, 0.125, and 2-μg samples of WT51 DNA (lanes 1–7), and 2 μg of LCL. 174 HLA class II deletion DNA (lane 8) were fractionated by agarose minigel electrophoresis, transferred to a Genetran membrane, hybridized to the DQα probe, and detected by the streptavidin-HRP conjugate. For size markers, we also included λ DNA digested with Bst EII and labeled with biotinylated psoralen (lane 9). Lanes 1–6 and 7–9 were on two separated agarose gels. The expected two bands of 4.8 kb and 2.5 kb can be seen even in the 0.25-μg samples (lane 5). A fainter 0.8-kb base band can be seen in the 4.0 and 2.0-μg samples (lanes 1 and 2).

Another method, one that depends upon changes in the mobility of duplex molecules in gradient denaturation gels, is also capable of detecting mutations.[37] A perfectly paired duplex between a genomic DNA segment and a labeled probe will migrate in the gel at a rate different from a heteroduplex containing even a single mismatch. In fact, this method has been used to analyze genomic DNA samples from four different forms of β-thalassemia,[38] although not all substitutions can be detected by its use.

Target Amplification

Very recently, a new technology has been developed that is likely to have a general impact on the use of DNA probes in diagnostics. The significance of this procedure lies in the fact that the target sequence to be analyzed can first be enzymatically amplified relative to the rest of the DNA present in the sample. All previous approaches toward making DNA probes a significant diagnostic tool have been aimed at improving the sensitivity of detection of the target, since the target is expected to be present at a very low concentration. The new amplification protocol, termed polymerase chain reaction (PCR),[39,40] is capable of substantially increasing the amount of target in the sample by enzymatically synthesizing many copies (10^5 to 10^6) of the original DNA segment. Significant amplification of the target, therefore, makes it possible to carry out the prenatal diagnosis on as few as 150 diploid cells in one day.[41] It may, in fact, allow the use of target detection methods such as nonradioactively labeled oligonucleotide probes, which are faster and easier to carry out.

The principle of PCR is shown in the series of figures below. The target genomic sequence to be amplified (......) and two small stretches of DNA that flank this target sequence are chosen first.

5′-----------catggt..agtgga-------------3′
3′-----------gtacca..tcacct-------------5′

Oligonucleotides (usually 20 bases but for the purposes of illustration shown here as 6) that are complementary to the sequences flanking the target and that will hybridize to opposite strands of the DNA are synthesized and used to prime DNA synthesis by DNA polymerase. The primer sequences (see below) are chosen so that when they form a duplex with the flanking sequences their 3′ ends face the target sequence.

Primers

5′ CATGGT 3′ 3′ TCACCT 5′

After denaturation of the genomic DNA, the primers are allowed to anneal to their complementary sequences flanking the target. DNA polymerase extension of the primers will produce newly synthesized DNA strands complementary to the target (xxxxxxx). These products (see below) are labeled L and they extend through the target for various distances (→), but in opposite directions.

First cycle

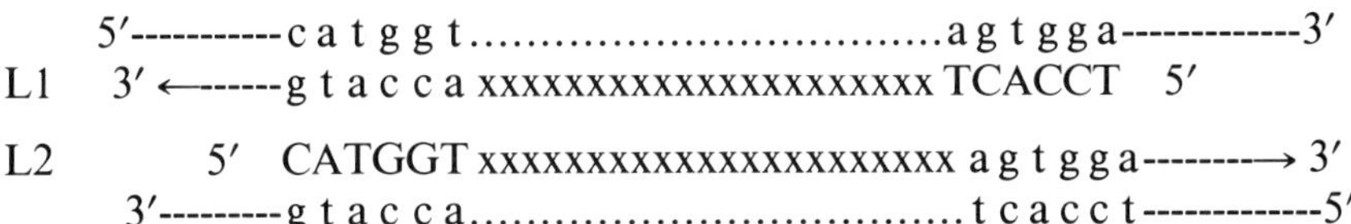

It is critical for the success of the method that each product extends far enough so that they will include the sequences complementary to the other primer. Following denaturation of the four strands and primer annealing, a second round of extension will again copy the target sequence. In the case of one of the strands (L2) formed after the first cycle, a product labeled S, which is exactly equal in length to the sum of the lengths of the two primers and the target DNA, is formed.

Second Round
(shown for L2 only)

L2 5′ CATGGTxxxxxxxxxxxxxxxxxxxxxxxxxxa g t g g a----------→ 3′
S 3′ g t a c c axxxxxxxxxxxxxxxxxxxxxxxxxxTCACCT 5′

Continuation of each cycle of denaturation, primer annealing and polymerase extension steps results in doubling the amount of target at each cycle. The products found after the fourth cycle are shown below.

Fourth Cycle
(All Products)

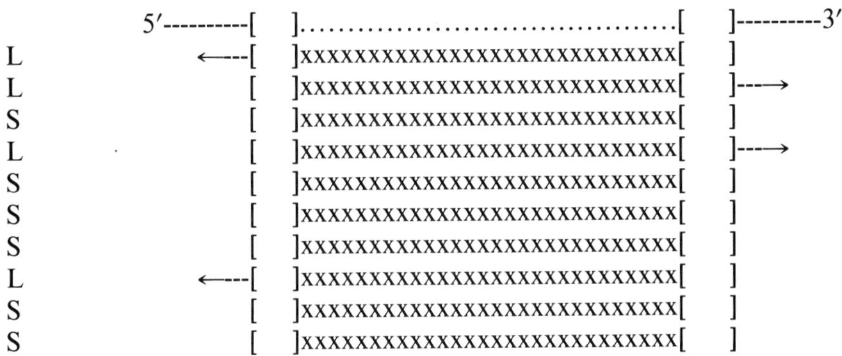

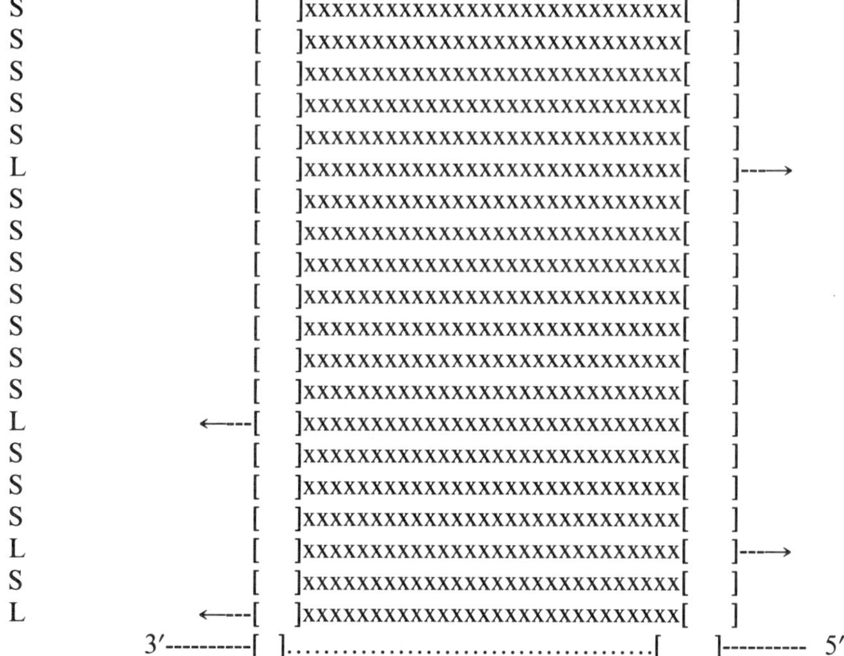

As can be seen, the number of target sequences found in the S forms accumulate rapidly and in an exponential fashion. For example, if this protocol were repeated 20 times and at 100% efficiency, the target would be expected to be amplified a millionfold (2^{20}).

The PCR amplification method has been applied to the diagnosis of sickle cell anemia in conjunction with the OR method discussed above.[40] In these experiments, the OR method (Fig. 9.3) involves a sequential digestion with not one, but two enzymes, *Dde*I and *Hinf*I. As shown, the cleavage of the hybridized oligonucleotide probe will produce a 3-base fragment with the sickle cell allele and an 8-base product for the wild allele. AA individuals will be expected to exhibit only 8-mer, SS individuals 3-mer, and heterozygotes both 8- and 3-mers. These probe cleavage products can be resolved from each other and the 40-base probe by polyacrylamide gel electrophoresis. If this procedure is carried out on genomic DNA without amplification, at least 10 μgs of DNA and 4 to 5 days of autoradiography are required to detect a signal.[34] On the other hand, if the PCR method is carried out first for 20 cycles, then the amount of DNA added to the gel can be reduced by three orders of magnitude.[40] The results of such an experiment are shown in Figure 9.4 where instead of a 4- to 5-day autoradiographic exposure, a 6-hour exposure was made and nanogram rather than microgram amounts of DNA were analyzed. The degree of target amplification was measured in independent experiments and found to be 220,000-fold after 20 cycles, an average efficiency of 85% per cycle. Using the sickle cell anemia test as a model system, decreasing amounts of genomic DNA were amplified for 20 cycles. As shown in Figure 9.5, a 24-hour autoradiographic exposure allowed the diagnosis of the AS genotype starting with as little as 20 ngs of nucleic acid. This amount is equivalent to a total of 6,000 molecules of the β-globin sequence in the sample.

Recently, the use of PCR to amplify specific genomic sequences prior to hybridization with synthetic oligonucleotide probes has allowed the analysis of allelic sequence variation in crude cell lysates of fewer than 100 cells in a dot blot format.[41] Thus, this approach eliminates simultaneously the need for DNA purification and gel electrophoresis while retaining the specificity of short oligonucleotide hybridization probes. This promises to be a simple and general method for clinical genetic diagnosis.

CANCER

Therapy

The worldwide market for cancer therapeutics is expected to be worth over $1 billion per year by the end of the century. Moreover, there are fewer regulatory barriers to the introduction of a new therapeutic drug for cancer than for other less life-threatening diseases. Consequently, many biotechnology companies have committed themselves to the development of new cancer therapeutics. The biologically complex nature of cancer and its relationship to the immune system has led to the concept that certain proteins involved in regulating the immune system might prove therapeutically valuable. Towards this end, a number of proteins that play a role in modulating the immune system (lymphokines) have been purified and their coding genes cloned. These genes have been expressed to produce large amounts of protein in order to test potential anticancer activity in a clinical setting. This category includes alpha, beta and gamma interferon, interleukins-1, -2, and -3, tumor necrosis factor, lymphotoxin, and a variety of colony stimulating factors.[42–51] One lymphokine, α-2a recombinant interferon, has already been approved by the FDA for therapy for hairy-cell leukemia.[52] A number of these gene products are currently in the early phases of clinical trials, but their eventual utility in cancer therapy remains to be documented. One

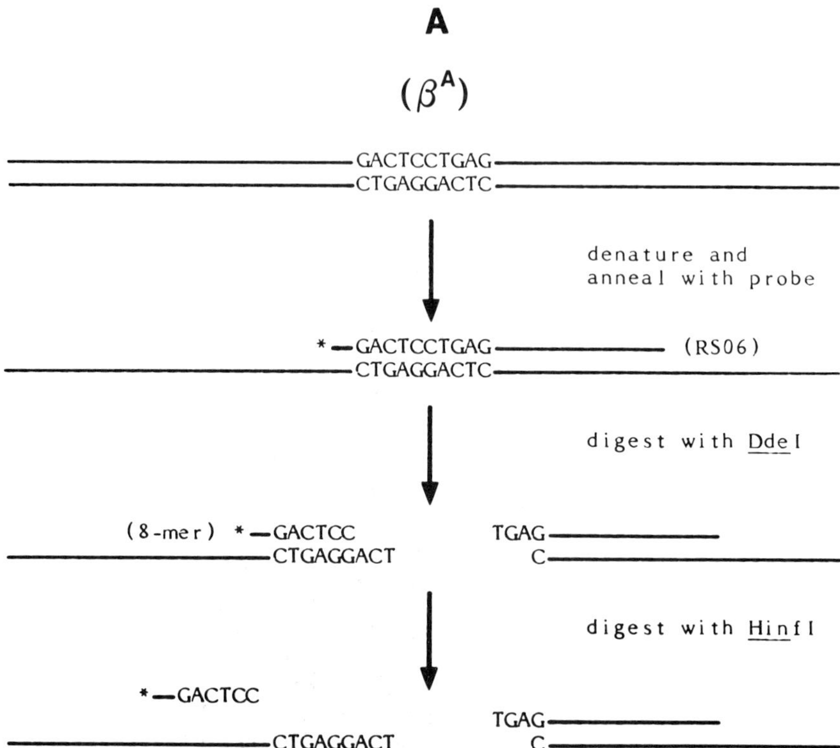

FIGURE 9.3 Schematic diagram of oligomer restriction by sequential digestion to identify β^A- and β^B-specific cleavage products. The DNA sequences shown are the regions of the β-globin genomic DNA and RS06 hybridization probe containing the invariant Hinf I site (GANTC, where N represents any nucleotide) and the polymorphic *Dde*I site (CTNAG). The remaining DNA sequences are represented as solid horizontal lines. The asterisk indicates the position of the radioactive ^{32}P label attached to the 5′-end of the RS06 probe with polynucleotide kinase. **A:** Outline of the procedure and expected results when RS06 anneals to the normal β-globin gene (β^A). After denaturation of the genomic DNA and hybridization of the labeled RS06 probe to the complementary target sequence in the β^A gene, digestion of the probe-target hybrid with *Dde*I

exciting preliminary result comes from studies using interleukin-2 in patients with advanced stages of usually refractory solid tumors of the lung and colon. The results of this study showed several examples of marked tumor regression when the IL-2 was used to stimulate a subset of killer T cells (lymphokine activated killer or "LAK") by adoptive immunotherapy.[53] This protocol involves the removal of white blood cells from the patient, in vitro culture and expansion of these cells in the presence of the lymphokine IL-2, and the reintroduction of these activated cells along with IL-2 into the

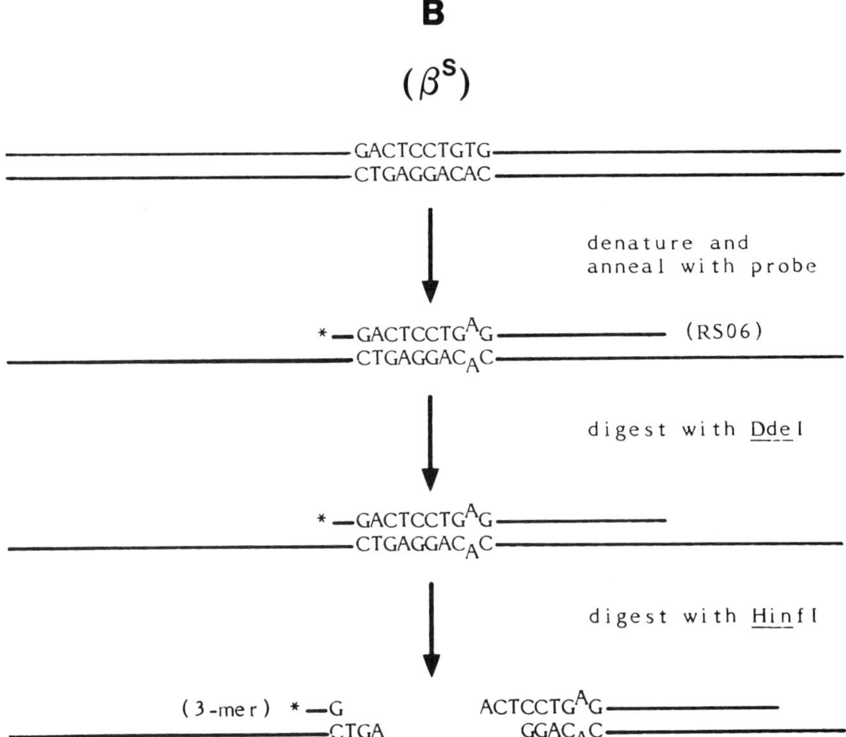

causes the release of a labeled (8-nt) cleavage product. Because of the relatively stringent conditions during *Dde*I digestion, the 8-nt cleavage product dissociates from the genomic DNA, and the subsequent digestion with Hinf I has no effect. **B:** Outline of *Dde*I and Hinf I digestion after hybridization of the RS06 probe to the sickle cell allele (β^S). As a consequence of the β^S mutation, the probe-target hybrid contains an A-A mismatch within the *Dde*I site and is not cleaved by the *Dde*I endonuclease. The Hinf I site, however, remains intact, and digestion with that enzyme generates a labeled 3-nt product. Thus, the presence of the β^A allele is revealed by the release of a labeled 8-nt fragment, whereas the presence of β^S is indicated by a labeled 3-nt fragment.

patient's circulation. Although toxicities are observed at high doses, this approach, combined with other lymphokines or chemotherapeutic drugs, holds considerable promise.

Recombinant DNA technology has also contributed to the immunotoxin approach to cancer therapy.[54–56] Immunotoxins consist of two covalently attached components, one conferring tumor cell specificity and the other toxicity. The toxic component, for example, may be a protein toxin of plant or bacterial origin which when introduced into a cell is capable of

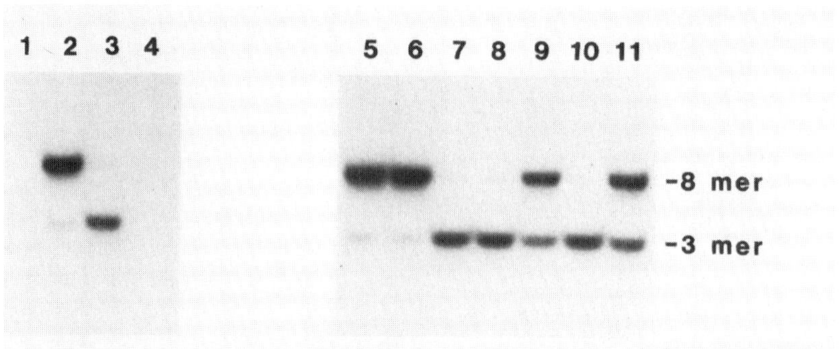

FIGURE 9.4 Determination of the β-globin genotype in human genomic DNA with PCR-OR. Samples (1 μg) of human genomic DNA were amplified for 20 cycles (as described above). The amplified DNAs (71 ng) were hybridized to the RS06 probe and serially digested with *Dde*I and Hinf I (as described in Fig. 9.3). Each sample (6 μl) was analyzed by 30% polyacrylamide gel electrophoresis and autoradiographed for 6 hours at −70°C with one intensification screen. Each lane contains 7 ng of genomic DNA; (Lane 1) unamplified Molt4 DNA (negative control); (lane 2) amplified Molt4 ($\beta^A\beta^A$); (lane 3) SC-1 ($\beta^S\beta^S$); (lane 4) GM2064 ($\Delta\Delta$); (lanes 5 to 11) clinical samples CH1 ($\beta^A\beta^A$), CH2 ($\beta^A\beta^A$), CH3 ($\beta^S\beta^S$), CH4 ($\beta^S\beta^S$), CH7 ($\beta^A\beta^S$), CH8 ($\beta^S\beta^S$), and CH12 ($\beta^A\beta^S$), respectively.

killing it with high efficiency. The specificity component is an immunoglobulin molecule directed against a cell surface antigen found preferentially on cancer but not normal cells, maximizing the likelihood that the toxin-antibody complex is taken up only by tumor cells. Large quantities of the specific immunoglobulin can be obtained by hybridoma technology while recombinant DNA methods have allowed the cloning and expression of toxin genes. The clinical efficacy of using toxins has been demonstrated in the removal of T cells from bone marrow, reducing the incidence of graft vs host disease in transplants[57] but in vivo demonstration of tumor specific killing in man awaits clinical trials.

Diagnosis

It is expected that, along with the growth of the cancer therapeutic markets, the commercial possibilities for sensitive and specific cancer diagnostic tests will also be expanded. Recombinant DNA technology has made a significant contribution toward providing new tools to be used in cancer diagnostics. An ideal cancer marker might be some specific antigen, detectable in serum, and unique to all types of tumors but absent from abnormal cells. Although a number of different serum cancer markers have been identified, they are far from this ideal.[58] Even though they play an important role in diagnosis and

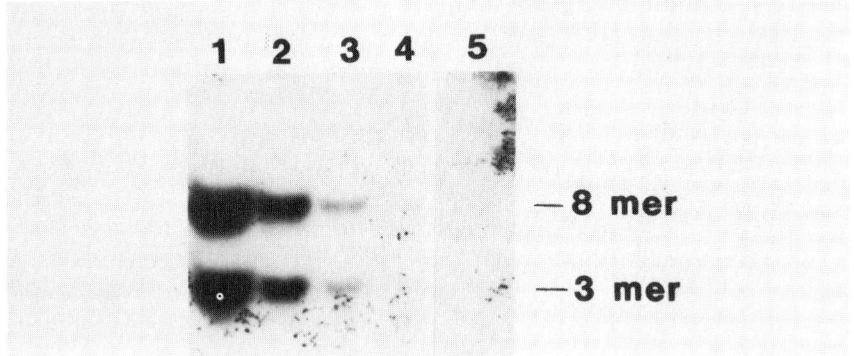

FIGURE 9.5 Detection threshold for PCR-OR. Fivefold serial dilutions of genomic DNA (500, 100, 20, and 4 ng) from the clinical samples CH12 ($\beta^A\beta^S$) were amplified by 20 cycles of PCR and one-tenth each reaction (50, 10, 2, and 0.4 ng) was analyzed by OR. The gel contained (lane 1) genomic DNA (12.5 ng); (lane 2) 2.5 ng; (lane 3) 0.5 ng; (lane 4) 0.1 ng; (lane 5) 12.5 ng genomic DNA from the globin deletion cell lines GM2064. Autoradiographic exposure was for 20 hours at −70°C with an intensification screen.

in monitoring tumor progression, they are not universally applicable to all cancers. The recent discovery of oncogenes, however, has led to the possibility of finding a more widely distributed cancer marker or new markers highly specific for some cancers. Proto-oncogenes, whose normal function in most cases is unknown, can aid in the progression of normal cells to tumor cells when they have undergone mutation, amplification, or translocation to the oncogene state.[59–60] In the case of human cancers, all three modifications have been observed in human tumors. For example, the genes encoding the ras family of proto-oncogene products can undergo single nucleotide substitutions capable of aiding the transformation of normal cells to tumor cells.[59,60] The specific mutations that cause this transformation have been localized at two predominant sites in this approximately 188-bp polypeptide: positions 12 and 61. The detection of ras protein which is mutated in either of these sites in clinical samples therefore might suggest the presence of tumor cells. Since all normal cells contain the ras proteins, the distinction between normal ras and oncogene-activated ras polypeptides altered at position 12 or 61 in serum or tissue samples is required. The production of antibodies capable of this has recently been reported[61] using a synthetic peptide of 17 amino acids that included the position 12 amino acid as immunogen. Antibodies specific for four of the six possible amino acid substitutions resulting from a single base change at position 12 are available as research reagents in order to have their diagnostic utility examined. It is significant that the detection of ras protein in urine has been recently reported.[62] With the availability of oncogene-specific anti-ras antibodies, it should be possible to determine whether the ras proteins found in urine are the products of the normal protoncogene or whether they represent the products of oncogenes present in tumor cells.

The activation of protoncogenes to oncogenes by gene amplification and translocation have also been reported. Amplification of the N-myc oncogene in neuroblastoma cell lines and clinical samples has been observed.[63] Translocation of the c-myc gene on chromosome 8 to the immunoglobin heavy-chain cluster region on chromosome 14 has been associated with Burkitt's lymphoma[64,65] and is just one example of the many chromosome rearrangements associated with malignancy.[66,67] The cloning of these genes has not only led to new insights into the basic molecular biology of cancer but has also led to the application of this information to cancer diagnostics and therapy. The most dramatic example of the clinical utility of these probes comes from studies on the amplification of the N-myc gene in childhood neuroblastoma[63] and c-myc in small-cell lung carcinoma.[68] The extent of N-myc amplification in tumors at the five recognized clinical stages (I through IVS) was analyzed by using an N-myc probe. A statistically highly significant correlation was found between the degree of amplification and stage of the disease. More recently, the association of the degree of amplification with rapid tumor progression has been established.[69]

The diagnosis of certain leukemias may also benefit from the use of recombinant DNA probes in that specific translocations associated with well defined diseases can be identified. For example, in the case of certain follicular lymphomas, translocations between the immunoglobin heavy-chain loci on chromosome 14 and another locus on chromosome 18 (Bcl 2) have been observed.[70-72] The cytologically well-characterized Philadelphia chromosome associated with chronic myelogenous leukemia has recently been found to result from a translocation of the oncogene c-abl on chromosome 22 to a locus on chromosome 9 called Bcr.[73,74] The translocated gene segment produces a larger than normal c-abl polypeptide which results from a fusion at the DNA level.[75] Antibodies to the resulting fusion protein might prove diagnostically valuable.

INFECTIOUS DISEASE DIAGNOSIS

Cloned Gene Products. In general, the diagnostic use of the protein products of genes cloned from infectious organisms depends on their ability to function as specific immunogens for the production of a diagnostic antibody or as specific antigens for the detection of human serum antibody. Genes which encode proteins specific for a given infectious disease pathogen can be expressed in bacterial or mammalian hosts and the purified protein used to raise monoclonal or polyclonal antibodies. The large amounts of protein product that can be obtained from bacterial expression systems facilitates significantly the purification of the pathogen protein. In some cases, fusion proteins produced by inserting cloned DNA fragments containing open reading frames (a nucleotide sequence containing no termination codons and thus capable of encoding a polypeptide) of unknown function into a bacterial gene have been used as immunogens. Recently, this approach has been used to identify polypeptides encoded by the pre-S open reading frame of Hepatitis B virus,[76] as well as to analyze HTLV-III (ORF) gene segments.[77] A recent study of the syphilis pathogen, *T. pallidum*, reported that a rabbit antiserum to a 190-kD protein encoded by cloned *T. pallidum* DNA and expressed in *Escherichia coli* bound to the surface of the pathogen in the trepaneme immobilization (TPI) test.[78]

A pathogen-specific protein encoded by a cloned gene can also serve in the diagnosis of infectious disease by detecting the serum antibody response to the pathogen infection. Such an approach, which is obviously limited to protein antigens, is particularly useful when the pathogen is difficult to grow in culture (eg, *T. pallidum*) or when the specific protein antigens are difficult to purify. Genomic libraries of pathogen DNA cloned in vectors that allow the production of pathogen protein sequences can be screened with a variety of sera from infected patients or with antisera to identify genes encoding antigens of a particular specificity. For example, the antibody response to some individual antigens may be diagnostic of acute vs chronic infection or of primary rather than later stages of an infection. In a study of serum antibodies in individuals with acute and chronic toxoplasmosis, an antigen-specific IgM antibody response uniquely associated with acute infection was revealed by Western blot analysis.[79] Thus, in principle, libraries could be screened with sera from both acute and chronically infected patients and clones that reacted differentially could be analyzed further.

T. pallidum is not readily propogated in culture and is grown only in rabbit testicles; moreover, syphilis represents an infectious disease for which serodiagnosis, the detection of the patient's immune response to infection, is the standard diagnostic test. A variety of protein antigens, encoded by cloned *T. pallidum* genes, have been shown to function effectively as a specific antigen in the analysis of serum panels from controls and patients. The sensitivity and specificity in RIA and ELISA tests based on cloned syphilis antigens are comparable to results obtained with the standard confirmatory serologic tests based on the whole pathogen.[80,81] The ELISA screening test for HTLV-III specific serum antibodies represents another potential use of cloned pathogen antigens. The env polypeptide, synthesized in *E. coli*, has been used[82-83] and found to yield comparable results to the ELISA tests performed with virus purified from infected cell lines. Diagnostic tests based on cloned pathogen gene products should reduce potential health hazards to which clinical laboratory workers may be exposed. In addition, the comparative analysis of cloned pathogen nucleotide sequences allows identification of conserved regions and those that may be type specific, eg, HSV-I vs HSV-II. Thus, synthetic peptides or fusion proteins encoding potentially type-specific epitopes might be produced and used to detect serum antibodies for the differential diagnosis of HSV-I and HSV-II infections.

Cloned Gene Hybridization Probes. Cloned DNA fragments from infectious disease pathogens can also serve as specific hybridization probes to detect pathogen nucleic acid sequences present in the clinical sample. This approach does not require that the cloned fragment encode a protein, but only that it be capable of hybridizing to all the clinically relevant strains or isolates (range) and that it discriminate between the pathogen and other microorganisms likely to be in the clinical sample (specificity). The application of DNA probes was first reported by Falkow and colleagues in their pioneering analysis of toxigenic *E. coli.*[84] The initial work in this area utilized ^{32}P-labeled probes and autoradiography. Herpesvirus and chlamydial infections of cultured cells have been detected recently using modifications of the Ward biotinylated probe system.[85] Some of these probes are now commercially available as research reagents (Enzo). This approach to the analysis of pathogen infected cells may prove very useful in the diagnosis of certain infectious diseases, particularly if this procedure can be simplified or automated. Radioactive DNA probes specific for *Salmonella* and toxic *E. coli* have also been used to detect bacterial contamination of foodstuffs.[86,87] This latter analysis, like all infectious disease probe applications, would benefit greatly from the use of nonisotopic labels.

The first commercial DNA probe kit for infectious disease is based on the ingenious idea of detecting pathogen specific sequences in ribosomal RNA (Gen-Probe). These sequences would be expected to be present in approximately 10,000 copies per cell and allow more sensitive detection of the pathogen. A test for *Mycoplasma* contamination in tissue culture cells, as well as a *Legionella* clinical test, utilized the solution hybridization of a radioactive DNA probe with ribosomal RNA present in the clinical sample and the subsequent separation of the probe/target duplex from the unbound probe using hydroxylapatite.[88] The strategy of using ribosomal RNA as a target, although powerful and elegant, is not in general use because the evolutionary conservation of rRNA sequences may preclude distinguishing between some closely related pathogens and will also not be applicable to virus detection.

The ability of an infectious disease diagnostic test to detect very small amounts of pathogen in the clinical sample is crucial in determining clinical sensitivity (the fraction of infected patients scored as positive). In this regard, the capability of enzymatically amplifying specific pathogen DNA sequences using PCR (discussed above) may prove useful. Recently, Sninsky and his colleagues have applied the newly developed techniques of PCR and OR to the analysis of HTLV-III in cell lines infected with patient material;[89] their results indicate this approach has great diagnostic potential in this area.

In general, the requirements for clinical diagnosis of infectious disease are that the test be simple, fast, and inexpensive, in addition to meeting the standard diagnostic criteria of specificity and sensitivity. The challenge for DNA probe detection is to develop commercial tests that can meet these stringent criteria. The tests will have to be nonradioactive and either simple or capable of automation for this market.

VACCINES

Although the major focus of this chapter is on the diagnosis and therapy of genetic diseases and chronic diseases with a genetic component, the significant potential of recombinant DNA technology for vaccine production warrants at least a brief mention. The cloning and expression of pathogen genes makes possible the use of purified pathogen proteins (eg, viral coat proteins) in vaccines, thereby eliminating the health hazards associated with either killed virus vaccines or attenuated viral vaccines. The challenge in the development of such subunit vaccines is to identify those viral proteins capable of eliciting a strong protective immune response. Generally, subunit vaccines are less immunogenic than those based on attenuated virus or killed virus, but the increased safety and economy of recombinant protein production as well as the decreased hazards of their use suggest that this technology may play an important role in vaccine production. A hepatitis B vaccine, based on recombinant hepatitis surface antigen, has been developed by Merck, Sharp, and Dohme, in collaboration with Chiron, and has recently been approved by the FDA.[90] Recombinant HTLV-III antigens, as well, have been shown to elicit antibodies to the virus envelope capable of in vitro neutralization.[91]

Vaccines, based on the use of cloned gene products, may also be useful in the protection against pathogens that produce protein toxins. Here, the gene encoding the toxin can be cloned and subjected to site-specific mutagenesis, allowing the production of an immunogenic and potentially protective protein which has lost its toxic properties. The genetic engineering of toxin proteins for potential vaccine use has been reported for diphtheria toxin[92] and pertussis toxin.[93]

An important additional strategy for vaccine development involves subcloning pathogen sequences into the vaccinia viral vector. In this case, the actual vaccine consists of an attenuated recombinant vaccinia virus that will produce potentially protective pathogen antigens after infection. This approach combines the immunogenic advantages of an attenuated viral vaccine, namely that the virus can replicate and stimulate the immune system, with the safety aspects of specific purified subunit vaccines. The vaccinia vector approach has been used in the production of a protective vaccine for mouse Friend leukemia virus[94] and parasites.[95]

Although recombinant DNA technology is ideally suited to the production of human vaccines, the commercial development of recombinant DNA vaccines has lagged behind the development of therapeutic and diagnostic products. This may reflect issues of product liability and financial return on investment associated with preventative health measures. Marketing analyses suggest that people are willing to pay substantially more for a therapeutic drug when sick than they are for a preventative measure while still healthy. In addition, many of the populations who might benefit from, for example, the impressive recent progress on a recombinant DNA vaccine for malaria[96,97] live in relatively poor countries. Unfortunately, in this case, the economic incentives that motivate the biotechnology industry may not prove sufficient to develop such products. Thus, it remains to be seen whether the significant potential of recombinant DNA technology to produce safe and economical vaccines will be fully realized.

CONCLUSIONS/FUTURE DIRECTIONS

Recently, human proteins of known therapeutic value have been produced by recombinant DNA technology and are already on the market and in clinical trials. It is clear that the ability to clone and express human genes will ultimately lead to the production of therapeutically valuable proteins whose functions are still poorly defined or currently unknown. This capacity to economically produce foreign proteins in bacterial or mammalian cells will continue to have a major impact on therapeutic and preventative medicine. In addition, recombinant DNA technology has significant potential in the areas of genetic disease, cancer, and infectious disease diagnosis, using either the protein products of the cloned genes or the cloned DNA sequences themselves as specific hybridization probes. Given the recent development of automated synthetic chemistries, oligonucleotides and peptides whose sequence is based on the analysis of cloned genes can be used in nucleic acid hybridization and in immunological-based detection systems. The recent emergence of sensitive nonradioactive DNA probe systems removes many of the barriers to widespread clinical applications while the newly developed ability to enzymatically amplify specific DNA segments enables the detection of very few target sequences. This amplification procedure has important implications for all nucleic acid based diagnostic systems.

The commercial products developed by biotechnology companies using recombinant DNA technology should help realize the enormous promise and potential of molecular biology for progress in clinical medicine.

REFERENCES

1. Platz P, Jakobsen BD, Morling N, et al: HLA-D and DR antigens in genetic analysis of insulin dependent diabetes mellitus. *Diabetologia* 1981;21:108–115.
2. Goeddel DV, Kleid DG, Bolivar F, et al: Expression in *Escherichia coli* of chemically synthesized genes for human insulin. *Proc Natl Acad Sci USA* 1979;76:106.
3. McKee PA: Hemostasis and disorders of blood coagulation, in Stanbury JB, Wyngaarden JB, Fredrickson DS, et al (eds): *The Metabolic Basis for Inherited Disease*, ed 5. New York, McGraw-Hill, 1983, p 1531–1560.
4. Gitschier G, Wood WI, Goralka TM, et al: Characterisation of the factor VIII gene. *Nature* 1984;312:326–330.
5. Wood WI, Capon DJ, Simonsen CC, et al: Expression of active human Factor VIII from recombinant DNA clones. *Nature* 1984;312:330–336.
6. Toole JJ, Knopf JL, Wozney JM, et al: Molecular cloning of a cDNA encoding human antihaemophilic factor. *Nature* 1984;312:342–347.
7. Goeddel DV, Heyneker HL, Hozumi T, et al: Direct expression in *Escherichia coli* of a DNA sequence coding for human growth hormone. *Nature* 1979;281:544–548.
8. Norman C: News and comment: virus scare halts hormone research. *Science* 1985;228: 1176–1177.
9. Kurachi K, Chaudra T, Dengen SJF, et al: Cloning and sequence of cDNA coding for α1-antitrypsin. *Proc Natl Acad Sci USA* 1981;78:6826–6830.
10. Kidd VJ, Wallace RB, Itakura K, et al: α1-antitrypsin deficiency detention by direct analysis of the mutation in the gene. *Nature* 1983;304:230–234.
11. Courtney M, Jallat S, Tessier L-H, et al: Synthesis in *E. coli* of α1-antitrypsin variants of therapeutic potential for emphysema and thrombosis. *Nature* 1985;313:149–151.
12. Rosenberg S, Barr PJ, Najarian RC, et al: Synthesis in yeast of a functional oxidation resistant mutant of human α1-antitrypsin. *Nature* 1984:312:77–80.
13. Gadek JE, Crystal RG: α1-antitrypsin deficiency, in Stanbury JB, Wyngaarden JB, Fredrickson DS, et al (eds): *The Metabolic Basis for Inherited Disease,* ed 5. New York, McGraw-Hill, 1983, p 1450–1467.
14. Mark DF, Lu SD, Creasey AA, et al: Site-specific mutagenesis of the human fibroblast interferon gene. *Proc Natl Acad Sci USA* 1984;81:5662–5666.
15. Wang A, Lu SD, Mark DF: Site-specific mutagenesis of the human interleukin-2 gene: Structure-function analysis of the cysteine residues. *Science* 1984;224:1431–1433.
16. Kan YW, Golbus MS, Dozy AM: Prenatal diagnosis of α thalassemia: Clinical application of molecular hybridization. *N Engl J Med* 1976;295:1165–1167.
17. Kan YW, Dozy AM: Polymorphism of DNA sequence adjacent in human beta-globin structural gene: Relationship to sickle mutation. *Proc Natl Acad Sci USA* 1978;75: 5631–5635.

18. Botstein D, White RL, Skolnick M, et al: Construction of a genetic linkage map in man using restriction fragment length polymorphisms. *Am J Hum Genet* 1980;32:314–331.
19. Orkin SH, Markham AP, Kazazian HH, Jr: Direct detection of the common Mediterranean β-thalassemia gene with synthetic DNA probes: An alternate approach for prenatal diagnosis. *J Clin Invest* 1983;71:775–779.
20. Cox DW, Woo SLC, Mansfield T: DNA restriction fragments associated with αl-antitrypsin indicate a single origin for deficiency allele PIZ. *Nature* 1985;316:79–80.
21. Pirastu M, Kan YW, Cao A, et al: Prenatal diagnosis of β-thalassemia: Direct detection of a single nucleotide mutation in DNA. *N Engl J Med* 1983;309:284–287.
22. Geever RF, Wilson LB, Nallaseth FS, et al: Direct identification of sickle cell anemia by blot hybridization. *Proc Natl Acad Sci USA* 1981;78:5081–5085.
23. Wilson JT, Milner PF, Summer ME, et al: Use of restriction endonucleases for mapping the allele for β^S globin. *Proc Natl Acad Sci USA* 1982;79:3628–3631.
24. Chang JC, Kan YW: A sensitive new prenatal test for sickle cell anemia. *N Engl J Med* 1982;707:30–32.
25. Orkin SH, Little PFR, Kazazian HH, Jr, et al: Improved detection of the sickle cell mutation by DNA analysis. *N Engl J Med* 1982;307:32–36.
26. Conner BJ, Reves AA, Morin C, et al: Detection of sickle cell β^S-globin allele by hybridization with synthetic oligonucleotides. *Proc Natl Acad Sci USA* 1983;80:278–282.
27. Langer PR, Waldrop AA, Ward DC: Enzymatic synthesis of biotin-labeled polynucleotides: Novel nucleic acid affinity probes. *Proc Natl Acad Sci USA* 1981;78:6633–6637.
28. Leary JJ, Brigati DJ, Ward DC: Rapid and sensitive colorimetric method for visualizing biotin-labeled DNA probes hybridized to DNA or RNA immobilized on nitrocellulose: Bio-blots. *Proc Natl Acad Sci USA* 1983;80:4045–4049.
29. Garbutt GJ, Wilson JT, Schuster GS, et al: Use of biotinylated probes for detecting sickle cell anemia. *Clin Chem* 1985;31:1203–1206.
30. Chan VT-W, Fleming KA, McGee JO: Detection of subpicogram quantities of specific DNA sequences on blot hybridization with biotinylated probes. *Nucleic Acids Res* 1985; 13:8083–8091.
31. Sheldon EL, Kellogg DE, Watson R, et al: Use of nonisotopic M13 probes for genetic analysis: Application to HLA class II loci. *Proc Natl Acad Sci USA* 1986;83:9085–9089.
32. Sheldon EL, et al: Nonisotopic M13 probes for the detection of the beta-globin gene: Application to the diagnosis of sickle cell anemia. *Clin Chem* to be published.
33. Pinkel D, Gray JW, Trask B, et al: Cytogenetic analysis by *in situ* hybridization with fluorescently labeled nucleic acid probes. *Molec Biol Homosapiens* 51, *Proc CSHSQ Biol.* In press.
34. Saiki RK, Arnheim N, Erlich HA: A novel method for the detection of polymorphic restriction sites by cleavage of oligonucleotide probes: Application to sickle cell anemia. *Biotechnology* 1985;3:1008–1012.
35. Myers RM, Larin Z, Maniatis T: Detection of single base substitutions by ribonuclease cleavage at mismatches in RNA:DNA duplexes. *Science* 1985;230:1242–1246.
36. Winter E, Yamamoto F, Almoguera C, et al: A method to detect and characterize point mutations in transcribed genes: Amplification and overexpression of the mutant c-Ki-ras allele in human tumor cells. *Proc Natl Acad Sci USA* 1985;82:7575–7579.
37. Fischer SG, Lerman LS: DNA fragments differing by single base-pair substitutions are separated in denaturing gels: Correspondence with melting theory. *Proc Natl Acad Sci USA* 1983;80:1579–1583.
38. Myers RM, Lumelsky N, Lerman LS, et al: Detection of single base substitutions in total genomic DNA. *Nature* 1985;313:495–498.
39. Mullis K, Faloona F: Specific synthesis of DNA *in vitro* via a polymerase catalysed chain reaction. *Meth Enzymol* 1987;55, to be published.

40. Saiki RK, Scharf S, Faloona F, et al: Enzymatic amplification of β-globin genomic sequences and restriction site analysis for diagnosis of sickle cell anemia. *Science* 1985; 230:1350–1354.
41. Saiki RK, Bugawan TL, Horn GT, et al: Analysis of enzymatically amplified β-globin and HLA-DQα DNA with allele-specific oligonucleotide probes. *Nature* 1986;324:163–166.
42. Gray PW, Leung DW, Pennica D, et al: Expression of human immune interferon cDNA in *E. coli* and monkey cells. *Nature* 1982;295:503.
43. Goeddel DV, Yelverton E, Ullrich A: Human leukocyte interferon produced by *E. coli* is biologically active. *Nature* 1980;287:411–416.
44. Taniguchi T, Mantei N, Schwarzstein M, et al: Human leukocyte and fibroblast interferons are structurally related. *Nature* 1980;285:547–549.
45. Derynck R, Gutent J, DeClercq E, et al: Isolation and structure of a human fibroblast interferon gene. *Nature* 1980;285:542–547.
46. Rosenberg SA, Grimm EA, McGrogan M, et al: Biological activity of recombinant human interleukin-2 produced in *E. coli. Science* 1984;223:1412–1414.
47. Fung MC, Hapel AJ, Yuer S, et al: Molecular cloning of cDNA for murine interleukin-3. *Nature* 1984;307:233–237.
48. Kawasaki ES, Ladner MB, Wang AM, et al: Molecular cloning of a complementary DNA encoding human macrophage-specific colony-stimulating factor (CSF-1). *Science* 1985; 230:291–296.
49. Lee F, Yokota T, Otsuka T, et al: Isolation of cDNA for a human granulocyte-macrophage colony-stimulating factor by functional expression in mammalian cells. *Proc Natl Acad Sci USA* 1985;82:4360–4364.
50. Pennica D, Nedwin GE, Hayflick JS, et al: Human tumor necrosis factor: Precursor structure, expression and homology to lymphotoxin. *Nature* 1984;312:724–729.
51. Gray PW, Aggarwal BB, Benton CV, et al: Cloning and expression of cDNA for human lymphotoxin, a lymphokine with tumor necrosis activity. *Nature* 1984;312:721–724.
52. Quesada JR, Hersh EM, Manning J, et al: Treatment of hairy cell leukemia with recombinant α-interferon. Blood 1986;68:493–497.
53. Rosenberg SA, Lotze M, Muul LM, et al: Observations on the systemic administration of autologous lymphokine-activated killer cells and recombinant interleukin-2 to patients with metastatic cancer. *N Engl J Med* 1985;313:1485–1492.
54. Vitetta EA, Uhr JW: Immunotoxins. *Ann Rev Immunol* 1985;3:197–212.
55. Frankel A, Issell B, Ramakrishnan S, et al: Prospects for immunotoxin therapy in cancer. *Ann Rev Med* to be published.
56. Vitetta ES, Krolick KA, Miyama-Inaba M, et al: Immunotoxins: A new approach to cancer therapy. *Science* 1983;219:644–650.
57. Filipovich A, Youle R, Neville D, et al: Ex vivo treatment of donor bone marrow with anti-T-cell immunotoxins for prevention of graft-vs-host disease. *Lancet* 1984;1:469–472.
58. Sell S: Cancer markers: Past, present and future in monoclonal antibodies and cancer therapy. Reisfeld RA, Sell S (eds): Proceedings of the Roche-UCLA Symposium. New York, Alan R. Liss, 1985; p 3–21.
59. Bishop JM: Viral oncogenes. *Cell* 1985;42:23–38.
60. Varumus H: The molecular genetics of cellular oncogenes. *Ann Rev Genet* 1984; 18:553–612.
61. Clark R, Wong G, Arnheim N, et al: Antibodies specific for amino acid 12 of the ras oncogene product inhibit GTP binding. *Proc Natl Acad Sci USA* 1985;82:5280–5284.
62. Niman HL, Thompson AMH, Yu A: Anti-peptide antibodies detect oncogene-related proteins in urine. *Proc Natl Acad Sci USA* 1985;82:7924–7928.

63. Brodeur GM, Seeger RC, Schwab M, et al: Amplification of N-myc in untreated human neuroblastomas correlates with advanced disease stage. *Science* 1984;224:1121–1124.
64. Taub R, Kirsch I, Morton C, et al: Translocation of the c-myc gene into the immunoglobulin heavy chain locus in human Burkitt lymphoma and murine plasmacytoma cells. *Proc Natl Acad Sci USA* 1982;79:7937–7941.
65. Dalla-Favera R, Martinotti S, Gallo RC, et al: Translocation and rearrangements of the c-myc oncogene locus in human undifferentiated B-cell lymphomas. *Science* 1983; 219:963–967.
66. Rowley JD: Identification of the constant chromosome regions involved in human hematologic malignant disease. *Science* 1982;216:749–751.
67. Rowley JD: Human oncogene locations and chromosome aberrations. *Nature* 1983; 301:290–291.
68. Little CD, Nau MM, Carney DN, et al: Amplification and expression of the c-myc oncogene in human lung cancer cell lines. *Nature* 1983;306:194–196.
69. Seeger RC, Brodeur GM, Sather H, et al: Association of multiple copies of the N-myc oncogene with rapid progression of neuroblastomas. *N Engl J Med* 1985;313:1111-1116.
70. Tsujimoto Y, Finger LR, Yunis JJ, et al: Cloning of the chromosome breakpoint of neoplastic B cells with the t(14:18) chromosome translocation. *Science* 1984;226: 1097–1099.
71. Tsujimoto Y, Cossman J, Jaffe E, et al: Involvement of the bcl-2 gene in human follicular lymphoma. *Science* 1985;228:1440–1443.
72. Bakhshi A, Jensen JP, Goldman P, et al: Cloning the chromosomal breakpoint of t(14:18) human lymphomas: clustering around J_H on chromosome 14 and near a transcriptional unit on 18. *Cell* 1985;41:899–906.
73. Groffen J, Stephenson JR, Heisterkamp N, et al: Philadelphia chromosomal breakpoints are clustered within a limited region, bcr, on chromosome 22. *Cell* 1984;36:93–99.
74. deKlein A, VanKessel AG, Grosveld G, et al: A cellular oncogene is translocated to the Philadelphia chromosome in chronic myelocytic leukemia. *Nature* 1982;300:765–767.
75. Konopka JB, Watanabe SM, Witte ON: An alteration of the human c-abl protein in K562 leukemia cells unmasks associated tyrosine kinase activity. *Cell* 1984;37:1035–1042.
76. Wong DT, Nath N, Sninsky JJ: Identification of hepatitis B virus polypeptides encoded by the entire pre-s open reading frame. *J. Virol* 1985;55:223–231.
77. Chang NT, Charda PK, Barone AD: Expression in *Escherichia coli* of open reading frame gene segments of HTLV-III. *Science* 1985;228:93–96.
78. Rehniger TE, Walfield AM, Cunningham TM, et al: Purification and characterization of a cloned protease-resistant *Treponema pallidum* specific antigen. *Infect Immun* 1984; 46:598–607.
79. Erlich HA, Rodgers G, Vaillancourt P, et al: Identification of an antigen-specific immunoglobulin M antibody associated with acute *Toxoplasma* infection. *Infect Immunol* 1983;41:683–690.
80. Coates SR, Sheridan PJ, Hansen DS, et al: Serospecificity of a cloned protease-resistant *Treponema pallidum*-specific antigen expressed in *Escherichia coli. J Clin Microbiol* 1986;23:460–464.
81. Rodgers G, Laird WJ, Coates SR, et al: Serological characterization of an *Escherichia coli*-expressed 37-kilodalton *Treponema pallidum* antigen and gene localization. *Infect Immunol* 1986;53:16–25.
82. Chang PW, Cato I, McKinney S, et al: Detection of antibodies to Human T-cell Lymphotropic Virus-III (HTLV-III) with an immunoassay employing a recombinant *Escherichia coli*-derived viral antigenic peptide. *Biol Technol* 1985;3:905–909.
83. Cabraclilla CD, Groopman JE, Lanigan J, et al: Serodiagnosis of antibodies to the human

AIDS retrovirus with a bacterially synthesized *env* polypeptide. *Biol Technol* 1986; 4:128–133.
84. Moseley SL, Huq I, Alim ARMA, et al: Detection of enterotoxigenic *Escherichia coli* by DNA colony hybridization. *J Infect Dis* 1980;142:892–898.
85. Goltz S, Todd J, Kline S, et al: DNA probes for diagnosis of sexually transmitted diseases. *Am Clin Prod Rev* 1986;5:30–35.
86. Fitts R, Diamond M, Hamilton C, et al: DNA-DNA hybridization assay for detection of *Salmonella* spp. in foods. *App Environ Microbiol* 1983;46:1146–1151.
87. Hill WE, Madden JM, McCardell BA, et al: Foodborne enterotoxigenic *Escherichia coli*: Detection and enumeration by DNA colony hybridization. *Appl Environ Microbiol* 1983;45:1324–1330.
88. Kohne DE: Application of DNA probe tests to the diagnosis of infectious disease. *Am Clin Prod Rev* 1986;5:20–29.
89. Kwok S, Mack DH, Mullis KB, et al: Identification of HIV viral sequences using *in vitro* enzymatic amplification and oligomer cleavage detection. *J Virol,* to be published.
90. Beardsley T: Genetic engineering: Hepatitis vaccine wins approval. *Nature* 1986;322:396.
91. Putney SD, Matthews TJ, Robey WG, et al: HTLV-III/LAV-neutralizing antibodies to an *E. coli*-produced fragment of the virus envelope. *Science* 1986;234:1392–1395.
92. Tweten RK, Barbieri JT, Collier RJ: Effect of substituting aspartic acid for glutamic acid 148 on ADP–ribosyltransferase activity. *J Biol Chem* 1985;260:10392–10394.
93. Locht C, Barstad PA, Coligan JE, et al: Molecular cloning of pertussis toxin genes. *Nucleic Acids Res* 1986;14:3251.
94. Earl PL, Moss B, Morrison RP, et al: T-lymphocyte priming and protection against friend leukemia by vaccinia-retrovirus *env* gene recombinant. *Science* 1986;234:728–731.
95. Smith GL, Cheng KC, Moss B: Vaccinia virus: An expression vector for genes from parasites. *Parasitology* 1986;92(suppl):S109–S117.
96. Kemp DJ, Coppel RL, Stahl HD, et al: Genes for antigens of *Plasmodium falciparum. Parasitology* 1986;91:S83–S108.
97. Nussenzweig RS, Nussenzweig V: Development of a sporozoite vaccine. *Parasitol To* 1985;1:150–159.

CHAPTER **10**

The Future of Genetic Testing

Neil A. Holtzman, MD, MPH

The ability to move segments of DNA in vitro from one species to others in which they can be produced in large quantities, was made possible by government support for research in universities. It did not take long before the practical applications of this recombinant DNA technology were appreciated, spawning a new industry. Medical uses constitute only one facet of biotechnology, and not necessarily the most lucrative. The availability of diagnostic and therapeutic products based on recombinant DNA technology will depend not only on continued advances in our understanding of disease, but on commercial interest in developing and marketing them. In the first part of this chapter, I will examine the current state of research and development related to medical uses of recombinant DNA technology. This chapter deals only with the situation in the United States.

Many of the medical products currently being developed by recombinant DNA technology will enter the domain of primary care providers. This is particularly likely for genetic tests, the principal topic of this chapter. In the second part, I will address problems related to the entrance of genetic tests into the mainstream of medical practice. Can primary care providers be confident of the validity of these tests? Can they be assured that the laboratories performing them are reliable? Do they have the training to use them appropriately?

Tests for the alleles that cause or predispose to many diseases will precede by many years the development of effective therapies or interventions to prevent their manifestations. In the interim, interventions of unproved safety or effectiveness could be attempted. Insurance companies and employers could use tests that predict increased risk of untreatable disease to deny or limit coverage or employment. In the absence of treatment, avoidance of the conception or birth of offspring destined to be affected could become a major consequence of genetic testing not only for rare, early-onset diseases but for common adult-onset conditions as well. In the third and final part, I will consider some of the implications of the time lag between diagnosis and conventional therapy.

RESEARCH AND DEVELOPMENT

Support for Research Related to Biotechnology

Chapter 4 lists 26 diseases for which recombinant DNA probes are available as potential tools for diagnosis. The gene loci responsible for the vast majority of mendelian, and virtually all polygenic, disorders remain unknown. The nucleotide sequences of only a handful of genes, including the loci responsible for Duchenne's muscular dystrophy (DMD) and chronic granulomatous disease, have been identified by recombinant DNA methodology. The gene products for these few remain to be elucidated. Further advances depend on basic research.

Federally funded basic research in university laboratories provided the foundation of recombinant DNA technology as well as knowledge of the human genome. As a result of uncertainties regarding federal support for basic biologic research, the universities have sought financial gain from the discoveries of their own faculties, and turned to industry for direct support.

Patents

Recent changes in the Patents and Trademark Act,[1] which give universities and other federal grantees the right to obtain patents and grant exclusive licenses on work supported with federal funds, may lead universities to encourage work that has practical value. Prior to 1980 the federal government held most of the patents on such work and offered licenses on them freely.[1] By denying competing companies access to the discovery, the amendments to the patent law increased commercial interest in the acquisition of licenses from universities. In the area of genetic testing, the Massachusetts General Hospital has licensed the probes for markers of Huntington's disease exclusively to Integrated Genetics, Inc. Stanford University has applied for a patent to cover the use of RFLPs to detect gene loci implicated in human diseases. If the patent is granted, Stanford has agreed to give exclusive rights to Collaborative Research, Inc.[2]

Commercial Support

At the present time, both small and large companies with an interest in biotechnology are investing in university-based research. Multimillion-dollar agreements have been signed between Monsanto, a chemical company, and Washington University, and between the German pharmaceutical manufacturing firm of Hoechst and Massachusetts General Hospital. Funds derived from the Technicon Corporation established the Whitehead Institute, affiliated with the Massachusetts Institute of Technology.[3] The agreements give the industrial partners the opportunity to review manuscripts before publication, and obtain exclusive license for patents, which would be obtained by the University. The corporate partners have some input into faculty selection as well. Six corporations have combined to form the Engenics Corporation, which channels money for biotechnology research to universities. Michigan State University created Neogen to seek venture capital for limited partnerships for developing and marketing discoveries made at the University; the University receives money from successful commercialization of products.[2]

From a survey of biotechnology companies, investigators at Harvard University estimated that 46% of all firms support research in universities. Between 16 and 24% of all funds for biotechnology research and development at universities was supplied by industry in 1984.[4] From a parallel survey of faculty members at 40 universities, the Harvard group determined that 23% of faculty members engaged in biotechnology research received industrial support. This compares to 43% in chemistry and engineering.[5]

Implications for the Universities

Growing dependence of universities on support from the commercial sector might steer university research into areas with greater commercial potential and destabilize the research being conducted. To the Harvard investigators, the short duration of grants given to universities by small biotechnology companies "raises questions about whether some of these relationships shift the focus of university research toward applied work."[4] Thirty percent of faculty members receiving support from biotechnology companies reported that commercial application influenced their choice of research topic; 70% of them thought that industrial support could place too much emphasis on applied research, and 44% thought that it posed "the risk of undermining intellectual exchange and cooperation within departments." About one-quarter of faculty members receiving support from biotechnology companies reported that the results of their research supported by the companies were "the property of the sponsor and cannot be published without their (sic) consent."[5]

Growing interest in commercial applications of biotechnology could also reduce the pool of talented young scientists committed to basic research in universities. The loss of scientists to industry was described in a recent report in the *New York Times* that an entire laboratory of National Cancer Institute scientists formed their own company. While at the NIH they had to chronicle their work in professional journals. If they continued to do so, their work "would soon be taken over by private companies." Rather than let others capitalize on their discoveries, they were willing to postpone publication until they could capture the commercial rights. The report cites other examples.[6]

Realization of the dangers posed to basic research at universities by industrial support hinges to a great extent on the commitment of federal funds to basic research and training at the universities. Despite growing concern about balancing the federal budget, research support for work related to recombinant DNA has continued to increase. The number of NIH extramural projects for which a key descriptor was "genetic manipulation" rose from 546 in 1978 to 1,588 in 1982 with a commensurate tripling to $185 million in their support.[2] From both within the government and without pressure is being exerted to increase federal support for work with practical applications. The House of Representatives Committee on Appropriations wanted to know, for instance, how NIH efforts could expand the biotechnology industry.[7] Representatives of the biotechnology industry have also called on NIH to expand its support of commercial applications more rapidly.[8] The Small Business Innovation Development Act passed by Congress in 1982 requires the NIH and other agencies to set aside a small percentage of their budgets for grants to small businesses.[9]

Research related to human diseases continues to receive strong federal support. But if federal funds should decline, or be directed into areas with greater commercial payoff, it is by no means clear that increased reliance on industry as a source of support will assure the continued stream of investment in learning more about human diseases.

Commercial Interest in Human Diseases

In 1985, I began to determine the interest of biotechnology companies in the use of human recombinant DNA. This survey continued under the auspices of the U.S. Congress Office of Technology Assessment. Information has now been obtained on 83 (70%) of 118 companies. Six were visited; the remainder were surveyed by mail. Fifty-nine percent of the companies are using or planning to use probes of human DNA sequences, but only one-quarter (n = 21) have any interest in diagnostics for genetic or chromosomal diseases. Only six companies are limiting their work in the diagnostic area to these two categories of disease. All six have interests in nondiagnostic areas as well. Very few companies expect more than 20% of their sales to come from genetic tests. Eighteen percent of respondents to the survey said they abandoned or rejected plans to construct human recombinant DNA probes. The reasons most frequently given were small market, high costs, and the controversial nature of some of their uses (for instance, prenatal diagnosis).

The companies working on diagnostics for genetic disorders are interested primarily in common diseases from which they can expect high sales volume. At each of the six companies I visited, representatives responded affirmatively to the question, "Is it possible that diagnostic kits will *not* be developed for rare disorders because of lack of profit?" Lack of interest in the development of therapeutic products for rare diseases promoted passage of the Orphan Drug Act in 1982. No funds have yet been appropriated for its implementation, although the FDA does make grants for clinical studies on the safety and effectiveness of drugs and devices for orphan diseases.

Most companies working on the diagnosis of common genetic diseases would like eventually to market direct tests for disease-causing or susceptibility-conferring alleles that can be used to test entire populations for the carrier state or latent disease. The search in a population for persons possessing certain genotypes is defined as *genetic screening.*[10] To facilitate screening, genetic tests must be reduced in complexity and cost. Toward this end over half of the companies I surveyed are attempting to simplify recombinant DNA technology.

Very recently, two companies were reported to be developing tests for DNA markers for common, multifactorial diseases. A representative of California Biotechnology told *Science* magazine that his company would

> devise a blood test that can tell who is susceptible to cardiovascular disease. By looking at a battery of markers, each of which provides some information on risk, he expects to have an accurate test that will cost, if used on a large scale, about $50. Information from this test, he believes, could be used by individuals "for early prevention. They can control their diets, exercise, stop smoking, go on cholesterol-lowering diets, and use blood pressure-lowering drugs."[11]

Focus Technologies, a new company, was reported to be ready soon to use tests at the DNA and protein level to detect individuals at risk for common diseases. Those identified would, presumably, be more likely to adopt behaviors that are more healthful. Focus's managing director told the *Washington Post* that

> they are studying 187 markers that indicate the risk of getting 160 different diseases and are conducting cost-benefit analyses on which to use. A marker for an extremely rare disorder, or a marker that required complicated and expensive processing for a minor problem, would not be cost-effective.[12]

The company has arranged with the Equitable Life Assurance Society for a pilot program in which employees of the company and group insurance clients could volunteer to be tested. The results will be given to the employee, and, if desired, to the employee's physician, but not to employers or the insurance company. Equitable has committed more than $1 million to the program.

Malignant melanoma, breast cancer, Alzheimer's disease and bipolar affective disorder sometimes occur in multiple family members. In some of these instances, the disease may be due to the presence of alleles at a single gene locus, while in others to alleles at a small number of loci. Scientists associated with biotechnology companies are attempting to locate the genes that play a role in the familial forms of these disorders. Identifying these loci may prove helpful not only in predicting risk of disease in such families, but also in learning more about the disorders in all their forms. However, the optimism expressed by California Biotechnology and Focus Technologies, that they will soon have tests to predict those at risk for multifactorial diseases, is not shared by many scientists.

GENETIC TESTS IN THE MAINSTREAM OF MEDICAL CARE

With the exception of newborn and some carrier screening, most genetic testing is performed today in university laboratories, with medical geneticists or their associates often conveying the results directly to family members. (With screening, geneticists are frequently consulted when a subject's results are positive.) Even a significant growth of the specialty of genetics is unlikely to keep pace with the increased availability of genetic tests. Moreover, with simpler, inexpensive methods, routine medical laboratories—including those in physicians' offices—will be able to perform the tests. Scientists at one company told me that eventually their direct tests for disease-causing alleles would be so simple that "people could do them at home if the interpretation was as simple as the test." The test methodology will be simplified and the tests will be marketed to primary care providers if not to consumers directly. The problems of interpretation will be formidable. At the present time, there are insufficient safeguards against inadequate performance and inappropriate interpretation of genetic tests.

The Interpretation of Test Results

The Validity of Genetic Tests

Elsewhere in this volume some of the possible errors in test interpretation have been described, and I will discuss them only briefly. When linkage is used to indicate the presence and dosage of a disease-causing allele, crossing over will occasionally result in erroneous predictions. Linkage studies also depend on accuracy of clinical diagnosis in family members who are needed to permit prediction in others. Diagnosing an affected individual as unaffected, which is more likely to happen for late-onset than for early-onset diseases, will confuse interpretation, perhaps leading to the conclusion that prediction within the family is not possible when in fact it is. False paternity also can confuse the picture.

The predictive ability of direct tests for disease-causing mutations does not depend on clinical diagnosis in family members. Direct tests can, therefore, be used for genetic screening. If more than one mutation at the locus for which probes are available causes the disease, tests capable of detecting only one of them will fail to predict all cases of disease. The use of oligonucleotide probes directed against all *known* mutations may alleviate the problem, but rare mutations for which such probes have not been constructed could still occur. Efforts to develop more general methods, capable of detecting several unspecified mutations, are currently being made. Direct probes (or linked marker probes) for mutations at one locus will fail to detect disease-causing alleles at other loci that are capable of causing phenotypically indistinguishable disease.

Individuals in whom a disease-causing mutation is found in sufficient gene dosage to cause disease will not always develop the disease. Even within families in which a disease appears to follow mendelian patterns of inheritance, the disease-causing mutation will not always be expressed. Families with high expressivity are likely to be the ones that are used investigationally to discover the mutation in the first place. The frequency of expressivity in others can be determined only by testing populations.

For some diseases, independent tests for abnormalities in gene *product* can be used to confirm whether a positive test at the DNA level really means that disease will appear. For many diseases, however, the DNA test will be the only one available; the gene product may not even be known. Even when it is, the abnormality of gene product may not be manifest until long after the DNA test is used. This is particularly important in prenatal diagnosis; confirmatory evidence of the pathogenic effects of the mutation may be present only after the stage at which abortion is legally necessary. In other instances, a gene product abnormality may be present in the fetus, but not in tissues accessible prior to pregnancy termination.

For multifactorial diseases, the association between a positive test result and the subsequent occurrence of disease will always be imperfect. For instance, the presence of markers near the apolipoprotein genes, some of which may be polymorphic, will not always mean that heart diseases will appear. The marker serves as a genetic *risk factor*; its presence increases the chance that disease will develop, but by no means makes it certain. It will be much harder to establish true associations for multifactorial than for mendelian disorders.

The Reliability of Tests

The problems discussed so far will occur even when the test is performed in the best of laboratories. When tests are performed in many general medical laboratories, reliability—the precision and reproducibility of an assay—is sure to suffer. Chapter 7 discusses two situations in which the use of restriction enzymes can lead to erroneous results. One of these—contamination of genomic DNA with probe DNA—can be corrected by the design of the probes, but the other—incomplete endonuclease digestion—can occur in any laboratory and could be overlooked. Sporadic failure of a probe to hybridize has also been encountered.*

In a recent study at the Centers of Disease Control (CDC), investigators found that most of the failures of newborn screening tests to detect infants with congenital hypothyroidism or phenylketonuria (PKU) could be attributed to error.[13] They estimated that one in 70 cases of PKU were missed, and one in 120 cases of hypothyroidism. About half of the errors occurred in the laboratory performing the test; the remainder occurred in the prelaboratory phase, such as failure of the specimen to reach the laboratory, or in the postlaboratory phase, such as failure to notify the infant's physician of a positive test result. The CDC has also conducted proficiency testing of laboratories routinely performing newborn screening tests, uncovering considerable interlaboratory variation in the proportion of specimens that would require additional study.[14,15]

Communicating Test Results

Geneticists are not always successful in communicating risks. In a study of counseling at 47 genetics clinics, Sorenson and colleagues found that numeric risks given by the counselor were incorrectly interpreted by half of the clients.[16] Eighty-seven percent of clients came with inaccurate knowledge of risk; 54% of them still had inaccurate knowledge after counseling. Of the 13% who came with accurate knowledge, 16% had inaccurate knowledge after counseling. Part of the problem may stem from the difficulties people have in their ability to interpret risk information. We found that 25% of predominantly white, middle class women interpreted "1 out of 1,000" to mean 10% or greater. Those who made this error were twice as likely as those giving the correct answer to state that the occurrence of a birth defect in 1 out of 1,000 pregnancies was "often or occasionally" rather than "rarely or very rarely."[17] The way in which risks are conveyed can also influence peoples' perception

*Kazazian HH, Jr: Personal communication.

of them. For instance, the choice of an intervention for a disease is heavily influenced by whether the outcome is put in terms of the chance of living rather than dying.[18]

Physicians also have a hard time conveying risks. Many of them do not appreciate the uncertainties of test results. During the course of medical school and postgraduate training there is a significant decline in ability to calculate correctly the predictive value of a positive test result; fewer than half of practicing physicians are able to do so.[19] Only one-half of pediatricians attending a continuing education course could correctly interpret a positive newborn screening test result for PKU.[20] Even after exposure to education on maternal serum α-fetoprotein (MSAFP) screening for fetal neural tube defects, over three-quarters of obstetricians did not recognize that the risk of such defects following one positive screening test result was less than 5%.[21]

The current level of genetics training in medical schools contributes to the low level of physician preparedness. Twenty-one schools still do not have formal courses in genetics, and geneticists judge many of the existing courses to be of poor quality.[22] The notion that genetics is unimportant is reinforced by the small portion of questions on genetics on the National Board examinations, which most physicians take.[23] To compound the problem, genetics is not often the subject of continuing medical education courses for practicing physicians.

Assuring Effectiveness and Quality

Considering problems in the validity, reliability, and accurate communication of genetic test results, we might expect that procedures to minimize them are in place. This is not always the case.

Premarket Control

Before kits or reagents can be sold in the United States for the purpose of diagnosing disease or risk of disease, the manufacturer must notify the Food and Drug Administration (FDA). The agency must then decide whether evidence of safety and effectiveness is sufficient to warrant approving the "device" (as it is legally called) for marketing. Devices, including DNA probes, can be used for clinical testing without FDA approval. The manufacturer can sell the product "for research purposes only" without notifying the FDA. It is ethically bound not to build in a profit, although it could inflate its costs. This approach may prove more lucrative in the short run than going through the process of having the product approved as a clinical device, which may entail considerable expense in demonstrating the product's safety and effectiveness. University laboratories, at which much genetic testing is currently performed, use "research" reagents for clinical testing. Although some of these laboratories have had extensive experience with recombinant DNA technology, others, which are eager to "get into the act," have not. Few university-based research laboratories participate in the quality-control programs that are required of commercial laboratories, including those in hospitals (see below). Thus a research laboratory could provide a new test for clinical diagnosis when neither the quality of the laboratory nor the validity of the test reagents has been demonstrated.

When a manufacturer decides to market its reagents as a diagnostic test it must first notify the FDA. If the manufacturer can show that the test is equivalent in safety and effectiveness to one already on the market there is little more required of it. For instance, a recombinant DNA test to detect the sickle cell allele might simply require evidence that it is as safe and effective as tests that achieve the same end that already are on the market. When no "substantially equivalent" test is available the FDA may require evidence of safety and efficacy if it determines that the device is going to be used for a new purpose or if it "is of substantial importance in preventing impairment of human health, or . . . presents a potential unreasonable risk of illness or injury."[24] The FDA usually makes such a determination for life-supporting or invasive devices such as pacemakers and intraocular lenses, but it has occasionally placed the same requirements on in vitro diagnostics. As of September 1986, the FDA has received no premarket notifications or requests for premarket approval of genetic tests based on recombinant DNA technology.

In its assessment of effectiveness, the FDA's interest is in the diagnostic device per se, that is, its intrinsic ability to give correct answers. For genetic tests, this will be difficult to establish without following subjects in whom tests predicted high risks to see if disease actually appeared. The FDA has never restricted a device—although it has the power to do so—because the way in which results, even when they are accurate, are interpreted could pose an "unreasonable risk of . . . injury." Despite urging by a number of professional and consumer groups that the marketing of MSAFP kits be restricted because the low predictive value of a positive test result increased the chance that unaffected fetuses would be aborted, the FDA refused to do so.[25]

Postmarket Control

The FDA has not vigorously exercised its authority over devices after they are sold other than by monitoring reports of erroneous results or other adverse outcomes. It has no authority over reagents that a laboratory prepares itself and does not sell across state lines. Nor does it have responsibility for approving the laboratories in which these devices are used. The assurance of laboratory quality rests with two other federal agencies, the Centers for

Disease Control (CDC) under the Clinical Laboratory Improvement Act (CLIA) of 1967 and the Health Care Financing Administration (HCFA) following enactment of the Medicare program in 1965. Some states have their own programs, but many rely on the federal programs.

Efforts by government agencies and professional groups (eg, College of American Pathologists) to assure quality include personnel requirements, performance standards, and proficiency testing. Proficiency testing usually involves distributing specimens to laboratories, which then determine the concentration or other value by performance of the laboratory test. This permits a comparison of the precision and accuracy of tests in the laboratories participating in the program. No proficiency testing program includes all of the tests a laboratory is capable of performing. There is no evidence that proficiency in the performance of one class of tests correlates with proficiency of others. In genetics, only New York State requires cytogenetics laboratories to participate in its proficiency testing program, which includes correctly karyotyping unknown specimens. There are no proficiency tests for DNA-based genetic tests.

In recent years there has been a strong trend toward physicians performing diagnostic tests in their office laboratories.[26] For the most part, these laboratories are exempt from quality assurance regulations.

> This exemption was based on the assumption that laboratory testing is an integral part of the practice of medicine, at least when carried out in the physician's office. In essence, the M.D. degree has been treated by voluntary and Federal quality assurance programs as a sufficient condition to assure acceptable levels of public health protection with respect to clinical laboratory testing performed in unregulated physicians' offices.[27]

Experience with proficiency testing thus far indicates that low volume laboratories, which would characterize most physicians' offices, do poorly in proficiency testing.[27] There is no reason to expect the situation will be different when reagents or kits for genetic tests are marketed for use in office laboratories.

Utilization of Genetic Tests

New technologies are not often rapidly adopted. We have shown, for instance, that physicians were slow to adopt MSAFP screening for fetal neural tube defects.[21] In fact, physician reticence is a greater deterrent to test use than consumer refusal.[28] The process may be speeded up by court rulings that make physicians culpable for bad outcomes that could have been avoided by genetic testing.

Other barriers are financial. Physicians do not receive as much reimbursement for the time they spend counseling a patient about a genetic test result as they would for the same time seeing more patients or performing procedures. Before Medicare or Medicaid will reimburse for a test, HCFA must decide that the test is meritorious.[29] The agency does not always rely on FDA determinations that tests are safe and effective, but may commission its own study by the Office of Health Technology Assessment, a branch of the National Center for Health Services Research. One of the reasons for this repetition is the exclusion from FDA considerations of cost effectiveness. Although the FDA may compare the validity and reliability of a new test to existing ones—if they are available—it does not consider relative costs; HCFA does. The evidence presented to the FDA on test performance is often gathered by experienced investigators. There is no assurance that the conditions of test use will be the same once the test is marketed.

Private insurers also may be reluctant to reimburse for new technologies. The genetics community has already encountered this problem in regard to reimbursement for counseling services. A unique problem in linkage studies is that the family members who are needed may not all be covered by the same insurance. Insurers may be reluctant to reimburse for the test in their client, when the results will not be of direct benefit to him or her, but to someone else covered by another insurer.

CONSEQUENCES OF THE TIME LAG BETWEEN DIAGNOSIS AND TREATMENT

The first practical spinoff after the gene for a disease has been located will be the ability to detect those at risk for the disease in families in which it has already appeared. Once the gene is identified, knowledge of the disease-causing mutation(s) will permit detection in populations of those at risk for disease or whose offspring will be at risk. For many disorders, the capability of diagnosis will precede by many years the capability to treat the disease effectively.

New Therapies

Identification of the locus at which a disease-causing allele resides is not tantamount to discovering the function of the normal allele(s) at that locus. If the gene is not transcribed, it may take considerable time to determine its regulatory role. On the other hand, if it codes for a polypeptide, discovery of the gene product will ensue fairly rapidly, contributing to our understanding of pathogenesis. Whether this will permit an effective intervention depends on the particular function of the gene product, and the organs in which it functions. Toxic substrates that accumulate due to an enzyme defect cannot always be removed or counteracted. Nor can essential products be delivered very often from without. In some diseases, both substrate toxicity and product deficiency can play a role. Blood proteins can be replaced, and vitamin cofactors can sometimes boost function of a defective enzyme in more remote tissues or organs, but these approaches work in only a handful of diseases. In other diseases, irreversible damage has occurred prenatally.

The difficulties of gene therapy have been described in Chapter 6. For multifactorial conditions, the way in which the malfunction of one of the implicated genes leads to disease will be difficult to elucidate; there are too many other variables with which to contend.

Without a clear understanding of pathogenesis, and in the absence of animal models, the effectiveness of an intervention designed on the basis of knowledge of the primary gene defect will have to be determined empirically. It is doubtful, moreover, that interventions that *prevent* the manifestations of disease will have much effect in reversing them after they appear. To determine their effectiveness, new preventive measures will have to be administered to presymptomatic people at risk for disease. Because the effects of a malfunctioning gene can accumulate insidiously, treatments probably should be started early in life. The beneficial effect of preventive interventions for diseases that take many years to manifest will not become evident for some time.

Genetic testing will be used to identify presymptomatic individuals. This in itself raises problems. As should be apparent from the foregoing, genetic tests are not perfect predictors; some individuals with positive test results might never develop the disease. When tests developed in a few families are applied to populations, the ratio of false positives to true positives could be substantial; with virtually any test, as the number of people tested increases, the incidence of false positives rises as well. A new treatment given to *all* asymptomatic individuals with positive test results might appear to be effective because many of those who remain asymptomatic would never have developed the disease in the first place.

Presumably the FDA would want a demonstration of efficacy and safety before approving new drugs. Some interventions, however, do not require FDA approval. Companies promoting tests for multifactorial disorders, such as coronary heart disease, have maintained that the presence of genetic risk factors provides added incentive for people to undertake life-style changes. Although these changes cannot be regulated by the FDA, their safety and efficacy have not been established in all of those at risk. Low-fat diets, exercise, and cessation of smoking may have less of a salutary effect in those with a specific genetic risk factor for coronary heart disease than in others; the evidence is not yet available. Moreover, the early identification and labeling of those suspected to be at risk genetically might have harmful effects.[30]

Discrimination

Until it is possible to prevent the manifestations of many genetic diseases, or treat them effectively once they do appear, their care will be costly, often extending over several years. Increasingly in the United States, these costs are borne by third parties, and not by the patient. Tests to detect those at risk for diseases for which no effective interventions have been developed can be used by third parties to lower their overall costs, much to the detriment of those found to be at risk.

Insurance

In the absence of known differences in risk, each insured person pays the same premium, which is set at a level that provides sufficient income to reimburse for the deleterious events that will occur, and permits insurance companies to make a profit. When, however, subgroups or individuals can be demonstrated to be at greater risk, insurers can charge them higher premiums or refuse to insure them. This applies to life and health insurance. Those at greater risk can also be denied enrollment in some HMOs. Such discrimination permits the underwriter to charge lower premiums to those in whom the risk factor is missing. Consequently, if one insurer establishes a rate differential, others are likely to follow suit or lose business.

Discrimination in insurance rate-setting is permissible, as long as the action can be justified actuarially, and is not specifically prohibited by law or regulation. Thus youthful drivers, or their parents, are charged higher premiums for automobile insurance. In the early 1970s, when sickle cell screening came into vogue, some insurance companies raised premiums or denied insurance to heterozygotes for the sickle cell allele. The practice was stopped by public pressure, and, in a few states, by laws prohibiting discrimination on a genetic basis. Most states do not have such laws. A few insurance companies deny coverage to individuals who have positive tests for antibodies to the human immunodeficiency virus. Very few jurisdictions prohibit this practice, although the frequency with which the test is falsely positive has not yet been determined.

By denying insurance to high-risk individuals, companies can argue, they are protecting the financial interests of the remaining rate payers. In cases of youthful automobile drivers, or motorcyclists who refuse to wear helmets, this practice might be justified because those at high risk have some control over the probability of injury. However, persons at risk for untreatable genetic disease have no power to prevent the disability. In most other western countries, they would be covered under national health insurance. In this country if they are denied insurance, they are denied medical care unless they can pay out of pocket or are covered by special funds. A few states have established special programs for high-risk groups, including young adults with genetic diseases who can no longer be covered under their parents' policy, and cannot obtain insurance of their own.

The argument that an individual who is himself at risk for an untreatable genetic disease cannot be held responsible does not apply so well for couples at risk of having offspring with untreatable genetic diseases. Insurance companies might deny such couples insurance or insist that they take steps to avoid the conception or birth of affected offspring (see below). In the current anti-abortion climate, such policies seem unlikely. Moreover, it is doubtful that the aggregate cost-savings will be very great for the few rare diseases for which avoidance is currently used. If carrier detection and prenatal diagnosis become possible for more common diseases, and health care costs continue to mount to an intolerable degree, such policies might find greater support.

Because genetic tests will seldom if ever be perfect predictors of disease, some people who are not destined to develop the disease will be mislabeled and denied insurance. It is already evident, for instance, that although some individuals possessing certain polymorphisms for apolipoprotein genes will develop coronary artery disease, others will not. Conversely, some people destined to become ill will have negative test results.

Employment

Although genetic tests, physical examination, or other laboratory studies are not used as a condition of insurability under group health or life policies that come as a benefit of employment, they could be used to screen out high-risk job applicants. Insurers base the premium for a particular group on its past rate of disabilities or death, or the rate in actuarially similar groups. By denying employment to applicants who are found by genetic testing to be at increased risk for future disease, employers will have a pool of employees who are at lower risk. This will reduce their health care costs.

Genetic screening of workers has been performed to detect inherited traits that allegedly increase susceptibility to chemical or physical agents to which they are exposed in the workplace. A survey conducted by the Office of Technology Assessment (OTA) in 1982 of the largest U.S. companies found that 5% were, or had been, performing genetic tests on employees. The actions taken in individuals with positive test results included transfer to other jobs.[31] For a while, the Air Force Academy was screening applicants for sickle cell trait and denying them entry because of alleged dangers to them.

That policy has been reversed.[32] In addition to screening employees already on the job, at least one company, duPont, screened prospective black employees for sickle cell trait. A spokesman for the company said that the program was voluntary and was for the employees' "education and edification." He admitted that the company had no education or counseling program.[33] As pre-employment physicals can be required of prospective employees it is not clear what opportunity those seeking employment have for refusing genetic tests. Genetic screening of workers, followed by exclusion of susceptible individuals from certain jobs, is permissible under existing federal laws provided that screening is a "business necessity" (eg, being the only way for the company to avoid tort liability or costly engineering controls), or if there was a reasonable probability of future harm as a result of employment. "Reasonable probability" has not been defined by the courts.[32] Four states have laws prohibiting employment discrimination based on genetic testing. New Jersey prohibits discrimination in employment based on an individual's "atypical hereditary cellular or blood trait" (defined as including *traits* for sickle cell, hemoglobin C, thalassemia, Tay Sachs, and cystic fibrosis), and laws in Florida, North Carolina, and Louisiana prohibit such discrimination based on sickle cell trait.[31]

In its 1983 report, the OTA concluded that there were no genetic tests that could predict harm from workplace exposures.[31] With recombinant DNA technology, the situation is likely to change. In some instances, multiple alleles that each confer a different degree of susceptibility to harm from environmental agents—leading to the appearance of a specific disease—will undoubtedly be found. In such cases, drawing a line between "susceptible" and "resistant" will be arbitrary. Some physical and chemical agents encountered in the workplace (or elsewhere; eg, cigarette smoke) will have multiple toxic effects. Persons genetically less susceptible to the harmful effect for which screening is performed may be more susceptible to others for which no screening is available. Reducing ambient levels of toxic substances in the workplace will be to the advantage of all workers. Screening for genetic susceptibilities will not.

Avoidance

The conception or birth of offspring who are at risk for genetic disorders for which effective interventions have not yet been developed can be avoided. When carrier screening is available, couples need not wait for the birth of an affected child; those at risk can use avoidance strategies before having *any* children. Some of the avoidance strategies are still novel. All of them are controversial, interfering as they do with the natural reproductive process.

Alternative Methods of Conception

Knowledge that one is a carrier of an allele for a severe genetic disease could, presumably, influence choice of mate. An early study of sickle cell screening, before prenatal diagnosis was available, found that carrier screening did not lead to a reduction in the birth of offspring with sickle cell anemia; some carriers either failed to disclose their status when they married other carriers, or couples decided to take the chance of conceiving affected offspring.[34]

After mate selection, a number of strategies are possible. They depend on substituting someone else's germ cells for those of the carrier. When both partners are carriers for an autosomal recessive disorder, or when the male partner has a dominant disorder, the couple can use artificial insemination of sperm from a donor (AID) to avoid affected offspring. In a survey of 91 adults who had a 50% chance of being carriers of Huntington disease, 69% of males 45 years or younger, and 40% of males over 45 years old said they would be willing to "conceive through AID" to avoid the risk to offspring.[35] Couples can use ovum donation or a surrogate mother when they both are carriers for a recessive disorder, the female partner has a dominant disorder, or when the woman is a carrier for an X-linked disorder. These new techniques have been used primarily for infertility problems, but they are likely to be used for genetic indications. About one-third of providers of AID perform it for genetic as well as other indications; the actual proportion of all inseminations used for genetic purposes has not been reported.[36]

Occasionally, the use of sperm donors has resulted in the birth of affected children; the donor was, unknowingly, a carrier of the condition whose avoidance was being sought. Genetic testing of both sperm and ovum donors can reduce such occurrences. Although sperm and ovum donors have no legal claim, or responsibility, to offspring they helped conceive, the question of a surrogate mother's claim to retain the infant she delivers has not yet been resolved.

Prenatal Diagnosis and Abortion

Prenatal diagnosis followed by abortion of affected fetuses is the only avoidance option that allows *both* members of an at-risk couple to pass some of their respective genes to their offspring. Couples who elect to abort affected fetuses following prenatal diagnosis can conceive again, eventually having infants without the disorder. Prenatal diagnosis is also possible for chromosome abnormalities and some conditions of complex etiology, such as spina bifida, for which prenatal screening is possible. The risk of polygenic disorders in which a small number of loci are implicated, could also be predicted prenatally when tests are available to detect the responsible alleles at some or all of the loci. The chance of disease will be lower than for single gene disorders. For instance, if single doses of specific alleles at three unlinked loci are needed for disease to appear, and testing demonstrates that between them the parents have one dose of each of the alleles, the chance that all three will be passed to any one child is 12.5%. This risk is still higher than the risk of a Down's syndrome fetus in a 40-year-old pregnant woman.

The most widely used method of prenatal diagnosis is still amniocentesis, which is usually performed between the 16th and 19th week of pregnancy. (Legal abortion is possible until the fetus is viable, usually taken to be the 24th week.) Although the chance of fetal death following amniocentesis performed by experienced physicians is less than 1%, the procedure has other drawbacks. It is performed so late in pregnancy that by the time the diagnosis is made, the mother already feels the fetus moving. Should the fetus be affected, abortion carries a higher risk than when induced earlier. By some methods, a fetus who is breathing may be delivered.

Chorion villus sampling (CVS) overcomes these drawbacks. Its safety and accuracy are still being evaluated. It is best performed between the 9th and 11th weeks. Until recently, a transcervical approach was used, but recent studies in Europe suggest that a transabdominal approach may be at least as safe. Both must be performed with ultrasound guidance. Chorion villus cells can be cultured, but direct analysis can often establish a diagnosis within a few days. This contrasts with a 3- to 4-week delay following amniocentesis.

Acceptance of prenatal diagnosis by pregnant women is quite high. When it is offered, between 60 and 80% of older pregnant women accept it for avoiding the birth of infants with Down's syndrome and other trisomies; race and socioeconomic status are not major factors.[37,38] About 90% of at risk couples in which both partners are identified as Tay-Sachs carriers by screening have utilized it.[39] The proportion accepting it for thalassemia is apparently culturally dependent, varying from 59% among East Indians at risk living in Great Britain to 94% among Greek Cypriots living there. In predominantly Catholic Sardinia, 77% of carrier couples identified by screening accepted monitoring by prenatal diagnosis. The proportion of couples at risk for offspring with sickle cell disease who accept it is lower.[40] Of those who accept prenatal diagnosis for Down's syndrome, thalassemia, and Tay-Sachs disease, over 90% elect abortion when the fetus is found to be affected.[39,40] Only about half of women who undergo prenatal diagnosis for sickle cell anemia abort affected fetuses,[40] perhaps because the outcome is not as severe as for the other disorders.

Acceptance of avoidance strategies may be greater among the individuals at risk than among physicians. In studies in New York State and Canada, obstetricians did not always make prenatal diagnosis available to older pregnant women.[41,42] Infertile couples hold more positive attitudes toward AID than medical students.[43] The picture could change as physicians become more familiar with the technology, and as legal pressures are exerted. At least one state, California, requires that physicians *offer* prenatal screening (for fetal neural tube defects) to pregnant women. The courts have held physicians liable for the birth of handicapped infants when they failed to inform the parents of the availability of prenatal diagnosis and abortion.[44,45]

The Extent of Avoidance Strategies

Prenatal diagnosis by means of RFLP linkage studies is already being used for one late onset disorder, Huntington's disease, for which treatment is unavailable. Despite early productivity—Woody Guthrie, for instance, became a legendary folk singer, as well as composer, before he succumbed—those who harbor the Huntington's allele, and their relatives, face prolonged uncertainty before the disease becomes manifest, and sustained suffering and expense when it does. Some people at risk would prefer not to know, but others would. Some families want prenatal diagnosis, with the option of aborting affected fetuses. This same dilemma will arise for other late-onset disorders when genetic tests become available for them. Although the neurologic component may not be as great, Alzheimer's disease is not dissimilar from Huntington's in its progressive and prolonged downhill course. Cures of malignant melanoma and breast and lung cancer are still the exception, and treatments for bipolar affective disorder and schizophrenia leave much to be desired. In some families, each of these disorders may be due to the presence of disease-causing alleles at single loci, and in others to the presence of susceptibility-conferring alleles at a few loci.

Huntington's disease is an unlikely candidate for population-based screening even after the disease-causing mutation(s) is discovered. This is not the case for other, more common late-onset disorders such as the ones mentioned in the last paragraph. Once they become available, direct tests for the mutations responsible for at least some of the cases could be used for carrier screening or prenatal diagnosis, even if their intended use is for presymptomatic diagnosis. Because of their prevalence, and the prolonged course of some of them, these disorders contribute significantly (certainly more than rare disorders) to health care costs. The relatively low costs of prenatal screening programs,[46] suggest that carrier screening, prenatal diagnosis and abortion would be less costly than allowing infants with late-onset disorders to survive and manifest the illness, even taking into consideration their productive years. (Avoidance of conception using AID might also be less expensive, but ovum donation is still quite costly.)

An important condition, however, must be appended to this economic pronouncement: The population at risk must comply to a large degree with the program. For example, the costs of screening pregnant women for fetal neural tube defects (followed by prenatal diagnosis when indicated, and abortion of affected fetuses) would cease to exceed the costs of caring for those born with such defects when fewer than 40% accepted screening and abortion of affected fetuses.* Regardless of the frequency of the disorder, its severity, or its age at onset, maximum economic benefits require maximum compliance.

Given its current preoccupation with health care costs (which, although still increasing, do not compare with military expenditures), and the potential savings from prenatal detection, society could exert strong pressure for carrier screening, prenatal diagnosis and abortion. As I have already mentioned, California requires obstetricians to offer prenatal screening for neural tube defects. Mandatory laws for newborn screening[10] already set a precedent for coercion. In the early 1970s, 17 states passed sickle cell screening laws; 8 made screening a requirement for admission to school.[47] Carrier screening in high schools could be amenable to elements of coercion in the form of appeals from authority figures and peer pressure.[48] Discriminatory insurance policies (as discussed earlier) are more overt. Finally, diminished government expenditures for chronic care could persuade people that avoidance is the least costly option for them personally.

Immediate health care costs are not the only justification for curtailing the right of people to reproduce as they choose. The prominent geneticist, Bentley Glass, said in his presidential address to the American Association for the Advancement of Science in 1970:

> in an overpopulated world it can no longer be affirmed that the right of the man and woman to reproduce as they see fit is inviolate . . . Genetic clinics will be constructed to which, before long, as many as 100 different recessive hereditary defects can be detected in the carriers, who may be warned against or *prohibited* from having offspring (emphasis added).[49]

(Glass, of course, seriously underestimated the number of "defects" for which genetic screening will eventually be possible.) Although overpopulation may be the serious problem that Glass maintains it is, it seems doubtful that even the most massive genetic screening program will have much of an effect. The fraction of all serious diseases with a straightforward genetic etiology is quite small. The evidence is not yet in that common diseases will prove due entirely or largely to genetic factors amenable to genetic testing and avoidance. Unless that proves to be the case, and I doubt it will, testing will lead to a percentage reduction of some common disorders, but certainly not eradicate them. There is the danger, moreover, as compulsory avoidance is extended to more and more conditions (in order to lower health care costs

*Holtzman NA: Unpublished.

or reduce population growth) of a growing intolerance of those with handicap or who differ from the norm.

Margery Shaw, geneticist and lawyer, maintains that mothers who refuse to abort fetuses discovered to have serious diseases by prenatal diagnosis are inflicting abuse, much as those who willfully neglect or beat their children:

> It should be incumbent upon the law to control the spread of genes causing severe deleterious effects just as disabling pathogenic bacteria and viruses are controlled. . . . Parents should be held accountable to their children if they knowingly and willfully choose to transmit deleterious genes or if the mother waives her right to an abortion if, after prenatal testing, a fetus is discovered to be seriously deformed or mentally defective.[50]

I find it difficult to equate with child abuse a conscious decision on the part of parents—perhaps because they oppose abortion—to nurture a child who is born with, or will develop, a disabling condition. Nor am I convinced, as Shaw apparently is, that there exists in society some repository of wisdom that can decide more justly than the parents what constitutes serious deformation or mental defect, or, as it is sometime put, "wrongful life." As Shaw correctly predicts, "*every* mendelian genetic trait will be diagnosable prenatally" (emphasis in original). When we reach that stage, how will it be decided, and by whom, what disease is serious enough? By taking such decisions out of the hands of parents—even if couched in the best interests of the unborn—a dangerous precedent for social control is established. When alleles that interfere with growth or some component of learning ability are discovered, their avoidance could also be "encouraged." Indeed, a society that fosters the myth that modern medicine can assure "perfect" babies might well embrace such strategies.

CONCLUSIONS

As a result of recombinant DNA technology, the identification of genetic factors involved in many diseases is within reach. The actual discoveries —and their utilization to learn more about pathogenesis and ultimately treatment—are heavily dependent on research yet to be done. Based on the current level of commercial interest in genetic testing, on its pitfalls (misdiagnosis), and on the controversies surrounding it (discrimination; providing alternatives to natural reproduction), few companies will support such research either "in house" or by grants to universities. Further progress depends on government support. Ironically, when the research bears fruit and companies decide to market genetic tests, financial survival may dictate that they promote them as widely as possible. Traditionally, industry has opposed government regulation and often tended to exaggerate the benefits of its products. Given the magnitude of the problems related to genetic testing, which I have delineated in the foregoing, we could be courting social misfortune unless a suitable framework is developed now into which expanded genetic testing can be placed. The framework is multidimensional.

1. The procedures and guidelines for approving genetic tests need to be revamped. There must be a greater recognition of the difference between efficacy—how the test performs under ideal conditions, and effectiveness—how it works in the real world of clinics, physicians' offices, and, eventually perhaps, private homes. Current FDA premarket approval focuses almost exclusively on efficacy, relying heavily on information gathered by skilled clinical investigators collecting information on behalf of manufacturers.
2. The proficiency of genetic test performance, as well as the ability to interpret results adequately, needs closer monitoring than is currently the case. Research laboratories in universities and physicians' office laboratories often operate without any external quality control.
3. New therapies administered to asymptomatic individuals presumed to be at high risk on the basis of positive genetic test results will require long term evaluation. There is little precedent for the lengthy randomized controlled trials that would best establish efficacy. The frequency with which those in the control group did *not* manifest the disease would indicate the false positive rate of the genetic test.
4. Genetic tests should not be used to generate additional inequities in employment and health care. An individual is not responsible for his or her genetic endowment and should not be blamed for it. If people are denied regular insurance or employment because they are found to be at risk for genetic diseases (and there is seldom a justification for doing so), they should be adequately compensated. Placing them in high risk insurance pools maintained by insurance companies, perhaps with state government support, and providing alternative employment are two approaches.
5. Health professionals must be trained in genetics, in the ability to interpret test results correctly and counsel people accordingly. Current undergraduate and postgraduate medical education accomplishes this inadequately. As genetic testing increases in volume, other health professionals, including nurses and medical social workers, can contribute to patient understanding if they are adequately trained.

6. Public understanding of genetics is critical. Some secondary school systems are incorporating sections on human genetics, but as a result of bureaucratic intransigence, and the opposition of creationists and anti-abortion groups, many graduates will be ill prepared to appreciate the implications of genetic tests with which they will be confronted.
7. Informed consent should be a touchstone of any genetic testing program. In families in which disease has already struck, individuals coming for testing will have some idea of the severity of the condition. Often, they will not appreciate the risks to their own offspring, or the options for avoiding the conception or birth of affected offspring. In population-wide screening, the vast majority of those coming for testing will have no personal experience with the condition, and will appreciate neither the severity, nor the risks to their offspring. Severity, risk, and therapeutic or avoidance options should all be covered in the disclosure in order to permit fully informed choices. Informed consent is consonant with individual autonomy, but does not guarantee it. Free choice is interfered with when, for instance, genetic testing is made a condition of employment (especially when jobs are hard to find), or when support for the care of infants born with avoidable handicapping conditions is withdrawn.

   There is little doubt that some people will refuse genetic screening after being fully informed. This means that the net savings to society will be lower than with a compulsory program. The dangers of coercion are too great, however, to allow economics to govern screening policies. The benefits of genetic testing must accrue primarily to individuals, and only secondarily to society. I suspect, however, that within an educated, well-informed citizenry most will choose genetic testing in the absence of *any* coercive pressure.
8. Genetic testing can be most effectively and safely carried out within the context of a continuing doctor-patient relationship, as is one of the ideals of primary care. For this to happen, however, all of the preceding seven parts of the framework must be in place. In addition, important changes in medical practice will be needed. Physicians will have to be adequately compensated for the time they spend talking to patients about the meaning of tests and their implications. In large group practices, genetic associates, who usually have master's degrees in human genetics, could be hired to provide much of the counseling; in smaller offices, nurses could be trained to counsel as one of their duties. Paternalism in deciding what is best for the patient should be avoided. In the quietude of the physician's office, patients are more likely to reach decisions consonant with their values than in a mass screening atmosphere or at the workplace. Moreover, there is greater assurance of confidentiality in the patient-doctor relationship.

One of the drawbacks to having personal physicians as the principal officers of screening for reproductive purposes is that many young adults do not have a regular doctor. Screening could be offered when women seek care in early pregnancy, but that deprives them of some avoidance options and may not give them adequate time to make a reasoned decision. Testing could be provided in childhood, but there is no assurance that the child or his or her parents will remember the results or comprehend them later in life. Recording results of genetic tests on a medical record, which the subject makes available to physicians who provide care subsequently, is one solution. In some instances, however, in order to reach a large segment of the target population, it may be necessary to offer screening in other settings (schools, churches), taking care to preserve the autonomy of the individual.

Genetic testing will be the first step in reducing the burden of many diseases. For some, effective interventions to prevent or treat the manifestations of the disorder will be developed. For others, effective therapy will prove elusive, and the burden will be reduced only by avoidance of the conception or birth of affected offspring. For both, significant problems are likely to accompany the wide dissemination of testing unless we begin to consider solutions now.

REFERENCES

1. Sylvester EJ, Klotz LC: *The Gene Age; Genetic Engineering and the Next Industrial Revolution.* New York, Charles Scribner's Sons 1983, p 128.
2. *Collaborative Research, Inc. Annual report,* 1984.
3. Office of Technology Assessment, Congress of the U.S. Commercial biotechnology: An international analysis. Washington, Government Printing Office 1984, 612 pp.
4. Blumenthal D, Gluck M, Louis KS, et al: Industrial support of university research in biotechnology. *Science* 1986;231:242–246.
5. Blumenthal D, Gluck M, Louis KS, et al: University-industry research relationships in biotechnology: Implications for the university. *Science* 1986;232:1361–66.
6. Berg EN: Small concerns battle cancer. *New York Times*, December 28, 1985, p 29.
7. Wyngaarden JB: *Report on Biotechnology.* National Institutes of Health, February 1985.
8. Culliton B: NIH role in biotechnology debated. *Science* 1985;229:147–148.
9. 97th Congress, Public law 97–219. 96 Stat 217–221, 1982.
10. Committee for the Study of Inborn Errors of Metabolism: *Genetic Screening: Programs, Principles and Research.* Washington, National Academy of Sciences, 1975, 388 pp.
11. Kolata G: Reducing risk: A change of heart? *Science* 1986;231:669–670.
12. Henderson N: Biomark program draws high-tech portraits of employees' health risks. *Washington Post* March 17, 1986.
13. Holtzman C, Slazyk WE, Cordero JF, et al: Descriptive epidemiology of missed cases of phenylketonuria and congenital hypothyroidism. *Pediatrics* 1986;78:553–558.
14. Ambrose JA: Report on a cooperative study of various fluorometric procedures and the

Guthrie bacterial inhibition assay in the determination of hyperphenylalaninemia. *Health Lab Sci* 1973;10:180–187.
15. *Neonatal Screening for Inborn Errors of Metabolism: Hypothyroidism Summary Report V.* Atlanta, Centers for Disease Control, 1986.
16. Sorenson JR, Swazey JP, Scotch NA: Reproductive pasts reproductive futures; genetic counseling and its effectiveness. *Birth Defects: Original Article Series* 1981;17:1–194.
17. Chase GA, Faden RR, Holtzman NA, et al: The assessment of risk by pregnant women: Implications for genetic counseling. *Soc Biol* 1986;33:57–64.
18. McNeil BJ, Pauker SG, Sox HC, et al: On the elicitation of preferences for alternative therapies. *N Engl J Med* 1982;306:1259–1262.
19. Holtzman NA: Medical de-education. Submitted for publication.
20. Holtzman NA: Rare diseases, common problems. *Pediatrics* 1978;62:1056–60.
21. Holtzman NA, Faden RR, Leonard CO, et al: Effect of education on physician knowledge of a new technology: Alpha-fetoprotein screening for neural tube defects. In preparation.
22. Riccardi V, Schmickel R: Survey for the American Society of Human Genetics, 1986. Unpublished.
23. Childs B, Huether CA, Murphy EA: Human genetics teaching in U.S. medical schools. *Am J Hum Genet* 1981;33:1–10.
24. Title 21 Code Federal Statutes, p 793.
25. Holtzman NA: Prenatal screening for neural tube defects. *Pediatrics* 1983;71:658–60.
26. Wildermann RF, Schnieder KA: Regulatory and legal influences on physicians' office laboratories. *JAMA* 1986;256:252–253.
27. Kenney ML: Final report of an assessment of clinical laboratory regulations. *USDHHS*, 1986;1–3.
28. Holtzman NA: *Genetic Testing in the Future.* Baltimore, Johns Hopkins University Press, to be published.
29. Bucci VA, Reiss JB: Technology assessment of medical devices under Medicare: Who should examine "safety and effectiveness"? *Food Drug Cosmet Law J* 1985;40:445–455.
30. Holtzman NA: Hyperlipidemia screening: A search for heffalumps? *Pediatrics* 1979; 64:270–71.
31. Office of Technology Assessment, Congress of the United States: *The Role of Genetic Testing in the Prevention of Occupational Disease.* Washington, Government Printing Office 1983, 243 pp.
32. Uzych L: Genetic testing and exclusionary practices in the workplace. *J Pub Health Pol* 1986;7:37–57.
33. Severo R: Du Pont defends genetic screening. *New York Times*, October 18, 1981.
34. Stamatoyannopoulos G: Problems of screening and counseling in the hemoglobinopathies; Motulsky AG, Lenz W (eds): in *Birth Defects*, Amsterdam, Excerpta Medica, 1974, pp 268–276.
35. McCormack MK, Leiblum S, Lazzarini A: Attitudes regarding utilization of artificial insemination by donor in Huntington disease. *Am J Med Genet* 1983;14:5–13.
36. Curle-Cohen M, Luttrell L, Shapiro S: Current practice of artificial insemination by donor in the United States. *N Engl J Med* 1979;300:585–90.
37. Marion JP, Kassam GR, Fernhoff PM, et al: Acceptance of amniocentesis by low-income patients in an urban hospital. *Am J Obstet Gynecol* 1980;138:11–15, 1980.
38. Ferguson-Smith MA: Prenatal chromosome analysis and its impact on the birth incidence of chromosome disorders. *Br Med Bull* 1983;39:355–64.
39. Holtzman, NA: Screening for congenital abnormalities. *Int J Tech Ass Health Care* 1985;1:805–19.

40. Rowley PT: Predicting patient receptivity: A need for pilot programs and cost-benefit analysis, in Willey A (ed): *Genetic disease: Screening and management.* New York, Alan R. Liss, 1986, pp 151–172.
41. Lippman-Hand A, Cohen DI: Influence of obstetricians' attitudes on their use of prenatal diagnosis for the detection of Down's syndrome. *Canad Med Assn J* 1980;122:1381–5.
42. Bernhardt BA, Bannerman RM: The influence of obstetricians on the utilization of amniocentesis. *Prenat Diagn* 1984;4:43–9.
43. Leiblum SR, Barbrack C: Artificial insemination by donor: A survey of attitudes and knowledge in medical students and infertile couples. *J Biosoc Sci* 1983;15:165–72.
44. Shaw MW: Presidential address: To be or not to be? That is the question. *Am J Hum Genet* 1984;36:1–9.
45. Coplan J: Wrongful life and wrongful birth: New concepts for the pediatrician. *Pediatrics* 1985;75:65–72.
46. Holtzman NA, Leonard CO, Farfel MR: Issues in antenatal and neonatal screening and surveillance for hereditary and congenital disorders. *Ann Rev Pub Health* 1981;2:219–51.
47. Reilly PR: *Genetics, Law, and Social Policy.* Cambridge: Harvard University Press 1977.
48. Holtzman NA: Genetic screening: For better or for worse? *Pediatrics* 1977;59:131–33.
49. Glass B: Science: Endless horizons or golden age? *Science* 1971;171:23–29.
50. Shaw M: Conditional prospective rights of the fetus. *J Legal Med* 1984;5:63–116.

Index